Palestinian Doctors

Palestinian doctors became a dynamic, vocal, influential, and fascinating professional community over the first half of the twentieth century, growing from roughly a dozen on the eve of World War I to 300 in 1948. This study examines the social history of this group during the late Ottoman and British Mandate periods, examining their social and geographic origins, their professional academic training outside Palestine, and their role and agency in the country's medical market. Yoni Furas and Liat Kozma examine doctors' interactions with the rural and urban society and their entangled relationship with the British colonial administration and Jewish doctors. This book also provides an in-depth description of how Palestinian doctors thought and wrote about themselves and their personal, professional, and collective ambitions, underlining the challenges they faced while attempting to unionize. Furas and Kozma tell Palestine's story through the acts and challenges of these doctors, writing them back into the local and regional history.

YONI FURAS is a senior lecturer in the Department of Middle Eastern and Islamic Studies at the University of Haifa. Furas is the author of *Write Down We are a Nation! Musa Kazem al-Husseini, a Political Biography* (in Hebrew, 2017) and *Educating Palestine: Teaching and Learning History under the Mandate* (2020). He studies Palestinian social history and the history of Arab pedagogy.

LIAT KOZMA is the Harry Friedenwald Chair in the History of Medicine at the Hebrew University. Her research focuses on the modern Middle East and the history of medicine in the region. Kozma is the author of *Policing Egyptian Women: Sex, Law, and Medicine in Khedival Egypt* (2011) and *Global Women, Colonial Ports: Prostitution in the Interwar Middle East* (2017).

Palestinian Doctors

Medical Practice and the Transformation of Palestine, 1900–1948

YONI FURAS
University of Haifa, Israel

LIAT KOZMA
Hebrew University of Jerusalem

CAMBRIDGE
UNIVERSITY PRESS

CAMBRIDGE
UNIVERSITY PRESS

Shaftesbury Road, Cambridge CB2 8EA, United Kingdom

One Liberty Plaza, 20th Floor, New York, NY 10006, USA

477 Williamstown Road, Port Melbourne, VIC 3207, Australia

314–321, 3rd Floor, Plot 3, Splendor Forum, Jasola District Centre,
New Delhi – 110025, India

103 Penang Road, #05-06/07, Visioncrest Commercial, Singapore 238467

Cambridge University Press is part of Cambridge University Press & Assessment,
a department of the University of Cambridge.

We share the University's mission to contribute to society through the pursuit of
education, learning and research at the highest international levels of excellence.

www.cambridge.org
Information on this title: www.cambridge.org/9781009463355

DOI: 10.1017/9781009463362

When citing this work, please include a reference to the DOI 10.1017/9781009463362

First published 2025

Cover image: Left to right standing: Mahmud Tahir al-Dajani, Nahil Habub al-Dajani, Akram Nuri, Beit Safafa Hospital, 1948, courtesy of Nuri Nuri's private collection.

A catalogue record for this publication is available from the British Library

A Cataloging-in-Publication data record for this book is available from the Library of Congress

ISBN 978-1-009-46335-5 Hardback

Dedicated to Palestinian Medical Personnel, Then and Now

Contents

Figures

Acknowledgments

The journey toward *Palestinian Doctors* began almost a decade ago, and its completion was made possible through the help, consultation, patience, cooperation, and love of friends, colleagues, and family.

We are deeply indebted to our generous colleagues who read, commented on, and significantly improved our work: Toufoul Abou-Hudeib, Naama Ben Zeev, Tawfiq Daʿadli, Sara Farhan, Dotan Halevi, Abigail Jacobson, Nicole Khayat, Hagit Krik, Ahmad Mahmud, Benny Nuriely, Itamar Radai, Yair Wallach, and Avner Wishnitzer. The thorough reading and wise comments of Hilary Falb Kalisman were invaluable to the completion of this project. Special thanks to Ido Shahar, Uri Simonsohn and Itzchak Weismann for their friendship and support.

The talented and promising Lily Eilan, Mustafa Hussin, Adam Anabosi, and Hamudi Abureesh greatly assisted us with collecting data, reading newspapers, and listening to hours of interviews. The professional work of Amir Simantov made our dream of an accessible online database come true, and our excellent, meticulous, and ever-prepared editor Ami Asher helped make this text coherent, lucid, and readable.

Nuri Nuri, Nakhleh Bishara, Ziad Deeb, Leon Erdekian, and Andre Dabdoub were gracious and generous in sharing the memories of their fathers and grandparents, who were Palestinian doctors. Their personal stories immensely contributed to our knowledge. We are grateful for Suzy Srouji's hospitality and generosity in inviting us into and teaching us about Nazareth Hospital EMMS. Srouji kindly introduced us to her father, the late Aziz Srouji, may God rest his soul, who shared his personal experience as a doctor in a Palestinian refugee camp. We also thank Muhammad ʻAql and Mahmoud Qaraqra, scholars of Palestinian medical history, who shared their experiences and studies of the field, enriching our knowledge.

Special thanks to the University of Haifa and its Department of Middle East and Islamic Studies, especially Yuval Ben Bassat and

Fruma Zachs, for their support and belief in this project. Funding from the Israel Science Foundation (grant no. 916/18, "A History of Arab Medicine in Mandate Palestine") also tremendously helped in pushing it forward.

Gady and Maya, our lifelong partners, and dearest Noga and Ori, Michael, Nuri, and Carmi, thank you for holding us in one piece, giving us care, treatment, and cure throughout this challenging period. None of this would have been possible without you.

Introduction

"During my last visit to my homeland, I sensed a new spirit, a spirit of progress and awakening that made me proud of my country. The conference I am currently attending sets a fine example for this awakening."[1] This testimony was given by a Palestinian who visited his homeland after three decades abroad. The conference mentioned was the first Congress of Arab Doctors in Palestine, convened in Haifa in June 1933. Twenty-seven doctors attended from across Palestine, and a similar number of doctors could not attend but sent letters of empowerment to the delegates. It would have been impossible to imagine an event such as this three decades earlier, the anonymous attendee noted in retrospect. The professional, personal, and communal challenges and demands facing these doctors would also have been inconceivable at the turn of the century. This book is about them.

Palestinian Doctors tells the story of the country's community of Arab doctors from its inception in the late nineteenth century until the catastrophe of 1948. It tells Palestine's story through the endeavors and challenges of doctors, writing them into local and regional history. The study of their origins and careers extends beyond the country's well-documented urban history and assembles cities, towns, and villages into one conceptual mosaic. The book examines the processes that enabled the emergence of this professional group and its positioning within the local community and the colonial hierarchy. It delves into doctors' relationships with British administration and their Jewish counterparts, their intellectual production, their attempts to unionize, and finally, their role in the 1948 war and the Nakba's immediate effect on their lives.

Doctors are a particularly compelling subject of historical research because, by the beginning of the twentieth century, they came to be regarded as the epitome of modern knowledge and virtue, called upon

[1] "Inʿiqad muʾtamar al-attibaʾ al-ʿArabi bi-Hayfa," *Filastin*, June 20, 1933, 7.

to heal both the individual and the social body. The rise of this professional community, the book argues, was determined by the Palestinian elite's effort to maintain its status amid a rapidly changing geopolitical, economic, and cultural reality, mediated by relations with fellow Arab medical students and doctors from across the region, a confining yet enabling colonial administration, and settler-colonial Zionist medical doctors and establishments. *Palestinian Doctors* traces the agency, potential, and limitations of this community.

Our analysis incorporates regional, national, and local scales. The *regional scale* is crucial for understanding the profession's formation and the connections forged with peers in neighboring countries. Before Israeli statehood, Palestine had no medical school of its own, requiring medical students to constantly migrate across countries and continents. For many of the book's protagonists, medical training meant a meaningful encounter with a foreign urban culture and the acquisition, alongside new knowledge, of new tastes, beliefs, and dispositions. Most doctors studied in Beirut, where they encountered a vibrant cosmopolitan student community that connected them to regional professional networks that would become part of their professional, intellectual, social, and national outlook.

The *national scale* enables us to look at this medical community's shared experiences within the particularities of Palestine. These included the colonial legal and political framework of the British Mandate and employment by the Department of Health (DoH). It also enables us to examine doctors' personal and collective interactions with those who gradually became their professional rivals, members of the Jewish medical community, which posed both a political and a professional challenge. On the national scale, the book also examines their countrywide unionization and the Palestinian Arab Medical Association's attempt to deal with the medical challenges of the 1948 catastrophe.

Finally, the *local scale* enables a nuanced understanding of how different socioeconomic and political developments in specific localities created different engagements with modern medicine. Some communities produced more physicians than did others, some became medical centers, while others did not, and local specificities help understand why. In some localities, a landowning household would send offspring to study medicine. Elsewhere, families of ulama sought to maintain their social status by converting cultural capital from religious education into formal university education. Other factors included the availability of missionary schools, which prepared some children better than others for Beirut's medical schools, or the choice of Mandate authorities to place a District Health Office in one town rather than another, creating employment opportunities and increasing both the supply of and demand for medical personnel.

Historicizing Professions in Colonial and Non-Colonial Contexts

Palestinian doctors were "modern doctors" in terms of their clinical training, acquaintance with the medical scientific canon, and proficiency in methods of treatment. It was their positioning in space, Palestine, and time, the Mandate period, and the attributes of their emergence as a community that made them a unique case study, one that urges us toward a reconceptualization of the professions in the colonized world.

Scholars have formulated a conceptual framework for the study of professions as an interaction between the university, state, professionals, and users. These four categories of actors and their interactions, they argue, can help us understand the resources and histories of professional communities. *Universities* train professionals and provide them with the cultural and practical capital on which their status and practice depend.[2] Education forms personal bonds and networks of people who perform interaction rituals and arrive at shared conceptions of identity and purpose.[3] *States* provide training, licensing, and employment and are involved in regulating the profession. *Professionals* unionize, self-regulate, and enhance their collective interests in relation to the other three actors. They are responsible for the profession's cohesion and continuity by creating formal and informal socialization mechanisms that enable the dissemination of knowledge. Finally, *users'* (or patients') material resources and demand for services are crucial to the profession's development. Medical insurance and

[2] Michael Burrage, Konrad Jarausch and Hannes Siegrist, "An Actor-Based Framework for the Study of the Professions," in *Professions in Theory and History: Rethinking the Study of the Professions*, eds. Michael Burrage and Rolf Torstendahl (London: Sage, 1990), 203–25, esp. 215.

[3] Randall Collins, "Market Closure and the Conflict Theory of the Professions," in *Professions in Theory and History*, 24–43.

state-sponsored health services expand demand and, with it, the users' community.[4]

Historians of the medical profession have noted the connection between university training and the rising power of the urban middle class, which demanded more medical services and higher standards of training. By the late nineteenth century, entry to the medical profession depended on extensive science-oriented secondary education and the ability to bear the financial burden of long years of study – thus limiting entry to the profession to the European and American upper middle classes.[5]

Historians of the professions in colonial societies challenge the validity of this theorization for its oversight of gender, race, ethnicity, and power relations outside the professional field. In her work on the Taiwanese medical profession under Japanese rule, sociologist Ming-Cheng M. Lo demonstrated how doctors' pursuit of market interests was qualified by ethnic solidarity with their consumers and how their organizational autonomy served alternately to protect their professional market and assist in the anti-colonial struggle. She therefore suggested studying the emergence of professions under colonial rule by examining, first, their internal organization, knowledge base, cultural system, and group interests; second, ethnic networks within the colonized society, its cultural traditions, and structural inequalities between colonizer and colonized; and finally, the context of the colonial state and colonized civil society.[6]

Professionals' education in colonial contexts was designed to create a cadre of intermediaries between the colonial power and the indigenous population. University graduates were integrated into the lower ranks of the colonial administration. Universities were rare, and those that did exist attracted students from neighboring colonies and facilitated the formation of group identities and networks that crossed colonial frontiers and a trans-imperial circulation of ideas, models, and experiences. The establishment of universities in the colonies was

[4] Burrage et al., "An Actor-based Framework," 207–13.

[5] Thomas Neville Bonner, *Becoming a Physician: Medical Education in Britain, France, Germany, and the United States, 1750–1945* (New York: Oxford University Press, 1995), 158, 203.

[6] Ming-Cheng M. Lo, *Doctors within Borders: Profession, Ethnicity, and Modernity in Colonial Taiwan* (Berkeley: University of California Press, 2002), 18, 81–82.

sometimes explicitly designed to prevent local students from traveling abroad and integrating into anti-colonial networks. Within the colonial apparatus, university education of colonized professionals created new racial distinctions between them and colonial colleagues, creating novel limitations on their professional mobility and salary.[7]

Professionals in colonial contexts were embedded in national, racial, or ethnic power relations that affected patients' trust in biomedicine and limited promotion tracks of colonized professionals within the government. Like many other university graduates, doctors often played key roles in both the anti-colonial movement and the colonial administration. In late nineteenth-century West Africa, for example, African doctors had difficulties finding employment outside the government because few African patients trusted Western biomedicine. Employment at the colonial medical service, however, came at the expense of sacrificing their professional autonomy and serving as the arm of the state among the colonized. In the early twentieth century, by contrast, private practitioners benefited from the emergence of an African elite willing to consult Western medicine.[8] In Taiwan, medicine was one of the only venues for upward mobility. However, since it entailed a long course of study, sometimes abroad, most doctors hailed from those elites and relied not only on their education but also on their family background for social prestige. Thus, in practice, the emergence of the new educated elites caused little disruption for the old.[9]

Our analysis examines the postcolonial critique within the Palestinian context. The Palestinian medical profession predated the direct colonial encounter and relied on foreign medical training outside Palestine, mainly in Beirut and Istanbul. From 1918 to 1948, Palestine was a colonial entity under British control: Palestinian doctors served as the backbone of the DoH but, as in other colonies, were denied

[7] Sara Legrandjacques, "L'enseignement supérieur en Asie française et britannique. Expériences croisées à l'âge des Empires (années 1850–1930)," *Revue Outre-Mer* 394–395 (2017): 30, 44; Van Tuan Hoang, "L'Université de Hanoi (1906–1945). Un outil de renouvellement des élites et de la culture vietnamiennes?" *Revue Outre-Mer* 394–395 (2017): 73, 81; Hélène Charton, "L'Homo africanus acadamicus: Les limites de la fabrique d'une élite universitaire africaine en Afrique de l'Est," *Revue Outre-Mer* 394–395 (2017): 133.

[8] Adell Patton, *Physicians, Colonial Racism, and Diaspora in West Africa* (Gainesville: University Press of Florida, 1996), 14–15, 122.

[9] Lo, *Doctors within Borders*, 37–39, 104.

decision-making positions. As for medical education, training outside Palestine, particularly in Beirut, integrated our protagonists into regional and transnational networks – which also posed a threat to the colonial state.

In addition to the colonizer-colonized dyad, the settler-colonial setting further problematizes the elements discussed in the fourfold model. The emergence and expansion of the Palestinian professional community paralleled a rapid expansion and institutionalization of a Zionist one, creating a bifurcated professional community. Palestinian doctors found themselves caught in an uneven competition with European immigrant doctors. The relationship between doctors and patients was consequently largely determined within the triangle of colonial, settler-colonial, and ethnic power relations. Elucidating these entanglements within Palestinian professional history enables a revision of our understanding of professions under colonialism.

Historicizing Medicine in the Middle East

The historiography of the medical profession in the Middle East is far from comprehensive. Several works have been dedicated to the Egyptian medical profession, which owes its emergence to Mehmet ʿAli Pasha's initiative to establish the Qasr al-ʿAini Medical School in 1827 to serve the needs of his new army. A second medical school was established in Istanbul the same year. During the same period, Egypt's viceroy and the Ottoman sultan dispatched students and interns to French, German, Italian, and British medical schools.[10]

Historians of the Egyptian medical profession have concentrated on Qasr al-ʿAini and the Egyptian Medical Association, founded in 1919. Egyptian doctors' intellectual production has also been given scholarly attention. From the 1920s onward, Egyptian doctors saw themselves as part of an intelligentsia committed to reforming the Egyptian nation,

10 Amira Sonbol, *The Creation of a Medical Profession in Egypt, 1800–1922* (Syracuse: Syracuse University Press, 1991), 21–80; Khaled Fahmy, *In Quest of Justice: Islamic Law and Forensic Medicine in Modern Egypt* (Berkeley: University of California Press, 2018), 39–80; Hibba Abugideiri, *Gender and the Making of Modern Medicine in Colonial Egypt* (London: Ashgate, 2010), 21–52; Najib Mahfuz, *The History of Medical Education in Egypt* (Cairo: Government Press, 1935).

yielding a corpus of publications aimed at that cause.[11] Palestinian doctors were involved in this social-intellectual discourse, consuming its textual productions and taking part in the Egyptian medical scene through participation in its conferences.

As for the Iraqi medical community, prior to the establishment of a local medical school in 1927, it had to rely on training abroad – particularly in Beirut, Istanbul, and Paris. Iraq's 1932 independence and the graduation of the first cohorts of Baghdad's Royal Medical College linked the Iraqi history of medicine to the state's policies on the one hand and to the college, its student body, and its administration on the other.[12]

The history of the Syrian medical profession concentrates on the Ottoman Imperial Medical School (later named the Arab Medical School) in Damascus and the relationship between its student body and staff, Syrian society, and Ottoman (and later French) authorities. The school's Ottoman Turkish curriculum was Arabized under Faysal's short rule and remained Arabic under the French. Fearful of French retribution, the school shunned nationalist activity throughout the 1920s.[13]

The history of the Palestinian medical profession is different. Lacking both a medical school and a state apparatus, its history cannot be that of an institution or a state-building process. Rather, it is a history of individual, familial, and collective efforts to obtain medical education, private practice, and employment in the DoH, the establishment of municipal and later national medical societies, and laying the foundations for a medical infrastructure. The British commitment to a

[11] Sylvia Chiffoleau, *Médecines et médecins en Egypte: Construction d'une identité professionnelle et projet médical* (Paris: L'Harmattan, 1997); Liat Kozma, "Health and Nation: The Egyptian Medical Profession under British Rule," and Soha Bayoumi, "Colonizing and Decolonizing Egyptian Medicine," in *The Oxford Handbook of Modern Egyptian History*, eds. Beth Baron and Jeffrey Culang (Oxford: Oxford University Press, 2024), 56–78.

[12] Omar Dewachi, *Ungovernable Life: Mandatory Medicine and Statecraft in Iraq* (Stanford: Stanford University Press, 2017), 29–103; Sara Farhan, *Medical Education and the Making of Iraqi Doctors, 1869–1959* (Edinburgh: Edinburgh University Press, 2025).

[13] Robert Ian Blecher, "The Medicalization of Sovereignty: Medicine, Public Health, and Political Authority in Syria, 1861–1936" (PhD diss., Stanford University, 2002), 167–212; Idir Ouahes, *Syria and Lebanon under the French Mandate: Cultural Imperialism and the Workings of Empire* (London: Bloomsbury, 2018), 128.

Jewish national home in the Mandate for Palestine made nation-building efforts overwhelmingly difficult for Palestine's Arabs, as the foundation of an independent Arab state was at the bottom of the British priorities. When comparing the community explored here with the Egyptian, Syrian, and Iraqi ones, the absence of a medical school and a state-building project are central to our analysis.

Against this backdrop, the history of medical education in nearby Beirut is central to both existing historiography and our own analysis. Doctors from the entire region studied in Beirut's two faculties of medicine: the Syrian Protestant College (est. 1866, the medical school – 1867, renamed the American University of Beirut (AUB) in 1920) and St. Joseph University (est. 1876, the faculty of medicine – 1883). In these schools, students gained not only medical training but also personal and professional connections and career opportunities throughout the region and beyond. Beirut's proximity encouraged hundreds of young Palestinian men and a few dozen women to complete their medical, pharmaceutical, dental, or nursing training there.[14] A group that received similar sociohistorical analysis is that of Armenian medical students, also heavily represented in Beirut, many of whom would proceed to practice in Mandate Palestine.[15]

As for European faculties, we only have limited research on the history of Arab, Turkish, or Persian students, except for Paris.[16] Students were dispatched to Europe by their respective governments, and some went there at their own expense. Geneva, for example, became a hub for Ottoman dissidents.[17] In European medical schools, Middle Eastern students also met Asian and African students who

[14] Chantal Verdeil, "Naissance d'une nouvelle élite ottomane. Formation et trajectories de médicins diplômés de Beyrouth à la fin du XIXe siècle," *Revue du Mondes Musulman et Méditerranée* 121–122 (2008): 217–37. For a broader social history of the AUB see Betty S. Anderson, *The American University of Beirut: Arab Nationalism and Liberal Education* (Austin: University of Texas Press, 2011).

[15] Hratch Yervant Kestenian, "A Portrait of Armenian Student Life at the Syrian Protestant College 1885–1920" (MA thesis, American University of Beirut, 2015).

[16] Daniel Panzac, "Les docteurs orientaux de la faculté de médecine de Paris au XIXe siècle," *Revue du Monde Musulman et de la Méditerranée* 75/76 (1995): 295–303.

[17] Ladislas Mysyrowicz, "Les étudiants 'Orientaux' en médecine à Genève (1876–1914)," *Gesnerus: Swiss Journal of the History of Medicine and Science* 34 (1977): 207–12.

arrived due to similar local limitations. Inter- and intra-imperial connections between Turkish-, Arab-, or Persian-speaking students and students from the colonized world are yet to be explored.

Besides educational venues, Palestinian doctors shared with other doctors in the region discursive tropes and real-life concerns. Arab, Turkish, and Armenian doctors often advised mothers on how to keep their homes clean and their children's nutrition hygienic and policymakers on how to contain or prevent the spread of epidemics and how to reform the countryside.[18] Facing the double challenge of British and Zionist presence, Palestinian doctors were no exception.

This study contributes to the understanding of the medical profession in the Middle East while adding its own specificities. Concentrating on medical education, historians have largely neglected to study doctors' professional communities. Focusing on luminaries, most historical work on the medical profession in the region ignores the hundreds or thousands of doctors who are not. Telling the profession's history through the less famous ones, this book attempts to shed light on their personal and communal stories.

Social Histories of Palestine

Our work builds on and contributes to the flourishing field of Palestine's social history in the late Ottoman and Mandate periods. In particular, it builds on existing scholarship on Palestine's urban Arab elites, bourgeoning middle classes, and histories of the professions. The Nakba created an archival rupture followed by a long process of silencing and erasure. Devoid of a state and with its institutions of memory and documentation under constant threat, Palestinian historiography, particularly for Palestinian historians, remains a methodological act of resistance. Personal archives, family photos, oral histories, autobiographies, and the published press complement the official filing of the Palestinian past at the British National

[18] See, for example, Nicole Khayat and Liat Kozma, "Medicine and Arabic Literary Production in the Ottoman Empire during the Nineteenth Century," *The British Journal for the History of Science* 55 (2022): 515–24; Omnia S. El Shakry, *The Great Social Laboratory Subjects of Knowledge in Colonial and Postcolonial Egypt* (Stanford: Stanford University Press, 2007); Cyrus Schayegh, *Who Is Knowledgeable Is Strong: Science, Class, and the Formation of Modern Iranian Society, 1900–1950* (Berkeley: University of California Press, 2009).

Archives or Israeli State Archive, enabling scholars to reconstruct particular Palestinian stories.

Histories of Palestinian villages, towns, and cities, those destroyed in the Nakba and those that remained, illustrate the historical transformations of the country from the turn of the twentieth century until 1948. Urban histories of Jerusalem, Haifa, and Jaffa have surveyed the emergence of modern urban classes.[19] These are often interlaced with the rise of notable families, whose members moved across the region for educational, professional, and business reasons. Many Palestinian professionals personified this mobility and these opportunities. Since they did not concentrate in one city, not even Palestine's largest cities, the current research offers a bird's-eye view of their formation as a professional class.

Histories of Palestinian towns highlight the social transformations occurring beyond the urban centers.[20] Jacob Norris' work on Bethlehem's Dabdoub household during the late Ottoman and Mandate periods illustrates how overseas travel, commerce, and connections transformed the town and its people and enabled the rise of

[19] Mahmoud Yazbak, *Haifa in the Late Ottoman Period, 1864–1914: A Muslim Town in Transition* (Leiden: BRILL, 1998); May Seikaly, *Haifa: Transformation of an Arab Society 1918–1939* (London: I. B. Tauris, 2002); Sherene Seikaly, *Men of Capital: Scarcity and Economy in Mandate Palestine* (Stanford: Stanford University Press, 2015); Itamar Radai, *Palestinians in Jerusalem and Jaffa, 1948: A Tale of Two Cities* (New York: Routledge, 2016); Maayan Hillel, "Constructing Modern Identity – New Patterns of Leisure and Recreation in Mandatory Palestine," *Contemporary Levant* 4 (2019): 75–90; Majdi al-Maliki and Salim Tamari, eds., *al-Madina al-Filastiniyya qadaya fi al-tahawulat al-hadariyya* (Beirut: Mu'assasat al-dirasat al-Filastiniyya, 2021).

[20] Mustafa Abbasi, "Mishpahot ha-nikhbadim ha-ʿAraviyot be-ʿAko be-shalhe ha-shilton ha-ʿOthmani u-bi-tkufat hamandat: Hemshekh o tmura?" *Cathedra* 130 (2008): 52; Mustafa Abbasi, *Zfat bi-Tkufat ha-mandat 1918–1948: ʿArvim vi-Yhudim be-ʿir meʿorevet* (Jerusalem: Yad Yishak Ben-Tsvi, 2015); Mustafa Abbasi, *Tverya ve-toshaveha ha-ʿArvim bi-yeme ha-shilton ha-Briti, 1918–1948* (Jerusalem: Yad Yitshak Ben-Tsvi, 2021); Tawfiq Daʿadli, "Walking with Ghosts along the Bazaar: Urban Life in Ludd, Palestine, at the Turn of the Twentieth Century," *Palestine/Israel Review* 1 (2024): 53–82; Leena Dallasheh, "Nazarenes in the Turbulent Tide of Citizenships: Nazareth from 1940 to 1966" (PhD diss., New York University, 2012); Liza Taraki, "Hayat ʿadiyya: Usul al-tabaqa al-wusta fi madina saghira fi Filastin fi matlaʿ al-qarn al-ʿishrin," in *al-Madina al-Filastiniya*, eds. al-Maliki and Tamari, 147–64; Beshara Doumani, *Rediscovering Palestine: Merchants and Peasants in Jabal Nablus, 1700–1900* (Berkeley: University of California Press, 1995); Dotan Halevy, "Toward a Palestinian History of Ruins: Interwar Gaza," *Journal of Palestine Studies* 189 (2018): 53–72.

Palestinian nouveaux riches with worldwide connections. The Dabdoubs made a fortune from crafting and exporting local Christian devotional objects,[21] enabling cousins Antoine and Michel to become doctors in the late 1940s. Antoine's brothers continued to work in the local family business with their father while he studied at the AUB. He returned to his hometown during the 1948 war and opened a clinic for the Deheisheh Camp refugees, later playing a central role in establishing Bethlehem's Caritas Baby Hospital.[22] Dr. Dabdoub's story is one example linking local Palestinian social developments to the history of the medical profession.

Palestinian society was predominantly rural, and documentation of most villages was scarce or nonexistent. Yet since the 1980s, historians have created a rich corpus of village histories.[23] Since the early 2000s, hundreds of interviews were conducted by projects such as PalestineRemembered.com and Zochrot and uploaded to open-access websites. These interviews were of tremendous value for this book, providing firsthand acquaintance with village realities and otherwise undocumented evidence about healthcare and doctors.

These testimonies complement existing studies on rural Palestine, which underline the entangled relationship between the upper classes and the countryside.[24] More recently, Basma Fahoum's study of peasants in the Palestinian tobacco industry illuminates their

[21] Jacob Norris, *The Lives and Deaths of Jubrail Dabdoub: Or, How the Bethlehemites Discovered Amerka* (Stanford: Stanford University Press, 2023).

[22] We are indebted to Andre Dabdoub for telling us his father's story.

[23] See, for example, Sharif Kana'na and Lubna 'Abd al-Hadi, *Lifta* (Bir Zayt: Markaz al-watha'iq wa-l-Abhath, 1991); Sharif Kana'na, *al-Lajjun* (Bir Zayt: Jami'at Bir Zayt, markaz al-watha'iq wa-l-abhath, 1987); Sharif Kana'na, *'Ayn Hawd* (Bir Zayt: Jami'at Bir Zayt, markaz al-watha'iq wa-al-abhath, 1987). A comprehensive study about this literature is Rochelle Davis, *Palestinian Village Histories: Geographies of the Displaced* (Stanford: Stanford University Press, 2011).

[24] Ylana N. Miller, *Government and Society in Rural Palestine, 1920–1948* (Austin: University of Texas Press, 1985); Issa Khalaf, *Politics in Palestine: Arab Factionalism and Social Disintegration, 1939–1948* (Albany: SUNY Press, 1991); Ted Swedenburg, *Memories of a Revolt: The 1936–1939 Rebellion and the Palestinian National Past* (Minneapolis: University of Minnesota Press, 1995); Amos Nadan, *The Palestinian Peasant Economy under the Mandate: A Story of Colonial Bungling* (Cambridge, MA: Harvard University Press, 2006); Rosemary Sayigh, *The Palestinians: From Peasants to Revolutionaries* (New York: Zed Books, 2007).

resourcefulness and agency amid stronger capitalist and colonialist forces.[25] Our focus on doctors adds another layer to our understanding of the distance between the city and the village, as doctors' national and professional calling was determined by their movement into or relationship with the rural periphery. Analyzing the community through this prism enables the incorporation of the local, urban, or rural with broader spatial perspectives.

The history of labor in Mandate Palestine was also given ample scholarly attention. Existing scholarship examines the unskilled labor market, mainly through the tensions and cooperation between Arab and Jewish workers.[26] The two communities were segregated politically, culturally, and economically but worked in shared spaces. The colonial infrastructure created encounters and challenges for both communities, which gradually grew apart as the conflict intensified. Still, as railroad workers or employees of the colonial bureaucracy, Arabs and Jews continued working together until the British departure. These shared spaces were pivotal in the evolution of each community's definition of national self, constantly forcing reevaluation while encountering the national other.[27] Employed by the DoH in its hospitals, clinics, and administration, Arab and Jewish doctors were part of this encounter. This direct interaction, alongside less direct interfaces as operators of neighboring clinics and members of a shared medical market, was formative in the evolution of the Palestinian medical community.

Local histories of professions during the Mandate are also gaining momentum. Nimrod Ben Zeev delved into Palestine/Israel's social and cultural history of construction, highlighting its ethnic and racial attributes.[28] Hilary Falb Kalisman's study of teachers sheds light on the

[25] Basma Fahoum, "Tobacco Cultivation and Production in Twentieth-Century Palestine/Israel" (PhD diss., Stanford University, 2023).

[26] See, for example, Zachary Lockman, *Comrades and Enemies: Arab and Jewish Workers in Palestine, 1906–1948* (Berkeley: University of California Press, 1996); Deborah Bernstein, *Constructing Boundaries: Jewish and Arab Workers in Mandatory Palestine* (Albany: SUNY Press, 2000); David De Vries, *Strike Action and Nation Building: Labor Unrest in Palestine/Israel, 1899–1951* (New York: Berghahn, 2015).

[27] Baruch Kimmerling, "A Model of Analysis of Reciprocal Relations between the Jewish and Arab Communities in Mandatory Palestine," *Plural Societies* 14 (1983): 45–68.

[28] Nimrod Ben Zeev, "Palestine along the Colour Line: Race, Colonialism, and Construction Labour, 1918–1948," *Ethnic and Racial Studies* 44 (2021): 219–212.

development of a community through a process of professionalization with the establishment of colonial or semi-colonial state education systems. As employees of the colonial government, teachers were at once in the service of the colonial apparatus and shared an emancipatory vocabulary. Like doctors, they were relatively mobile within and across state borders, shared a new professional language, and considered themselves pillars of the new society.[29] Similarly, Naama Ben-Zeev and Gal Amir's work on Palestinian lawyers underlined the role of this professional community in advocating Palestinian civil and judicial rights. Like Palestinian doctors, they numbered a few hundred, and many were prominent actors in the public sphere. Like doctors, they were centered in cities and evolved as a professional community under British rule. Like doctors, they were outnumbered by the Jewish professional community, and like healthcare, law was a central site of conflict between the two communities.[30]

Few works have been dedicated to Palestinian professional associations in the Mandate period. Sherene Seikaly's work on chambers of commerce examined men of capital's conferences and their professional and political lobbying, which included restricting Jewish immigration to ward off commercial competition.[31] Assaf Likhovski studied the legal thought and public advocacy of Palestinian lawyers, paying particular attention to their ongoing dialogues with their counterparts in other Arab countries and showing how they lobbied for more substantial representation for Arab lawyers and judges in the colonial legal system.[32] Our discussion of doctors' unionization will thus contribute to this scholarship on Palestinian professionals and professional associations.

Narratives of Modern Medicine in Palestine

Existing historiographies of medicine in Palestine underline the centrality of foreign missions and Jewish communities in the introduction of

29 Hilary Falb Kalisman, *Teachers as State-Builders* (Princeton: Princeton University Press, 2022).

30 Gal Amir and Naama Ben Zeev, "Lawyers in Transition – Palestinian Arab Lawyers in the First Decade of the Jewish State," *Continuity and Change* 35 (December 2020): 371–92.

31 Seikaly, *Men of Capital*, chapter 4.

32 Assaf Likhovski, *Law and Identity in Mandate Palestine* (Chapel Hill: University of North Carolina Press, 2006), chapter 8.

medical services while marginalizing the role of the Ottoman state, municipalities, and local actors. Studies have demonstrated the segregated nature of healthcare during the Mandate, mainly the Jewish community's relatively well-established healthcare system and its dedication to the national project, as opposed to the limited services offered to the Arab population by the colonial system and private practitioners.[33] Overshadowed by a larger Jewish-Zionist one since late Ottoman times, the Palestinian Arab medical community was overwhelmed by the mass migration of more than 2,000 German and Central European Jewish doctors after the Nazi rise to power in 1933, which made the Jewish medical community roughly ten times larger.[34] Histories of the Jewish medical profession and biographic studies of individual doctors abound.[35] Jewish doctors treated Arab patients and sometimes collaborated with Arab doctors. Our contribution to the history of Jewish doctors lies in our insistence on tracing their interactions with their Palestinian colleagues, which historians of the Jewish community in Palestine tend to ignore. A notable exception is Nisim Levi, whose comprehensive lexicon of local pre-1948 physicians includes roughly

[33] Nira Reiss, *The Health Care of the Arabs in Israel* (Boulder, CO: Westview Press, 1991); Nira Reiss, "British Public Health Policy in Palestine, 1918–1947," in *Health and Disease in the Holy Land: Studies in the History and Sociology of Medicine from Ancient Times to the Present*, eds. Samuel S. Kottek and Manfred Waserman (Lewiston, NY: Edwin Mellen Press, 1996), 301–27; Muhammad Qaraqra, *al-Khidamat al-sihiyyah al-hukumiyyah wa-l-ahliyya li-l-sha'b al-Filastini aban al-intidab, 1918–1948* (Shefa-ʿAmr: Jamʿiyyat al-Jalil li-l-buhuth wa-l-khidamat al-sihhiyyah, 2017); Frances S. Hasso, *Buried in the Red Dirt: Race, Reproduction, and Death in Modern Palestine* (Cambridge: Cambridge University Press, 2021); Sandra Sufian, "Arab Health Care during the British Mandate, 1920–1947," in *Separate and Cooperate, Cooperate and Separate: The Disengagement of the Palestine Health Care System from Israel and Its Emergence as an Independent System*, eds. Tamara Barnea and Rafiq Husseini (Westport, CT: Praeger, 2002), 9–30; Sandra Sufian, *Healing the Land and the Nation: Malaria and the Zionist Project in Palestine, 1920–1947* (Chicago: University of Chicago Press, 2007).

[34] Doron Niederland, "Hashpaʿat ha-rof'im ha-ʿolim mi-Germania ʿal hitpathut ha-refu'a be-Erets-Yisraʾel 1933–1948," *Cathedra* 30 (1983): 111–60.

[35] Nisim Levi, *Prakim be-toldot ha-refu'a be-Eretz Yisra'el* (Haifa: The Technion, 1998); Avishay Golz, *Refu'at Af-Ozen-Garon be-Eretz Israel, 1911–1948* (Zichron Yaʿakov: Itai Bahur, 2009); Tzipora Shehori-Rubin, *Rof'ot Rishonot be-Erets Israel 1900–1918* (Beersheba: Ben-Gurion University of the Negev Press, 2014); Michal Man, "ha-Tipul ha-refu'i ba-kibbutsim ba-shanim 1910–1948," *ʿAlei zait ve-herev* 17 (2018): 95–116.

4,000 short biographies of 400 Arab and Armenian physicians.[36] It was this list that started our journey.

European and American missionary doctors are also central to existing historiography. They established the first hospitals in Palestine.[37] This history is often narrated in conjunction with or as a prelude to the development of Jewish health services. Jewish doctors, mostly European immigrants backed by Jewish philanthropists and philanthropic organizations, managed to establish competing medical institutions and, from the second decade of the twentieth century, a medical infrastructure: a national sick fund, hospitals, and dispensaries.[38] English- and Hebrew-language histories of medicine describe the country's medical landscape in terms of a rivalry between Jewish communities and missionary initiatives in the late Ottoman period and a booming Zionist medical infrastructure in the Mandate period.

The Arabic-language historiography of medicine is mainly biographical, and leading physicians feature in general biographical dictionaries.[39] Muhammad ʿAql's three-volume study on Palestinian doctors surveys the historical development of medical professions in Palestine and includes an impressive lexicon of doctors, dentists, and pharmacists. ʿAql's use of Arabic, Hebrew, and English sources makes his work the most comprehensive one about the medical community.[40]

36 Nisim Levi, *Rofʾei Erets Yisraʾel*, 3rd ed. (Zichron Yaʿakov: Itai Bahur, 2017).

37 For example, Yaron Perry, *British Mission to the Jews in Nineteenth-Century Palestine* (London: Frank Cass, 2003); Yaron Perry and Efraim Lev, *Modern Medicine in the Holy Land: Pioneering British Medical Services in Late Ottoman Palestine* (London: Tauris Academic Studies, 2007); Nakhle Bishara, *Irus Vartani: Sipuro shel bet ha-holim Nazereth* (Zikhron Yaʿakov: Itai Bahur, 2011); Abraham Morgenstern, *Tsaraʿat u-metzoraʿim bi-Yerushalayim* (Zikhron Yaʿakov: Itai Bahur, 2019); Yali Hashash, "Gender, Religion, and Secularism in the English Mission Hospital of Jerusalem, 1844–1880," *Journal of Levantine Studies* 7 (2017): 9–34.

38 Shifra Shvarts, *The Workers' Health Fund in Eretz Israel: Kupat Holim, 1911–1937* (Rochester, NY: University of Rochester Press, 2002).

39 Kamil ʻAsali, *Muqaddima fi ta'rikh al-tibb fi al-Quds mundhu aqdam al-azminah hatta sanat 1918 M* (ʿAmman: al-Jamiʻah al-Urduniyya, ʻImadat al-bahth al-ʻilmi, 1994); Bashir Barakat, *Tarikh al-khidamat al-sihiyya fi Bayt al-Maqdis* (Istanbul: Dar al-nidaʾ, 2019); Salim ʿAbabinah, *Tarikh al-tibb al-Urduni al-hadith* (Irbid: Dar al-kitab al-thaqafi, 2019).

40 Muhammad ʿAql, *Muʿjam al-atibbaʾ wa-l-sayadlah al-Filastiniyyin* (ʿArʿara: self-published, 2021).

Muhammad Qaraqra's monograph concentrates on the DoH and is less concerned with the physicians themselves.[41]

Given the relatively small number and weaker organizations of Arab medical professionals, their historical significance is arguably marginal. As we demonstrate in this book, the history of medicine in late Ottoman and Mandate Palestine is incomplete without them. They were a crucial part of Palestine's emerging Arab professional class and the changing urban landscape. They were the backbone of the DoH and thus constituted, like teachers and other government employees, a crucial interface between the British authorities and Palestine's Arab society. The book also explores their interactions with Jewish doctors – sometimes collaborative, sometimes conflictual. The collapse of medical services to the Arab population in 1948 remains an unexplored aspect of this crucial historical moment, a lacuna we address in Chapter 7.

Methodology and Sources

The book's analytical framework combines qualitative and quantitative sources and methodologies. In the absence of official Palestinian archives for this period, it relies on Arabic, English, Hebrew, and French sources from Israeli, British, and French archives, as well as the Hebrew and Arabic press, publications of the DoH and the Palestine Arab Medical Association, biographies and autobiographies, and works on specific localities.

For mapping the profession's sociology, we created a database (mideastemed.org) compiled using biographical dictionaries, phonebooks, official indexes, newspaper advertisements, and more. It includes some 400 men and three women who worked as doctors in Palestinian cities and towns during the period under study. The database includes other medical professionals – dentists, pharmacists, nurses, and midwives – as well as thousands of medical professionals who worked in the Middle East, particularly the Levant and Egypt. Historians of medicine and the medical profession often turn to biographies of notable individuals because information on others is meager. Analyzed collectively, however, the research outcomes enable tracing the production of medical professionals as an intersection

[41] Qaraqra, *al-Khidamat al-sihhiyya.*

between global, regional, and local processes – for example, as part of global educational mobilities, regional networks of Arab doctors, and a town's relationship with its hinterland. Overall, the combination of sources and methods allows for both micro-level analysis of specific individuals or localities and macro-level analysis of the medical community. This database enables independent browsing and data analysis and encourages further research of this history. We find this possibility respectful of our academic community and the historical subjects.

Chapter Outline

Chapter 1 examines the development of the medical profession in late Ottoman Palestine, with a particular focus on Jerusalem. It argues that it was the encounter between the local elite and the myriad forms of imperial and missionary medical interventions that introduced modern medicine into Ottoman Palestine. The missionary involvement accounts for the presence of foreign doctors and the establishment of hospitals and clinics – providing care for the poor and employment to the first cohorts of Palestinian doctors.

Chapter 2 traces the sociological background of Palestinian doctors – their families, birthplaces, and education. It argues, first, that the Palestinian medical community was a regional phenomenon, as it attracted doctors from Anatolia and all parts of Greater Syria and relied mostly on Beirut's faculties of medicine and the networks students had forged there. Second, the chapter argues that this professional class was not uniformly of urban elite origin but was rather diverse in terms of origins and denomination. We show how the composition of the professional community changed over time in relation to these terms.

Chapter 3 positions the professional community's agency and challenges within the colonial context. The DoH employed eighty-three doctors throughout the Mandate years, making it one of the main employers and providers of medical services to Palestine's Arabs, particularly the lower classes. This chapter explores the ambivalent relationship between the colonial department and the medical community, arguing that while it provided employment to dozens of physicians and some rudimentary medical services, it offered limited promotion opportunities to its Arab employees. This policy led to the fragmentation of the professional community and reliance on private practice, compromising the development of a national Arab medical apparatus.

Chapter 4 delineates doctors' professional mobility. Different factors determined the size, nature, and reach of local professional communities. These included the size of the locality, its changing economic role within local and regional markets, and the presence of missionary, governmental, and Jewish institutions. Three categories are examined: the countryside, where very few doctors worked; small towns such as Acre and Nazareth, which housed small groups of doctors alongside a few pharmacists, dentists, and midwives; and Palestine's major cities – Jaffa, Haifa, and Jerusalem – which served as medical hubs for a few dozen doctors, who worked as private practitioners as well as in governmental and missionary hospitals and clinics.

Chapter 5 provides a labor-oriented analysis of the medical market as a microcosm of the Palestinian-Zionist settler relationship, whose specificities were connected to the intimate nature of medical treatment and the large disparity between the Jewish and Arab medical communities. With superior organization and funding, Jewish doctors constituted both a political and a professional challenge. The 1933 Nazi takeover brought about a massive migration of German Jewish doctors to Palestine. The occupational threat posed by the immigrant doctors intensified the politicization of the professional relationship between Jewish and Arab doctors. Palestinian doctors were not only affected by the conflict but became active in the national movement.

Chapter 6 takes us to the 1940s, which witnessed the maturation of the professional and political processes explored throughout the book. It examines doctors' role as public intellectuals criticizing the colonial government's meager investment in public health, proclaiming themselves as the nation's educators in matters of health and hygiene, and protesting the licensing of immigrant Jewish doctors. It then looks at doctors' unionization, their relationship with medical associations in neighboring countries, their central role in regional medical congresses, and the formation of city-based associations culminating in the establishment of the Palestinian Arab Medical Association in 1944. The 1940s were a decade of vibrant Palestinian public activism, in which doctors played a leading role, seeking to reform their society and using their personal skills and collective power to take part in a nation-building process.

Finally, Chapter 7 addresses the 1948 catastrophe through the medical prism. Within the space of several months, the British authorities withdrew their funding of public health, the fighting increased the demand for medical services, and many of Palestine's Arab doctors were displaced. This chapter follows the paths of those who remained, their efforts to save lives under wartime conditions, and the postwar fate of the medical community. It argues that the slow and belated unionization of the Palestinian medical profession and subsequent withdrawal of the meager British medical services resulted in limited Palestinian ability to cope with the huge numbers of wartime casualties, which was metonymic of the overall collapse of Palestinian civil society.

1 *Prelude: Jerusalem, circa 1903*

Dr. Emile Mauchamp was immortalized in historical scholarship as the one whose murder in Marrakesh in 1907 triggered the countdown to France's eventual takeover of Morocco in 1912.[1] In 1903, however, he was very much alive, concluding his first two years of service as the French government's physician in Jerusalem and director of St. Louis Hospital. He was also compiling a detailed report about his mission in the city, designed above all to showcase his achievements as the hospital's director, having managed to earn the confidence of all of Jerusalem's communities and attract patients of all creeds and nationalities. For historians, the report offers a detailed description of Jerusalem's medical institutions and personnel during the nascent twentieth century. Mauchamp details the composition of each institute's personnel and clientele, what patients had for breakfast, and how many family visits were allowed per week.[2]

Detailed surveys of the city during this period are numerous. Nevertheless, when it comes to the city's medical landscape, Mauchamp's meticulous handwritten document is unmatched in level

[1] Jonathan G. Katz, *Murder in Marrakesh: Émile Mauchamp and the French Colonial Adventure* (Bloomington: Indiana University Press, 2006); Ellen Amster, "The Many Deaths of Dr. Emile Mauchamp: Medicine, Technology, and Popular Politics in Pre-Protectorate Morocco, 1877–1912," *International Journal of Middle East Studies* 36 (2004): 409–28.

[2] Centre des Archives Diplomatiques de Nantes (CADN), 294PO/A, Emile Mauchamp, Rapport du Dr. Emile Mauchamp, médecin du gouvernement français, charge des services de l'Hôpital St. Louis, sur l'exercice de sa mission du 15 novembre 1900 au 11 janvier 1903 et sur la situation hospitalière de Jérusalem. Eleven years later, Jurji Zaydan wrote that the greatest concentration of health institutions in the Levant could be found in Jerusalem. Philippe Bourmaud, "Epidemiology and the City: Communal vs. Intercommunal Health Policy-Making in Jerusalem from the Ottomans to the Mandate, 1908–1925," in *Ordinary Jerusalem 1840–1940: Opening New Archives, Revisiting a Global City*, eds. Angelos Dalachanis and Vincent Lemire (Leiden, The Netherlands: Brill, 2018), 440–41.

of detail and comprehensiveness. The French doctor's intimate acquaintance with the city's medical institutions and professionals makes him, in Vincent Lemire's terms, one of those "best-informed observers,"[3] despite his obvious bias in favor of the French mission and self-proclaimed success in leading St. Louis. This chapter analyzes this report alongside other primary and secondary sources that situate medical institutions and professionals within their urban context, particularly the Palestinian Arab elite and the Ottoman administration.

The high availability of medical services in late Ottoman Jerusalem had no parallels in Palestine, but was also metonymic of processes taking place elsewhere in the region at the time. The Hamidian period (1876–1908) witnessed the dual processes of state centralization and European incursion. As a hub of a newly built road network, Jerusalem's increasing connectivity brought in representatives of foreign powers – consuls, merchants, and missionaries. Ottoman authorities' interest in public health and hygiene and the newly founded municipalities facilitated municipal intervention in the streets' cleanliness and epidemic control. Thus, during the last Ottoman decades, the city became a site of competition and cooperation in which foreign doctors and nurses, alongside local Arab and Jewish doctors, the municipality, and Ottoman officials, engaged in the development of medicine. Municipal doctors, public health measures, and missionary hospitals emerged in those years in Haifa, Jaffa, Nazareth, Gaza, and Nablus. However, Jerusalem preceded them all, becoming Palestine's medical hub, with one of the highest bed capacities in the entire empire.

At that point in time, most doctors in Jerusalem were foreigners – missionaries, representatives of foreign governments, and a handful of Jewish and/or Zionist immigrants. This demographic composition would change dramatically in the coming years. Very few Palestinian Arab doctors worked in Palestine at the beginning of the twentieth century. A younger generation of doctors, who would become the backbone of the medical profession in the Mandate years, were merely children then. Nevertheless, the medical landscape Mauchamp described shaped these men's worldview and vision of their future.

By focusing on Jerusalem, we argue that medical missions, late Ottoman administrative reform, Zionist immigration and funding, and local Palestinian initiative created an institutional and social

[3] Dalachanis and Lemire, *Ordinary Jerusalem 1840–1940*, 82.

setting that transformed Palestine's medical landscape. More medical services were available, and the Ottoman state required doctors to hold university degrees and aspired to make modern medicine the standard practice. The political and sociocultural transformations of the late Ottoman decades thus lay in the background for future generations of medical doctors explored in this book.

Late Ottoman Medicines

From the mid nineteenth century onward, the professionalization of medicine in the Ottoman Empire entailed the replacement of community-based training and supervision over the practice of medicine by government regulation and state monopoly over licensing. At the beginning of the nineteenth century, medical knowledge often passed within the family, medical practice relied on an apprenticeship system, and was regulated by a guild, the *muhtasib*, and in case of wrongdoings – the local court.[4] Mid nineteenth-century processes aimed at centralizing and improving imperial control over its provinces, sought to include medicine under its purview as well. Thus, the authority to educate doctors was transferred from the family, master, and guild to the medical school.

In 1827, two medical schools were established in the Ottoman Empire: the Imperial School of Medicine in Istanbul and Egypt's medical school, first located in Abu Zaʿbal, near Cairo, and later relocated to Qasr al-ʿAini. These faculties, however, attracted very few students from *Bilad a-Sham* or Greater Syria. Much more popular were Beirut's medical faculties, at the Syrian Protestant College (est. 1867 (SPC); renamed American University of Beirut (AUB) since 1920) and St. Joseph University (est. 1883). A new medical school opened in 1903 in Damascus, but was small and less relevant to our story. Others earned their degrees abroad – and some had to certify them in Istanbul. By 1903, hundreds of Ottoman medical doctors worked in municipalities, the Ottoman military, and missionary hospitals.

[4] Michael Winter, *Egyptian Society under Ottoman Rule, 1517–1798* (London: Routledge, 1992), 231–32, 243–44; Miri Shefer-Mossensohn, *Ottoman Medicine: Healing and Medical Institutions, 1500–1700* (Albany: State University of New York Press, 2010), 142–44; Sherry Sayed Gadelrab, "Medical Healers in Ottoman Egypt, 1517–1805," *Medical History* 54 (2010): 365–86.

An 1861 regulation allowed medical practice only to those holding a medical diploma from the Imperial School of Medicine or an external diploma from an institution recognized by the state.[5] Graduates of foreign institutions in Ottoman territories like St. Joseph and SPC were required to pass a final examination in Istanbul (and later in Beirut) to obtain an official state license.[6] Furthermore, Ottoman subjects needed to submit their license to local authorities, and foreigners to their consular representatives, and those were later sent to the Imperial Medical School. However, the lack of certified doctors in the provinces compromised the local authorities' ability and incentive to enforce this law.[7] Nevertheless, the 1861 regulation marked a shift in the empire's supervision over medical practice.

The Ottoman state rarely intervened in foreign doctors' medical practice in Palestine. Missionary or Jewish immigrant doctors did not always bother to receive a license from the state, and their reception depended on their interaction with local communities – which sometimes welcomed free medical care and sometimes resented missionary or foreign incursion.[8] After the 1908 coup, it did endeavor to limit municipal doctors' employment to Imperial Medical School graduates.[9]

The small number of university-trained physicians made traditional practitioners and practices the main solution for most subjects. These were, for example, the *mujabbir*, who set broken bones, the talisman writer, the herbalist, or simply homemade herbal medications. Dr. Subhi Ghusha noted that most Jerusalemites preferred traditional healing during the Mandate period as well, and doctors were usually the last resort.[10]

5 Philippe Bourmaud, "'Ya doktor': Devenir médecin et exercer son art en 'Terre sainte', une expérience du pluralisme médical dans l'Empire ottoman finissant (1871–1918)" (PhD diss., Aix-Marseille I, 2007), 13, 27, 42, 145–47, 208, 217.

6 Robert Ian Blecher, "The Medicalization of Sovereignty: Medicine, Public Health, and Political Authority in Syria, 1861–1936" (PhD diss., Stanford University, Ann Arbor, MI, 2008), 48–49.

7 Ceren Gülser İlikan Rasimoğlu, "The Foundation of a Professional Group: Physicians in the Nineteenth Century Modernizing Ottoman Empire (1839–1908)" (PhD diss., Bogazici University, 2012), 97–98, 101, 108, 112; Ceren Gülser İlikan Rasimoğlu, "Boundaries, Education, and License: The Nineteenth Century Ottoman Standardization of Medical Professions," *Trakya Üniversitesi Sosyal Bilimler Dergisi* 19 (2017): 227–46.

8 Bourmaud, "'Ya doktor'," 28, 77–78, 139.

9 Blecher, "Medicalization," 126–32.

10 Subhi Ghusha, *Shamsuna lan taghib* (Jerusalem: al-Matbaʿa al-ʿArabiyya al-haditha, 1994), 88–99.

Late Ottoman Jerusalem

In 1872, the Sanjak of Jerusalem became a separate administrative unit, subordinated directly to Istanbul rather than to the province of Damascus. This administrative change reflected and accelerated Jerusalem's integration into regional and global networks. By Mauchamp's arrival in Jerusalem, the city was much more connected regionally and globally than it had been just three decades before. Between 1872 and 1892, Ottoman authorities had built new roads, placing Jerusalem at the center of a grid connecting Jaffa, Jericho, Nablus, and Hebron. Inaugurated in 1892, the Jaffa–Jerusalem railroad made travel from the Mediterranean coast faster and safer. The clock tower built in 1907 on top of the city walls gave this speed a new visible presence.[11] At around the same time, Jerusalem began expanding beyond the Old City walls, and the population outside the walls increased from 6 percent in 1880 to 47 percent in 1897. Consequently, in 1896, the municipality relocated from the Old City to its new location outside Jaffa Gate. This move helped reinforce the centrality of the Jaffa Gate neighborhood and the rapidly growing modern city.[12] As we place the city's medical institutions on the map (see Figure 1.1), we can trace them along the newly established neighborhoods and the road to the Mediterranean port.

The 1871 Ottoman Municipality Law mandated the appointment of municipal doctors in the newly founded municipalities and encouraged the employment of university-trained physicians.[13] Consequently, in 1886, Jerusalem established a municipal clinic headed by the municipal doctor, who treated poor patients thrice a week.[14] The municipal doctor oversaw vaccination and the implementation of a cordon sanitaire during epidemic outbreaks. He also held an ex officio seat on the municipal council alongside a municipal veterinarian. From 1906, he

[11] Ruth Kark, *Jerusalem and Its Environs: Quarters, Neighborhoods, Villages, 1800–1948* (Detroit: Wayne State University Press, 2001), 30–36; Johann Büssow, *Hamidian Palestine: Politics and Society in the District of Jerusalem 1872–1908* (Leiden: Brill, 2011), 447–50, 496–97.

[12] Vincent Lemire, *Jerusalem 1900: The Holy City in the Age of Possibilities* (Chicago: The University of Chicago Press, 2017), 4, 21–22.

[13] Bourmaud, "'Ya doktor'," 27.

[14] "Yerushalayim," *Havazelet*, May 21, 1886, 1; "Yerushalayim," *ha-Tsfira*, June 14, 1886, 3.

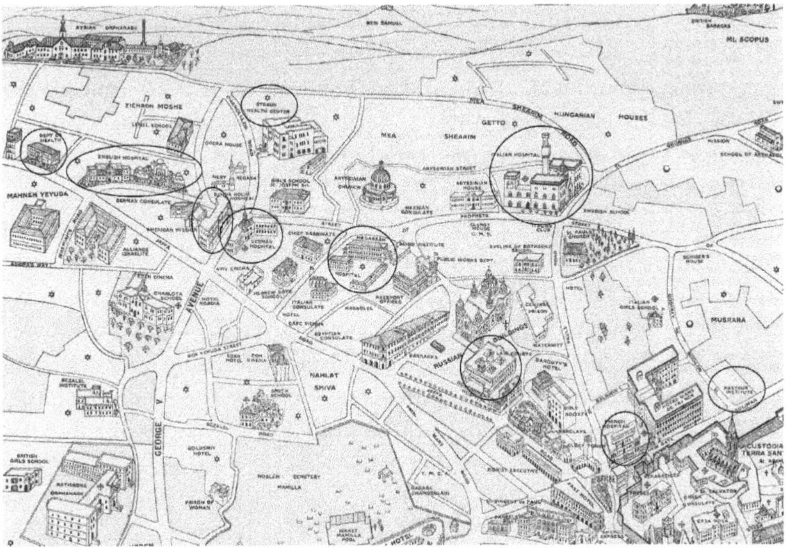

Figure 1.1 Spiridon's map of Jerusalem, 1935
The Eran Laor Cartographic Collection, National Library, Jerusalem.

oversaw postmortem examinations as well. The Municipal Hospital opened in 1891, and a municipal pharmacy opened the following year.[15]

During these decades, the city's streets began looking – and smelling – differently. The municipality paved new streets inside the Old City and dug new sewage canals. From the 1890s, its workers irrigated the streets several times a day to prevent the dust clouds caused by the constant movement of people and carriages. Later, the municipality also assigned workers to garbage disposal.[16]

As the Sanjak's capital was subordinated directly to Istanbul, Jerusalem became very attractive to representatives of foreign powers seeking a stronghold in the empire. As a holy city, it was also attractive

15 In 1895, the hospital was allowed to import surgical equipment. Lemire, *Jerusalem 1900*, 120–21.

16 Ruth Kark, "Pe'ilut 'iriyyat Yerushalayim be-sof ha-tkufa ha-'Othmanit," *Cathedra* 6 (1977): 74–94; Johann Büssow, "Ottoman Reform and Urban Government in the District of Jerusalem, 1867–1917," in *Urban Governance under the Ottomans: Between Cosmopolitanism and Conflict*, eds. Nora Lafi and Ulricke Freitag (London: Routledge, 2014), 97–141; Bourmaud, "Epidemiology," 445.

to missionaries seeking to evangelize Palestine's Jews and those seeking to walk in Christ's footsteps and heal Jerusalem's poor. The first consulates, missionary posts, and missionary hospitals opened in the 1830s. By the end of the century, Jerusalem's increasing accessibility accelerated the arrival of foreigners in the city.

These decades also witnessed transformations within Jerusalem's elite families, such as the Husaynis, Khalidis, and Dajanis. They held important religious and administrative posts in the city as waqf managers, muftis, and shariʿa court judges. By the end of the century, however, maintaining sociopolitical power required families to diversify their economic and cultural capital. Islamic learning maintained its importance, but it was now supplemented with technical and scientific skills acquired in specialized schools: missionary or Ottoman high schools and, for some – higher education in Beirut or Istanbul.[17] More broadly, missionary competition and initiatives of the Ottoman administration and local communities made Jerusalem densely inhabited by primary schools and, to a lesser extent, secondary ones as well.[18]

Mauchamp's Report

Alongside schools and churches, nurses, doctors, and hospitals became a central conduit of foreign influence in the city. Missionary doctors settled in Palestine's cities and towns as early as the 1840s, followed by French, German, Russian, British, Greek, Italian, and Ottoman hospitals that transformed Jerusalem's public space.[19] Described by Philippe Bourmaud as a "Medical Babel,"[20] by the beginning of the twentieth century, fourteen hospitals operated in Jerusalem, a city of

[17] Büssow, *Hamidian Palestine*, 318–23, 338–40, 454–57.

[18] Ibid., 458–60; Lemire, *Ordinary Jerusalem,* 139.

[19] See, for example, Amalie M. Kass, "Western Medicine in Nineteenth-Century Jerusalem," *Journal of the History of Medicine & Allied Sciences* 44 (1989): 447–61; Yaron Perry, *British Mission to the Jews in Nineteenth-Century Palestine* (London: Routledge, 2003); Elena Astafieva, "La Russie en Terre Sainte: Le cas de la société Imperiale Orthodoxe de Palestine (1882–1917)," *Cristianesimo Nella Storia* 24 (2003): 41–68.

[20] Philippe Bourmaud, "'A Son of a Country': Dr. Tawfiq Canaan, Modernist Physician and Palestinian Ethnographer," in *Struggle and Survival in Palestine/Israel*, eds. Mark LeVine and Gershon Shafir (Berkeley: University of California Press, 2012), 107.

55,000 people (35,000 Jews, 10,000 Christians, and 10,000 Muslims). Seven of those hospitals were established by various missions, six by Jewish doctors and organizations, and one by the municipality. Private clinics and pharmacies were also numerous.[21]

The most influential actors in this game were foreign governments and missionaries. Foreign representatives, official or nonofficial, collaborated to enhance political and economic influence in the Holy Land and the Ottoman Empire at large. They did so through consular assistance or privileges, the provision of religious services to their denomination, and, at times, by attempting to win over followers from among the local Christian communities.

The first initiative was British. In the 1830s, the London Society for Promoting Christianity among the Jews sent a physician and a pharmacist to Jerusalem. The Society later established the English Mission Hospital (1844), intending to convert Jerusalem's Jews to Christianity. In the early 1850s, the German Deaconess Sisters and the French St. Louis hospitals were established.[22] The Jewish incentive to promote modern health services was to curtail Christian proselytization efforts, considered a serious threat to the Jewish community. In 1843, Sir Moses Montefiore brought in the first (German) Jewish doctor, Simon Frankel (1809–1880), and funded his salary, medical equipment, and pharmacy for fifteen years. Trained in Munich and Berlin, Frankel collaborated with the second doctor in the city, British missionary Edward McGowan.[23]

Jewish institutions operated under European consular protection, but were funded and run almost entirely by Jews, a modus operandi enabling Jewish medical entrepreneurship to expand to meet the growing need for modern medicine and combat missionary influence. The Rothschild family established the Hôpital Israélite Meyer Rothschild in 1854, under Austrian protection. It was headed by Dr. Bernard Neumann, a Warsaw Jewish doctor who had studied medicine in

21 Norbert Schwake, "Toldot ha-refu'a bi-Yerushalayim ba-tkufa ha-ʿOthmanit ha-me'uheret," in *Sefer Yerushalayim be-shilhe ha-tkufa ha-ʿOthmanit (1800–1917)*, eds. Israel Bartal and Haim Goren (Jerusalem: Yad Yitzhak Ben-Tsvi, 2010), 283–300.

22 Ibid.; Nissim Levi, *Prakim be-toldot ha-refu'a be-Erets Yisra'el, 1799–1948* (Tel Aviv: ha-Kibbuts ha-Meuhad, 1998), 25–42, 103–14.

23 Kass, "Western Medicine"; Levi, *Prakim be-toldot*, 43–51.

Kraków and Vienna.[24] Bikur Holim, another Jewish hospital, was established in 1857.[25] The Jewish battle against the missions within the general European competition for influence in the city increased the politicization of every aspect of modern medicine in Jerusalem.

The many hospitals that adorned the new neighborhoods were all built in the fifteen years preceding Mauchamp's text. Following Jerusalem's expansion beyond the walls, some of its older hospitals also relocated into spacious new buildings. Built from the 1880s to the early 1900s, the impressive architecture of hospitals remains a unique feature of Jerusalem's landscape to this day. The streets surrounding Prophets Street (then, Consuls' Street) offer a time tunnel to the vibrant medical landscape Mauchamp describes. Rothschild Hospital, which had operated inside the city walls since 1854, relocated to its new building in 1888. The German Hospital moved to its new location in 1894. The English Mission Hospital moved to its new spacious building surrounded by a garden in 1897. The new Sha'are Zedek Hospital, directed by Dr. Moshe Wallach, opened in 1902, and its modern facilities impressed Mauchamp – they included a heater, well-ventilated patient halls, a modern operation room, a comfortable ward for the hospital's personnel, an isolation ward, bathrooms, and a house for the doctor.[26]

The Municipal Hospital opened in 1891. It included thirty-two beds (later expanded into forty), a clinic for the free treatment of peasants, a doctor, a surgeon, a pharmacist, and nursing staff.[27] Its staff represented the multiethnic, multireligious nature of late Ottoman

[24] Yaron Perry and Efraim Lev, *Modern Medicine in the Holy Land: Pioneering British Medical Services in Late Ottoman Palestine* (London: I. B. Tauris, 2007), 152; Shifra Shvarts, "Histadrut nashim le-ma'an imahot be-Erets Yisra'el: Pe'ilutan shel Hadassah, Histadrut Nashim 'Ivriyyot ve-WIZO le-hakamat tahanot em va-yeled be-Erets Yisra'el ba-shanim 1918–1948," *Bitahon Sotsiali* 51 (1998): 57–62.

[25] Yehoshua Ben-Arieh, *'Ir bi-re'i tkufa* (Jerusalem: Yad Ben-Tsvi, 1977), 300, 378–79.

[26] Mauchamp, "Report," 4–5, 7–10, 12–15; Levi, *Prakim be-toldot*, 90–102; David Kroyanker, *Sippur mitham Rotschild: Yerushalayim: Rehov ha-nevi'im, biographiya refu'it ve-hinnukhit* (Jerusalem: Keter, 2001), 9–28; David Kroyanker, *Rehov ha-nevi'im, shehunat ha-habashim, ve-shhunat Musrara: Sippuro shel makom, dyokana shel 'ir*, Yerushalyim, 1850–2000 (Jerusalem: Yad Ben-Tsvi, 2000), 22.

[27] Vital Cuinet, *Syrie, Liban et Palestine: Géographie administrative, statistique, descriptive et raisonnée* (Paris: Ernest Leroux, 1896), 553.

Jerusalem, including its Anatolian Greek doctor and Catholic nurses from the Daughters of Charity.[28] Born in Bursa and trained at Athens University, Photios Efklides (1864–1916) served as Jerusalem's municipal doctor but was dismissed from this post, like all Greek doctors, following the 1897 Greco-Turkish War. However, his connections with the Greek Patriarch enabled him to keep his position as head of the Municipal Hospital until his death from typhus in 1916.[29] Funding for the Municipal Hospital was guaranteed by a tax levied on horse carriages entering the city with goods or passengers. This income plunged following the expansion of the Jaffa–Jerusalem railway and the subsequent coachmen's demand to abolish the tax due to their reduced income. Having no other revenue to fund the hospital, it was suggested that the tax levied on the crossing of the Jordan River would be used for this purpose.[30] The Municipal Hospital's capacity had only 40 out of 565 and 592 beds in the city's hospitals in 1896 and 1903, respectively, and mainly served the poor Muslim population.[31] Its establishment embodied cross-denominational shared efforts and vision but also underlined the municipality's limitations in health provision and the socioeconomic and sectarian patterns of health service distribution in the city.

Mauchamp listed twenty-two hospitals, hospices, and dispensaries in Jerusalem, most of which were under European patronage, directed

[28] Zalman Greenberg, "Bet ha-holim ha-ʿironi ha-Turki, bi-Yerushalayim," *Cathedra*, n78 (1995): 49–64; Cuinet, *Syrie, Liban*, 554; Bourmaud, "Epidemiology," 440–56; Mauchamp, "Report," 5.

[29] Mauchamp, "Report" ; Jaffa's municipal doctor also graduated from Athens University: Yehushuʿa Shami, *mi-Zihronot ha-rofe ha-sfaradi ha-Yerushalmi ha-rishon* (Jerusalem: Miryam Kotev, 2015), 60–61. Jewish doctor Helena Kagan (1889–1978) worked under Efklides at the Municipal Hospital. After Efklides's death, Kagan headed the hospital for a few months. Helena Kagan, *Reshit darki bi-Yerushalayim* (Tel Aviv: Vitso, 1983), 39–40, 56–57.

[30] "Yom yom," *ha-Tsvi*, November 5, 1908, 2; see also correspondence between the municipality, the Ottoman Ministry of the Interior and the Ministry of Finance: November 29, 1908, TR-BOA/DH-MKT/2670–61, https://www.openjerusalem.org/ark:/58142/2wlMD#?c=0&m=0&s=0&cv=0; December 18, 1908, TR-BOA/DH-MKT/2686–49, https://www.openjerusalem.org/ark:/58142/2jGSL; December 24, 1908, TR-BOA/DH-MKT/2691–5, https://www.openjerusalem.org/ark:/58142/6Tjv6, accessed April 30, 2020; a document from early 1909 reports the hospital's shut down, January 21, 1909, TR-BOA/DH-MKT/2714–87, www.openjerusalem.org/ark:/58142/1Ncr6#?c=0&m=0&s=0&cv=0, accessed June 7, 2025.

[31] Cuinet, *Syrie, Liban*, 553

by a European, and maintained by European nurses. Particularly noteworthy was St. John Ophthalmic Hospital, founded in 1882 by the English section of the Order of St. John. The hospital employed two English ophthalmologists, and had eight hospitalization beds and an outpatient clinic frequented by 100 patients thrice a week. Unfortunately, Mauchamp noted, the hospital was situated on the dustiest road in Jerusalem, particularly unpleasant for eye patients.[32]

Treatment and medication were free for all in some of these hospitals and only for the local population in others. Some hospitals did not charge fees to a specific denominational or religious group. Some refused to treat patients of specific denominations. For example, since the Greek Hospital refused to treat Catholic patients, Mauchamp explains, the French Hospital refused Orthodox patients – a practice that Mauchamp abolished. The French doctor also credited himself with attracting new patients to the hospital, including Italian, Ethiopian, Armenian, Russian and Greek consulate workers, Ottoman officials, influential Muslim families, and members of the Bedouin tribes surrounding Jerusalem.[33] This universalist pretension in healthcare underlined the segregated reality of the time. Modern medicine was, by and large, provided and consumed within denominational borders.

Some of Jerusalem's medical institutions, however, also offered religiously mixed spaces. Many of the hospitals listed in the report provided hospitalization services exclusively to specific religious or denominational communities, but their outpatient clinics were open to other communities. The hospitals' operations also relied on diverse personnel: Greeks and Jews worked as physicians, and members of the Catholic Daughters of Charity order served as nursing staff at both the French and the municipal hospitals.[34] Greek Dr. Nikafuri Mazaraki was the physician of the Misgav Ladach Jewish Hospital and worked as a substitute physician for the French Hospital. The German Hospital reportedly did not admit Jewish patients, but it employed Jewish Dr. Abraham Abu Shadid, who graduated from SPC in 1899 and also worked in one of the Jewish hospitals.[35]

[32] Mauchamp, "Report," 17–18. See also Rika Izhaki, "Hakamato ve-hitpathutu shel bet ha-holim le-mahalot ʿenayim St. John," *Cathedra* 67 (1993): 114–35; Charles Savona-Ventura, "The Hospital of the Order of St. John in Jerusalem," *Historia Hospitalium* 24 (2004): 25–35.

[33] Ibid., 36. [34] Bourmaud, "Epidemiology," 445.

[35] Mauchamp, "Report," 5, 7, 11.

Although Jerusalem was home to local Jewish, Muslim, and Christian doctors, most doctors working in the city were foreigners. Mauchamp listed thirty-six doctors working in Jerusalem and its surroundings. The French, Russian, British, and Greek hospitals employed compatriots. Other institutions employed Austrian, German, and Italian doctors. Two of the city's doctors were local Christians who had graduated from St. Joseph: Dr. Philippe Barakat (graduated in 1899), worked in the French Hospital in Bethlehem, and Dr. Bernardin Damiani (1895), worked in the Latin dispensary in Jerusalem. Two others were Turkish-speaking Ottomans: government physician Dr. Salah al-Din and military physician Dr. Salih. Two were Armenian: municipal physician Dr. Armenag and Dr. Vahan Pascal, Montpellier graduate (1900), worked for the Armenian Convent. Finally, ten Jewish doctors worked in three of Jerusalem's four Jewish hospitals.[36]

Little has changed in the urban medical geography depicted by Mauchamp until the outbreak of WWI. Jerusalem's small community of medical doctors continued to grow as more Jewish doctors immigrated to the city, some Palestinian Arab doctors returned to Jerusalem after studying abroad, and more Palestinian students left to pursue medical training.

Among those who returned to Jerusalem in later years, one can find Muhammad Tawfiq Sulayman Nusayba (1885–1917),[37] and Husam al-Din Abu al-Sa'ud (1874–1939), members of notable Muslim families,[38] and Yeshu'a Shami,[39] son of a prominent Jewish family from Istanbul, who were trained in Istanbul.[40] Tawfiq Canaan (1882–1964) completed his primary education at the German missionary Schneller School and medical training at SPC. The Halabi brothers, Dr. Ilyas and pharmacist Anton, who graduated from SPC in 1908 and 1912, respectively, were born and raised in Jerusalem and worked there, as were Wadi' and Kamil Haddad.[41]

36 Ibid., 28–29.

37 Salim 'Ababina, *Mu'jam a'lam al-tibb fi al-tarikh al-'Arabi al-Islami* (Amman: Dar al-Bayruni lil-Nashr wa-l-tawzi', 2010), 257.

38 Kamil 'Asali, *Muqaddima fi ta'rikh al-tibb fi al-Quds mundhu aqdam al-azminah hatta sanat 1918 M* ('Amman: al-Jami'ah al-Urduniyya, 'Imadat al-bahth al-'ilmi, 1994), 247–48.

39 *Salname nezaret-i ma'arıf-i umumiye* 1318 (Istanbul: Dar al-Tiba'a al-'Amira, 1318h), 635, 641, 651.

40 "ha-Shavu'a," *Hashkafa*, July 3, 1903, 2.

41 The American University of Beirut, *Directory of Alumni, 1870–1952* (Beirut: American University of Beirut, 1953), 66, 89.

The French Medical Faculty at St. Joseph also attracted the city's elite. In 1909, three doctors and one pharmacist from notable Jerusalemite Jewish families completed their studies there. These included the sons of two prominent religious figures, Rabbis Haim Elyashar and Sulayman Mani.[42] The St. Joseph graduates' list includes at least thirteen doctors and pharmacists born in Jerusalem, mostly Jews, but also members of Christian denominations.[43]

The proliferation of hospitals, clinics, and doctors not only changed the city's landscape but also turned doctors into celebrities whom Jerusalemites could read about in the emerging Arabic press.[44] Ilyas Halabi, for example, contributed articles to the local press on medical and religious issues.[45] He wrote extensively on tuberculosis (TB) in *Filastin* and *al-Muqtataf*, utilizing the disease as a platform from which he proclaimed an entire cultural manifesto. Halabi pointed a finger at the damp, dark, and suffocating homes of both rich and poor, "that are not that different from graves." Moreover, he harshly criticized people's laziness, eating, and leisure habits. While wishing for clean cafés and an end to the germ-spreading greeting customs and narghile smoking, Halabi not only wanted to prevent the spread of TB but envisioned the rebirth of Jerusalem as a modern city, cured of its oriental ills. He did not spare the municipal administration, condemning its indifference toward public places, which he depicted as "poisonous swamps." Instead of "ornamenting the city and its exterior scenery," Halabi lamented, the municipality should invest in parks with fresh air and shaded spaces for sports.[46]

42 "Pri ha-arets," *Ha-Herut*, November 12, 1909, 2.

43 Université Saint-Joseph, *Faculté française de médecine et de pharmacie, Liste officielle de MM. les médicins et pharmaciens diplômés de la faculté Française Beyrouth* (Session de mars 1887 – Session de juillet 1922) (Beirut: Université Saint-Joseph, [1922]).

44 Phillippe Bourmaud, "Experts at Large: Physicians, Public Debate and the Press in Late Ottoman Palestine," *Archív Orientální* 80 (2012): 295–305; Yoni Furas, "'What Did the Ottomans Ever Do for Us?' Modern Medicine and Administration in Late Ottoman Jerusalem," in *From the Household to the Wider World: Local Perspectives on Urban Institutions in Late Ottoman Bilad a-Sham*, eds. Yuval Ben-Bassat and Johann Büssow (Tübingen: Tübingen University Press, 2022), 247–49.

45 Bourmaud, "Experts," 295–337.

46 Ilyas Halabi, "al-Sill fi-l-Quds al-sharif," *al-Muqtataf* 39, no. 3 (September 1, 1911): 217–21; Ilyas Halabi, "al-Sill fi-l-Quds wa-asbab intishariha fiha," *Filastin*, August 16, 1911, 2–3; August 16, 1911, 2.

Zooming Out: The Medical Landscape beyond Jerusalem

Since the Ottomans did not publish regular licensing lists as the British did, data about doctors working across late Ottoman Palestine is far from comprehensive. Available data includes twenty-four doctors employed in Palestine at some point during the decades preceding WWI. Their employers were mainly missionary hospitals (e.g., in Tiberias, Jerusalem, Jaffa, and Gaza) and municipalities (e.g., Haifa, Bethlehem, and Safad). At least a third were born in what would become Lebanon, and another third in the larger cities of Palestine – Haifa, Jaffa, and Jerusalem. Two-thirds were educated at SPC, and three at St. Joseph. Some of them, such as Jibra'il Abyad of Haifa, George Da'das of Nablus, and Ilyas Sawabini of Jaffa, would become pillars of Palestine's medical community in decades to come.

The provision of public and private health services outside Jerusalem evolved sporadically. Born in Istanbul and trained in Edinburgh, the Armenian Dr. Kaloost Vartan reached Nazareth in the 1860s and inaugurated the Edinburgh Medical Mission Society clinic, which would later become a hospital. An Austrian hospital opened in the city in 1884.[47] Elsewhere in the Galilee, Safad was a site of competition between the London Society for Promoting Christianity among the Jews and Jewish doctors, who worked in the city for short periods. The former dispatched a physician to the city in 1884 and opened a hospital in 1904. A Jewish Rothschild Hospital was eventually opened in Safad in 1910.[48] In nearby Tiberias, similar competition began after the arrival of Scottish doctor David Torrance and the subsequent establishment of the Scottish Mission Hospital in 1894.[49]

The mission employed a few local doctors alongside their predominantly foreign staff. The overwhelming majority of doctors before WWI held institutional positions, and private practice was rare. Outside Jerusalem, Bourmaud identified ten to fifteen Arab physicians working in Nablus, Nazareth, Gaza, Bethlehem, Tiberias, and Safad. Arab doctors

[47] Yaron Bar-El and Nissim Levi, "Reshita shel ha-refu'a ha-modernit be-'are ha-Galil, 1860–1900," *Cathedra* 54 (December 1989), 96–98; Nakhla Bishara, *Irus Vartani: Sippuro shel bet ha-holim Natseret* (Zikhron Ya'akov: Itay Bakhur, 2001).

[48] Bar-El and Levi, "Reshita shel," 96–102; Perry, "le-Korot bet ha-holim ha-Briti bi-Tsfat," *Cathedra* 103 (2002): 69–84.

[49] Bar-El and Levi, "Reshita shel," 103–06.

also worked in municipal hospitals, and several municipalities employed municipal doctors. Church Mission Society (CMS) hospitals initially recruited SPC graduates, but from the late 1880s, they only hired European doctors. By 1904, the organization replaced all its local doctors with European ones. The London Society for Promoting Christianity Amongst the Jews' hospital in Safad employed two Lebanese SPC graduates in the 1880s. A few Arab doctors were also employed in Jewish settlements. Dr. Shahdan Nuhra, for example, worked in Rosh Pina in the mid 1880s.[50] In Metula, Dr. Mujalli Masʿud Jabarah from Jdeidat Marj-Ayun (SPC, 1892) was employed as the colony's doctor, others worked in Zikhron Yaakov.[51]

Conclusion

Drawing an administrative self-portrait, Mauchamp detailed the achievements and innovations introduced during his tenure in the French Hospital. His earnest depiction of the need to maintain order in the external clinic and prevent patients from "invading" was a case in point. He achieved such order by installing an indoor pedal turnstile at the entrance to the consultation room and an outside window to the pharmacy to force patients to wait their turn. He also issued every patient a medical card that they were to present at every visit and at the pharmacy. "I was surprised to discover," he wrote, "that I was the only one in Jerusalem who cared about these things!" Moreover, hospital patients had to take a bath upon admission and wear only hospital clothes inside the facility. Upon discharge, they received their clothes back – clean and ironed.[52] Mauchamp's emphasis on maintaining order, bathing, and dressing patients underlined, at least in his mind, the boundaries between the city and hospital.

At the turn of the twentieth century, the provision of modern medicine in Jerusalem could already be a subject worthy of a lengthy report by one of its foreign doctors. Its author is only one example of the many dedicated doctors who cured people, saved lives, and inspired the locals to pursue a similar path. Jerusalem was expanding rapidly, becoming a site of a cosmopolitan community, an administrative

[50] Perry, "le-Korot," 75; Nakdimon Rogel, "ʿOd ʿal reshit ha-refuʾa ba-Galil," *Cathedra* 63 (1992): 179, 182.

[51] Levi, *Prakim be-toldot*, 259; *Directory of Alumni, 1870–1952*, 25.

[52] Mauchamp, "Report," 38–39.

center, and, as we have seen, Palestine's medical hub. Jerusalemites witnessed professionals – engineers, lawyers, teachers, financiers and physicians – accumulate power, wealth, and social capital in their city. Elite families demanded their share in the game, and sending their sons to a medical faculty was also a means to this end. It was the urban elite who could afford modern medical treatment, it was they who encountered foreign medical personnel the most, and it was they who eventually produced the city's first generation of native doctors.

Becoming doctors meant claiming space, power, and wealth in this quickly evolving market. It was a market dominated and motivated by foreign interests with clear, and yet sometimes pervious boundaries. Still, whether French, Anglican, or municipal, Jerusalem's hospitals offered roughly the same medical treatments, and their personnel were of similar standards. Doctors and nurses of different, even rival, denominations cooperated and often treated patients of other denominations. This relative flexibility enabled the absorption of the first local doctors into these institutions.

Modern medicine was foreign, pricy, and, for the most part, urban. At the turn of the twentieth century, treatment was almost impossible to find outside Palestine's cities and larger towns. The provision of public health to the countryside proved frustrating and, as we shall see, remained a central preoccupation of the professional community until the end of the Mandate. In late Ottoman Palestine, pursuing a medical career was a path available only to the fortunate few. But within a few decades, their numbers multiplied tenfold. Chapter 2 builds on the seeds sown by these few, revealing the life stories of Palestinian doctors, their triumphs and setbacks.

2 *Class Matters: The Sociology of the Profession*

In 1910, students of the Syrian Protestant College (SPC, from 1920: the American University of Beirut, AUB) produced Alfred Tennyson's famous play *The Foresters: Robin Hood and Maid Marian*. "The actors lost themselves almost entirely in the parts they were playing, and that always means success," proclaimed the college journal *al-Kulliyyah*. The cast included almost thirty students from all faculties and origins, from eastern Anatolia to Cyprus. Some will play central roles in the following chapters as doctors in Mandate Palestine. ʿAziz Marmura and Vahan Kalbian played Robin's followers, Krikor Krikorian played a forester, Wadiʿ Nasir a mercenary, Kamil ʿId a beggar, and Salim Salama the Sheriff of Nottingham. Marmura came to Beirut from Nazareth, ʿId from Ramleh, Salama from Ramallah, and Nasir from the rapidly developing port city of Haifa. Armenian students Kalbian and Krikorian came to the SPC from Diyarbakır and Jerusalem, respectively. These six students represent the colorful mosaic of the emerging Palestinian professional community.[1]

The Middle East was gradually becoming part of a regional and global network of cultural exchange and people on the move. The Foresters acted in a play written by a famous Victorian poet who had gained popularity in the United States, on an American stage, in an Arab city that was part of the Ottoman Empire. Before World War I (WWI), it was plausible to lose oneself in a nationalist English tale about righteous Anglo-Saxons fighting crooked and foreign Normans while their true king was on a crusade in Palestine. The cry for justice of Robin Hood, a nobleman who stole from the rich and gave to the poor, was something the future doctors, around twenty years old at the time, could relate to. Despite their differences, they all shared several social characteristics and cultural dispositions. Representing a

[1] William T. Bliss, "The Dramatics of 1910," *Al-Kulliyyah* 1, no. 5 (1910): 149–53.

professional community that grew more than tenfold over the first half of the century, they formed part of a sociological phenomenon within Palestinian society and the Levant more broadly. This chapter ties their personal and collective stories, exploring this phenomenon by mapping Palestinian doctors' social origins and subsequent educational trajectories.

This chapter builds on a quantitative analysis of the biographical data of around 400 doctors who worked at some point in Palestine. Most stayed in Palestine throughout their adult lives, while some worked there for a few years before proceeding elsewhere. Others passed away in the early years of the Mandate or graduated toward its end. At its peak, in early 1948, this community numbered around 250 doctors. Sources include the British mandate indexes and reports, telephone books, newspaper advertisements, biographic dictionaries, biographies, and autobiographies. When discussing family background, we complement our analysis of the other medical professionals – pharmacists and dentists – as they often originated from the same social and even familial background.

The chapter first situates Palestine's professionals within the context of a changing class structure in late Ottoman Syria and mandatory Bilad al-Sham. It then examines the doctors' geographic origins and their changes over time – and thus maps the different categories of doctors and their social mobility. Finally, it looks at their secondary and higher education as a meeting ground for the formation of lifelong professional and personal networks on a regional scale, as doctors were one of the only groups educated outside of Palestine.

Class and Classes

In the introduction to his three-volume study about Palestine's doctors and pharmacists, Muhammad ʿAql briefly outlines their social origins as follows: "Most of them were from the rich notability, which enabled their admission to the medical faculties and colleges in Istanbul, Beirut, and a few European countries."[2] Toward the end of the Mandate, Yacov Shimoni made a similar observation: "If we take, for example, the list of doctors, and particularly the list of Arab lawyers, we find

[2] Muhammad ʿAql, *Muʿjam al-atibbaʾ wa-l-sayadila al-Filastiniyyin (1758–1948)*, vol. 1 (Ararah: self-published, 2021), 7.

that the vast majority are members of the known and privileged families and all own property and capital." He likewise observed that the same individuals or families were invested in land ownership, land industry, and municipal politics – while their sons would turn to the professions. A limited circle of notable families, he concludes, controlled Palestine's cultural, political, and economic spheres.[3]

These preliminary observations situate our protagonists within the Mandate's Palestinian class structure. They require, however, some qualifications. Most doctors originated from the urban upper-middle classes, and indeed, from the late Ottoman period until 1948, Palestinian society was largely stratified, maintaining a class division that separated the more wealthy, powerful, and educated from the less fortunate poor. A small class of urban and rural notability owned most of the land, controlled the emerging industry, and manned the high-ranking government bureaucracy. The same families also had a firm grip on the municipal administration and national movement.[4]

However, confining our analysis to a perpetuation of the existing class structure ignores those professionals who were not part of these strata. Power was gradually shared with an expanding list of families and individuals who gained mobility through sociocultural and economic capital. As Issa Khalaf argues, "family ties and personal followings competed with clearly newly emerging social groups and classes." Especially in the 1940s, Khalaf notes, these groups posed a challenge to the traditional notability in all social spheres.[5] The diversification of the expanding professional community in terms of ethnicity, denomination, class and geographic origin was related to urbanization processes that further challenged the hegemony of urban notability. The Palestinian urban labor market attracted educated professionals from across the country and region, including doctors, who gradually integrated into and diversified the upper middle classes of Haifa, Jaffa, and Jerusalem.[6]

[3] Yaacov Shimoni, *'Arviye Erets-Yisra'el* (Tel Aviv: Am Oved, 1947), 198–201.

[4] Issa Khalaf, *Politics in Palestine: Arab Factionalism and Social Disintegration, 1939–1948* (Albany: SUNY Press, 1991), 16–22; Kenneth W. Stein, *The Land Question in Palestine, 1917–1939* (Chapel Hill: University of North Carolina Press, 1985), 25–30.

[5] Khalaf, *Politics in Palestine*, 236–39.

[6] Naama Ben Zeev, "'I Came Naïve from the Village': On Palestinian Urbanism and Ruralism in Haifa under the British Mandate," *British Journal of Middle Eastern Studies* 47 (2020): 264–81.

ʿAql and Shimoni's observations, moreover, overlook processes within Palestine's upper classes from the late Ottoman period onward. Donald Reid argues that Egyptian professionals originated from families of Islamic religious learning, who converted and sometimes supplemented their sons' Islamic education and cultural capital with a professional one. Johann Büssow makes a similar observation regarding Jerusalem's late Ottoman bureaucratic and religious elites as well.[7] We also find a conversion of financial or landed capital into an educational and professional one. This conversion enabled Palestine's notable families to mitigate what Michael Provence saw as their eclipse and curb the rise of new professionals originating from more modest backgrounds.[8]

In addition, becoming a doctor was one facet of the changing balance of power between the Christian and Muslim notability. In the late Ottoman Empire, Muslims more easily found employment in the state's bureaucracy, dominated the judicial and religious positions, and controlled the endowments, therefore having less need for modern education for social mobility compared to their Christian counterparts. As we shall see, however, although the early generations of doctors were predominantly Christian, the urban Muslim notability enthusiastically jumped on the bandwagon in the early 1900s, gradually taking over a greater chunk of the medical job market during the Mandate, yet still far from representing their demographic share.

Greater provision of primary education was essential for the formation of new professions. Literacy was far from universal until the British departure, but its expansion was dramatic, especially for previously predominantly illiterate communities.[9] What Lucie Ryzova defined as "effendification," or acquiring middle-class living standards, distinctions, and possibilities, was a passion that cut across class divisions but maintained class-related attributes.[10] For many,

[7] Donald M. Reid, "Educational and Career Choices of Egyptian Students, 1882–1922," *International Journal of Middle East Studies* 8 (1977): 349–78; Johann Büssow, *Hamidian Palestine: Politics and Society in the District of Jerusalem 1872–1908* (Leiden: Brill, 2011), 447–50.

[8] Michael Provence, *The Last Ottoman Generation and the Making of the Modern Middle East* (Cambridge: Cambridge University Press, 2017), 45–46.

[9] Ami Ayalon, *Reading Palestine: Printing and Literacy, 1900–1948* (Austin: University of Texas Press, 2004), 16–42.

[10] Lucie Ryzova, *The Age of the Efendiyya: Passages to Modernity in National-Colonial Egypt* (Oxford: Oxford University Press, 2014), 178–236.

elementary education opened new occupational horizons in the lower ranks of the local and colonial industries or institutions. Senior positions, however, required secondary education or beyond, which were affordable only to a minority.

First in Mount Lebanon and its immediate environment, then in Palestine, and first in the cities, followed by smaller towns – educational opportunities created prospects for medical careers. Government secondary education under the British was free, but its highly selective and exclusive nature kept private missionary schools in the lead until 1948. This meant that for most Palestinians, completing a university education required costly private schooling prior to admission to even more costly academic training. In medical education specifically, educational experience, in and outside the classroom, was considered a must for acquiring the profession and for building essential networks. Arriving from different parts of the Ottoman Empire and later the Mandate territories, our protagonists forged professional networks and friendships that followed them throughout their careers.

Class Transformation in Late- and Post-Ottoman Greater Syria

The emergence and development of the Palestinian medical profession were related to the transformations within the late Ottoman elites and to the emergence of urban middle classes. Historians' critique of the paradigm of the "politics of the notables" in Greater Syria and their examination of its transformation in the late Ottoman decades are particularly pertinent to our analysis.[11] Keith Watenpaugh argues that by the early twentieth century, a new middle class emerged in the urban centers of Greater Syria, which defined itself against the urban notables and the city's poor. Their status in urban life was defined by wealth, profession, education, and new manners, tastes, and ideas. Watenpaugh argues that this class was drawn from previous generations of merchants, landowners, and clerics and from the cities' religious and ethnic minorities. This new middle class came to occupy a position of power disproportionate to its demographic share of the population due to its new skills and ability to integrate into the

[11] See, for example, Philip S. Khoury, "The Urban Notables Paradigm Revisited," *Revue des mondes musulmans et de la Méditerranée* 55–56 (1990): 215–30; James L. Gelvin, "The 'Politics of Notables' Forty Years After," *Middle East Studies Association Bulletin* 40 (2006): 19–29.

Western-dominated global economy and politics. At the same time, their power also relied on their ability to master the organizing principles of the politics of notables. This new generation of middle-class men differed from the older generations, who had been educated in Istanbul and aspired to integrate into the Ottoman officialdom. Their political and cultural aspirations were directed westward at an imaginary version of the European bourgeoisie.[12]

Toufoul Abou-Hodeib examines Beirut's middle class and shows how the second half of the nineteenth century gave rise to professionals who were invested in the new order. Middle-class Beiruti men, she argues, shared several characteristics: education, upward mobility, and investment in the city's position. They worked in new state institutions and were intimately connected to institutions such as the municipal council, customs, and police – and, in the case of doctors – the municipal and missionary hospitals and quarantine services. These men's position, Abou-Hodeib argues, was related to the city as an economic hub, a provincial center, and an intellectual melting pot.[13]

Watenpough and Abou-Hodeib take the city's social dynamics, elites, and middle classes as a point of departure. They focus on the middle classes as formed in the urban context – from within local notable families or after families had already immigrated to the city. By contrast, when Sherene Seikaly examines Palestine's businessmen in the 1940s – the heyday of Palestinian economic development – she shows that only a few of them had originated from the established urban notability, while many originated from and kept their connection with smaller and inland cities and towns.[14] Similarly, Yosef Waschitz underlines the connections and reliance of successful urban entrepreneurs, some of whom were of rural origins, to the village economy.[15]

[12] Keith David Watenpough, *Being Modern in the Middle East: Revolution, Nationalism, Colonialism, and the Arab Middle Class* (Princeton: Princeton University Press, 2006), 19–26; Keith David Watenpough, "Middle-Class Modernity and the Persistence of the Politics of Notables in Inter-War Syria," *International Journal of Middle East Studies* 35 (2003): 260–63.

[13] Toufoul Abou-Hodeib, *A Taste for Home: The Modern Middle Class in Ottoman Beirut* (Stanford: Stanford University Press, 2017), 15–16, 21.

[14] Sherene Seikaly, *Men of Capital: Scarcity and Economy in Mandate Palestine* (Stanford: Stanford University Press, 2015), 15.

[15] Yosef Waschitz, "Tmurot hevratiyot ba-yishuv ha-ʿArvi shel Hefa bi-tkufat ha-mandat ha-Briti: Soharim ve-yazamim aherim," *ʿIyunim* (2003): 393–438.

In late Ottoman Palestine, economic hegemony was shifting from the mountain to the coast. Greater Syria's economy was integrated into the global economy, and Mediterranean port cities connected the rural hinterland with the outside world. Growing maritime trade and an influx of European merchants, diplomats, and missionaries made cities such as Beirut, Jaffa, and later Haifa hubs of migration for work, education, and financial pursuits. Palestine's coastal towns became bridgeheads for European economic and political influence and intervention. This process increased these cities' populations and economies and marginalized the hinterland. In turn, it gave rise to new coastal urban middle classes, culturally different from their inland counterparts. Port cities gave rise to new municipal structures and power relations, and their rapid development meant they lacked established elites, thus enabling social mobility for new professional classes.[16] Haifa and Jaffa were emblematic of this development. Haifa's population grew from 15,000 in the early 1900s to around 145,000 by 1948.[17] Jaffa's grew from 40,000 in 1907 to around 100,000 in 1946. The outcome was an urban upper class less bound by the politics of notables and clientele networks and thus able to introduce reforms, new lifestyles, and modern consumption patterns.[18]

The economic shifts and growing Western encroachment also affected smaller towns. Mustafa Abbasi urges us to expand our perspective to include them, as the politics of notables was not merely an urban phenomenon but also relevant in smaller localities, shaping their sociopolitical lives and relations with their rural hinterland. These changes, alongside nineteenth-century Ottoman reforms, opened new employment opportunities in the private job market and the Ottoman administration, bringing them closer to the Ottoman orbit. These

[16] Beshara Doumani, *Rediscovering Palestine: Merchants and Peasants in Jabal Nablus, 1700–1900* (Berkeley: University of California Press, 1995), 23–27, 45; Salim Tamari, *Mountain against the Sea: Essays on Palestinian Society and Culture* (Berkeley: University of California Press, 2008), 22–27.

[17] Mahmud Yazbak, *Haifa in the Late Ottoman Period, 1864–1914: A Muslim Town in Transition* (Leiden: Brill, 1998), 103.

[18] Tamari, *Mountain*, 22–35; Leila Fawaz, "The Changing Balance of Forces between Beirut and Damascus in the Nineteenth and Twentieth Centuries," *Revue des mondes musulmans et de la Méditerranée* 55–56 (1990): 208–14; Cyrus Schayegh, *The Middle East and the Making of the Modern World* (Cambridge, MA: Harvard University Press, 2017), 5–14.

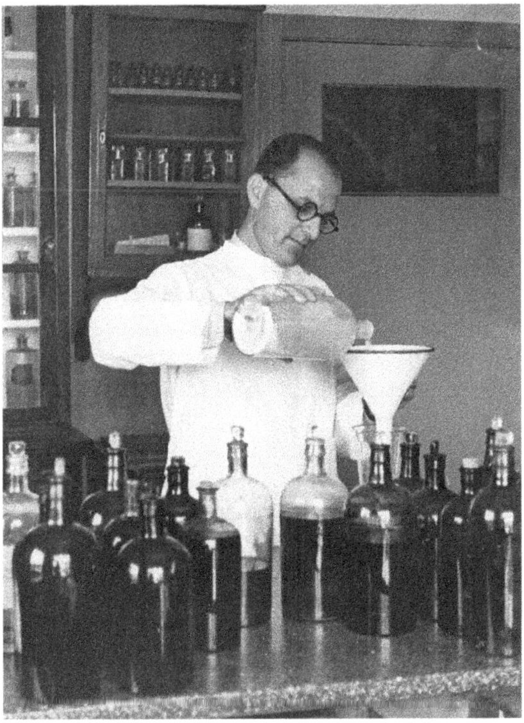

Figure 2.1 A pharmacist in Ramleh's government hospital
TS-3024/58, Public Information Office, ISA.

dynamics continued and intensified during the Mandate years, with greater and more diverse opportunities available to the younger generations.[19] As we show later, the sons of smaller-town notables entered the professions (see Figure 2.1), which now required university training, alongside Jerusalem and Jaffa's more established families.

[19] Mustafa Abbasi, "Mishpahot ha-nikhbadim ha-ʿAraviyyot be-ʿAko be-shalhe ha-shilton ha-ʿOthmani u-bi-tkufat ha-mandat: Hemshekh o tmura?" *Cathedra* 130 (2008): 52; Mustafa Abbasi, *Sfat bi-tkufat ha-mandat 1918–1948: ʿArvim vi-Yehudim be-ʿir meʿorevet* (Jerusalem: Yad Ben Zvi, 2015); Mustafa Abbasi, *Tverya ve-toshaveha ha-ʿArvim bi-yeme ha-shilton ha-Briti, 1918–1948* (Jerusalem: Yad Ben Zvi, 2021). See also Mahmoud Yazbak, "Comparing Ottoman Municipalities in Palestine: The Cases of Nablus, Haifa, and Nazareth, 1864–1914," in *Ordinary Jerusalem 1840–1940*, eds. Angelos Dalachanis and Vincent Lemire (Leiden: Brill, 2018), 240–61.

Geographical Origins

The genesis of the medical community was somewhat haphazard. The first university-trained Arab doctors in Palestine, for whom there is available data, came from villages such as ʿAzur, Mashghara, or Jabaʿ al-Shawf in the Beqaa Valley; from Shweir or Abey in Mount Lebanon; or from al-Nabk north of Damascus. Those born in Palestine include Alexander Aranki (b. 1869) from Bir Zeit, George Daʿdas (b. 1870), Iskandar Halabi (b. 1874) from Jaffa, and Nasif Qaʿwar (b. circa 1866) from Nazareth. They were all Christians, sons of a local landowning or merchant notability.

Existing sources provide the birthplace of 296 out of 400 doctors, and 24 more have been deduced based on their family names, family histories, or other biographical data.[20] The comprehensive lists of licensed medical personnel published by the Department of Health (DoH) in 1920, 1930, and 1946 offer three snapshots of the medical community at a given time. The 1920 list includes 68 Arab and Armenian doctors, 56 of whom with known birthplaces: 38 (68 percent) were native to Palestine, 13 (23 percent) were Lebanese-born, and 5 (9 percent) originated in Anatolia. The 1930 list includes 126 Arab, Armenian, and Greek doctors, 103 of whom have known birthplaces: 70 (68 percent) were born in Palestine, 19 (18 percent) in Lebanon, and the rest (14 percent) in Anatolia, and what became Syria, and Transjordan. The 1946 list includes 203 Arab and Armenian doctors, of whom the birthplace of 172 is known: 118 (68 percent) were born in Palestine, 21 (12 percent) in Lebanon, and the rest (20 percent) in Anatolia, Syria, or Jordan, or outside the Middle East. The lists indicate a slight decline in the reliance on Lebanon-born doctors and a persistence in the rate of Palestine-born doctors.

The largest category is composed of doctors born in Palestine's medium-to-large cities and towns (157 doctors, or 49 percent): Jerusalem (43) and Jaffa (36), followed by Nablus (28), Nazareth (18), Ramallah (18), and Haifa (14). The largest communities of practicing doctors were concentrated in Jerusalem, Jaffa, and Haifa, the main urban centers, indicating a partial overlap between the cities

[20] The core 320 are those who have worked in Palestine for more extended periods or left bureaucratic, social, or professional marks. This amplifies the comprehensiveness of the following survey despite the absence of available data about some eighty doctors who are rarely mentioned in the sources.

with a larger community of practitioners and those from which doctors originated. This gap can be explained by the centrality of Palestine's established notability in producing early generations of professionals. Haifa, for example, was a small town in the late Ottoman decades and gained its prominence only in the early Mandate years; thus, it had but a small established notability of its own. Nablus and Nazareth, by contrast, were homes for landed notable families. Nazareth was known as a center of missionary education,[21] and Nablus was also known for families of apprenticeship rather than university-trained doctors and pharmacists. Both towns had marginal administrative significance in the Mandate years and were thus less attractive as employment hubs.

Zooming out of the cities to smaller towns and villages and shifting to a regional perspective reveals an additional layer. Despite its unquestioned centrality, Jerusalem's semi-urban periphery did not produce future doctors. Southern Palestine was likewise poor in this respect, with only nine doctors originating from Gaza (5), Hebron (3), and Beersheba (1). This contrasts with the Galilee region, the birthplace of at least fifty-seven doctors. Alongside Haifa and Nazareth or towns such as Acre, Safad, and Tiberias, many doctors had their roots in villages such as Kafr Yasif, Shefa-ʿAmr, Biʿna, Rama, Tarshiha, and Kafr Birʿim – all home to strong Christian communities, a distinction reviewed in depth later.

A second category would be Lebanon-born doctors: sixty-three (19.6 percent) whose place of birth is known. Although Lebanon did not constitute a separate political unit in the Ottoman period, the distinct educational developments of Mount Lebanon and neighboring Beirut make Lebanese doctors a separate analytic unit. Their presence in Palestine is linked first to its geographic proximity. Since the 1880s, northern and central Palestine came under the administrative control of the Ottoman Beirut district, which included northern and central Palestine. Palestine was close geographically and culturally and gradually better connected transportation-wise. The relative abundance of doctors from Mt. Lebanon was linked to the development of the area's education system from the mid nineteenth century onward, as well as

21 Hanna Abu Hanna, *Dar al-muʿallimin al-Rusiyya fi al-Nasira "al-Siminar" 1886–1914 wa-atharuha ʿala al-nahda al-adabiyya fi Filastin* (Nazareth: Wizarat al-maʿarif wa-l-thaqafa, 1994).

to the importance of Beirut's faculties of medicine, particularly the SPC/AUB. The faculties of medicine were producing more Lebanese medical doctors than Lebanon required and equipped them with transportable skills in great demand elsewhere. The immigration of Mt. Lebanon-born physicians to Palestine began in the 1880s and continued into the Mandate years. Unlike doctors born in Palestine's cities and towns, Lebanon-born physicians originated in dozens of villages around Mt. Lebanon.

Lebanese doctors were overrepresented in the DoH and became significant in the professional community. Naif Hamzeh, born in Abey, had his official duties both as the director of the native department of Haifa's governmental hospital and as a mediator of disputes within Palestine's Druze community. Mikha'il Ma'luf, born in Kafarakab, was the director of Bethlehem's mental hospital for twenty years and an integral part of Bethlehem's social community. Tyre-born Ibrahim Zuʿrub, one of Haifa's first Arab doctors, was elected the honorary president of the Haifa Medical Association upon its establishment in 1928.

Two other groups in the Palestinian professional community included a handful of Arab doctors from Syria and Egypt. They were few in number, however, since Syria and Egypt offered many employment opportunities and because a degree from the Damascene Medical School was not recognized in Palestine.

A more substantial group that constituted a category in itself was Armenian doctors (25, or 7.8 percent). Some were born in Lebanon or Palestine, and some of the more senior ones came to Palestine from eastern Anatolia. Hovannes Torian and Khatcher Keshishian, two long-serving medical officers at the DoH, were born in Marash, while others hailed from Diyarbakır, Harpot, Elazığ, Urfa, Arabkir, and Aintab in today's Turkey. Like the Lebanese, they were overrepresented at the DoH and were integrated into Palestine's social and medical lives.

The entry or absorption of Anatolian-Armenian and Mt. Lebanon doctors into the Palestinian professional community was a product of late Ottoman and Mandate developments. Those from Lebanon benefited from educational development in their area and used the relative freedom of movement within the province to find job opportunities. Fleeing from genocide perpetrated by the Ottoman Empire, Armenians also moved within its territory and found refuge in

Palestine. Armenians and Lebanese experienced the demise of the multicultural, multiethnic Ottoman order and the materialization of a nation-state system with new borders. As we shall see, some became central members of the national or local associations. Some stayed in Palestine, and others left. They became assimilated into the Palestinian community during the Mandate as part of this community's materialization process.

Urban Notabilities

One family story succinctly exemplifies the notable connections between class and the medical profession. Statesman of Nablusi notability Ruhi ʿAbd al-Hadi (1885–1954) married Rifqa Nashashibi from the Jerusalemite dynasty. Rifqa's brother, Rashid Nashashibi, was a doctor, and three of the couple's four daughters married doctors: Leila married Dr. Akram Nuri from Haifa, the son of a prominent family of Ottoman officials; Samira married Dr. Khalil al-Budayri, of another powerful Jerusalemite household; and Suʿad married Dr. Hamdi al-Taji al-Faruqi of Ramleh's wealthy landowning family.[22] Five prominent Palestinian households from Jerusalem, Nablus, Haifa, and Ramleh were thus connected through matrimony and a noticeable preference for the son-in-law's professional calling. This family story centered on Jerusalem during the Mandate but had originated in the city and country's transformations decades earlier.

For Jerusalem's urban notability, medical education supplemented and sometimes replaced religious learning. Within a few decades, almost all of Jerusalem's notable Muslim families could boast at least one doctor among their members. Medicine became another path to preserve or enhance family power and prestige. The Husaynis, Dajanis, Abu-Saʿuds, Khalidis, Nusaybas, Budayris, and other prominent Muslim families held leading religious and administrative posts in the Ottoman state and continued to do so under the British. Since the mid 1800s, these families gained financial prominence by acquiring and

[22] We are indebted to Nuri Akram Nuri for this valuable information about his father's family. See also "Salma Ruhi basha ʿAbd al-Hadi," *al-Ghad*, October 20, 2023, https://bit.ly/44IK8dk, accessed May 22, 2025; Najwa Qaʿwar Farah, *wa-Kana sabah wa-kana masa': Amali al-dhikrayat* (Amman: Dar al-Bayruni li-l-nashr wa-l-tawziʿ), 267.

cultivating land outside the city and real estate inside it. Their capital enabled them to send their sons to private elementary, secondary, and university education, and the study of medicine fitted their social stature. The younger generation of these families, born around 1910, increasingly distanced itself from religious training and chose careers that facilitated their integration into the colonial administration or the growing possibilities of the private market.

The Dajanis, a prominent Jerusalemite dynasty, is one example.[23] Eight members of the family were medical professionals: two pharmacists, one dentist, and five doctors. Fu'ad Isma'il al-Dajani (1890–1940) was the first doctor in the family. Born in Jerusalem, he started his medical training at the SPC and completed it in the United Kingdom due to the war. His wife Fa'ika was also of local notable descent, the daughter of a Turkish mother and Gaza's mayor and jurist Fahmi al-Husayni.[24] According to his grandson, Dr. Fu'ad's villa was built in Jerusalem stone, and its gardens were decorated with Italian marble fountains. His five children were educated in private missionary schools and were "kitted out in the best of Italian and French fashion with shoes (invariably English) always polished and glistening."[25] Fu'ad returned from the United Kingdom to serve in Faysal's short-lived Syrian kingdom and, after its demise, worked in Jerusalem until 1926. A DoH employee, he continued to Jaffa's government hospital, later quitting his government position and establishing a hospital in the city – the only Palestinian-Arab private hospital before 1948.[26]

The Dajanis were invested in apprenticeship-based medicine before their ascendance in the modern trade. One prominent family member, 'Arif Daud Tahir al-Dajani (1895–1953), was a merchant of medicinal herbs (*'atara*), which he imported to Jerusalem from as far as India. Rifqa al-Dajani, 'Aref's sister-in-law (from the prominent Al-Sa'ud family), practiced traditional Arab medicine and specialized in treating trachoma.[27]

[23] 'Adil Mana', *A'lam Filastin fi awakhir al-'ahd al-'Uthmani (1800–1918)* (Beirut: Mu'assasat al-dirasat al-Filastiniyya, 1995), 174.
[24] Ibid., 5.
[25] Adel Dajani, *From Jerusalem to a Kingdom by the Sea* (London: Zuleika, 2021), 27–28.
[26] Rabiha al-Dajani al-Miqdadi, *Ida'at min khibrati wa-turath ummati* (Amman: Dar al-shuruq li-l-nashr wa-l-tawzi', 2010), 64–65.
[27] Ibid., 46–47, 52–53, 62, 172–73.

Mahmud Tahir al-Dajani married Dr. Nahil Habub, whom he met while studying medicine at the AUB. The two married in Beirut, settled in Jerusalem, and opened two adjacent clinics, forming a unique couple of two doctors.[28] Scion of a Sunni Beiruti notability, in 1931, Habub was the first Muslim woman to graduate in dentistry at the AUB and possibly the first female Muslim dentist in the region. Her older sister Saniya graduated from the Woman's Medical College of Pennsylvania the same year as Nahil.[29]

Dr. Saʿid al-Dajani and his dentist brother, ʿIsa, were from the family's Jaffa branch. Their father, ʿAbdallah, was a local judge and Jaffa's representative in the Ottoman Mutasarifiya Council in Jerusalem. Jaffa's Dajanis also converted the family's cultural capital into a modern one. ʿAbdallah studied *fiqh* from his father, a sheikh, and his uncle, Jaffa's mufti. Unlike his predecessors, he studied at the French Frères School in the city, marking a symbolic shift in the family's educational path.[30]

Notable families led the medical scene in Nablus as well. As Philippe Bourmaud demonstrates, by the mid nineteenth century, the Jabbars, Rahhals, Tuqans, and Abu Ghazalahs controlled the medical market before university education became a prerequisite for medical practice. From the early twentieth century, members of these families supplemented this family tradition with university degrees and official licenses in pharmacy and medicine.[31] In the following decades, other notable families followed their lead. The Tufaha family, who gave Nablus its first mayor and held prominent positions in religious institutions, also gave it two doctors: Dr. Jawdat Tufaha (1914–98) and Dr. ʿAli Shaykh Ahmad Tufaha.[32] Dr. 'Adnan Hassan Hammad

[28] "Alumni News," *Al-Kulliyyah* 19, no. 1 (November 1932): 32; "Alumni News," *Al-Kulliyyah* 19, no. 6 (July 1933): 207.

[29] "Dr. Saniyya Habboub, Fifty Years of Devoted Medical Service," *Al-Raida* 5, no. 22 (1982): 2.

[30] Manaʿ, *Aʿlam Filastin*, 177.

[31] Philippe Bourmaud, "'Ya doktor': Devenir médecin et exercer son art en 'Terre sainte,' une expérience du pluralisme médical dans l'Empire ottoman finissant (1871–1918)" (PhD diss., Université Aix Marseille 1, 2007), 94.

[32] Mahmud Yazbak, "Nabulsi Ulama in the Late Ottoman Period, 1864–1914," *International Journal of Middle East Studies* 29 (1997): 71–91; Bilal Muhamad Shalash, *Shayʾun ʿaʾbir: Nablus taht al-ihtilal* (huzayran/yunyu 1967–adhar/mars 1969) (Beirut: al-Markaz al-ʿArabi li-l-abhath wa-dirasat al-siyasat, 2023), 115.

(1920–2003) hailed from a prominent landowning family in Nablus; his father served as an Ottoman official and, in 1913, won the mayorship.[33]

Various doctors came from smaller towns' wealthiest families. Sabri and Jamal Qadura were members of a powerful Safad family. Their brother Salah was mayor, and their uncle As'ad was a prominent Azhari scholar, mufti, and qadi.[34] Khalil Khartabil, the father of Dr. Adib and veterinarian Drs. Muhammad and Shafiq, was the wealthiest man in Tiberias. After Adib's engagement, he entered the lavish modern house, which included a large clinic built by his father.[35]

For many, pursuing a medical career meant turning their back on the family business and favoring the more modest income of a private or even government doctor. Shortly after inaugurating his lavish house and clinic, Adib Khartabil chose to leave his hometown and escape his father's shadow. He relocated to different posts around Palestine as a DoH medical officer. His father, who inherited and expanded a fortune, failed to understand his son's altruistic motivations.[36]

A few doctors belonged to the local rural notability. Sa'id al-Nimr, of a landowning family in the village of Tubas, was an early and thus exceptional example. Nimr graduated from St. Joseph in Beirut in 1914 and served as a medical officer in the Ottoman army before joining the Arab Revolt in 1916 as Faysal's personal doctor. After Faysal's defeat, he returned to Palestine as a rich man. Nimr settled and worked in Jenin and later opened a second clinic in Bisan. Two of his sons were doctors, and one was a pharmacist.[37] In the 1940s, one could find doctors descending from wealthy families in the villages surrounding Nablus. Dr. Abd al-Majid Abu Hijla (b. 1919) and pharmacist Mamduh Abu Hijla (b. 1920) came from the village of

[33] Akram Zu'aytir, *Yawmiyat Akram Zu'aytir: Amal al-wahdah wa-alam al-inqisam 1949–1965* (Beirut: al-Markaz al-'Arabi li-l-abhath wa-dirasat al-siyasat, 2021), 316, fn. 71.

[34] Mustafa Abbasi, *Tsfat bi-tkufat ha-mandat 1918–1948, 'Aravim vi-Yehudim be-'ir me'orevet* (Jerusalem: Yad Yitshak Ben-Tsvi, 2015), 52–53, 55.

[35] Yusif Sayigh, *Yusif Sayigh: Arab Economist and Palestinian Patriot: A Fractured Life Story*, ed. Rosemary Sayigh (Cairo: The American University in Cairo Press, 2015), 103; Wadi'a Qadura Khartabil, *Bahthan 'an al-amal wa-l-wattan: Sittun 'aman min kifah imra'a fi sabil Filastin* (Beirut: Bisan li-l-nashr wa-l-tawzi', 1995), 47–48.

[36] Khartabil, *Bahthan*, 50–51.

[37] Sonia Nimr, "Sa'id Nimr's Stormy Career from the Dungeons of Istanbul to the Ranks of Faisal's Arab Army," *Jerusalem Quarterly* 30 (2007): 77–87.

Deir Istiya. Ali Kamal (b. 1918) was born and raised in the small village of Anabta before embarking on his journey to Beirut, the United Kingdom, and the University of Baghdad, where he became a prolific author in psychology.[38] This shift in occupational preference was not confined to the Muslim notability; the Christian Arab, Armenian, and Greek minorities had a hugely disproportionate share in the expanding community of trained doctors.

Church Connections and Professional Opportunities

Demographically speaking, Palestinian Christians were a small minority in late Ottoman Palestine and during the Mandate period.[39] Nevertheless, Christian Arab doctors represented roughly half of the local medical community.[40] The overrepresentation of Christian doctors originated in the communal transformations of the mid nineteenth century. A predominantly urban population, their exposure to and engagement with the era's socioeconomic and cultural shifts were momentous. The local Christian communities were most affected by Western encroachment and Christian missionary schools, as elaborated on later. Despite the presence of Muslim, Jewish, and Druze students in these institutions, they mainly served Christians. The instruction of foreign languages and sciences, alongside the encounter with educated foreigners, introduced new educational and training opportunities. Moreover, historically barred from high administrative posts in the Ottoman state, they were more likely to be drawn to Western education and the professional opportunities it could open. During the Mandate period, missionary education, urban affiliation, and commercial contact with Europe facilitated their upward mobility.[41]

[38] Khalil Ahmad Khalil, *Mawsu'at a'lam al-'Arab al-mubd'in fi al-qarn al-'ishrin*, vol. 3 (Beirut: al-Mu'assasa al-'Arabiyya li-l-dirasat wa-l-nashr, 2003), 1768.

[39] According to the 1922 census, out of 744,431 inhabitants, 79.15 percent were Muslims, 11.25 percent Jews, and 9.5 percent Christians. The 1945 survey counted 1,750,520 inhabitants, of whom 60.62 percent were Muslims, 31.62 percent Jews, and 7.74 percent Christians.

[40] Laura Robson, *Colonialism and Christianity in Mandate Palestine* (Austin: University of Texas Press, 2011), 1–43; *A Survey of Palestine*, vol. 1 (Jerusalem: Government Printer, 1946), 147–60.

[41] Noah Haiduc-Dale, *Arab Christians in British Mandate Palestine: Communalism and Nationalism, 1917–1948* (Edinburgh: Edinburgh University Press, 2013), 13; Merav Mack, "Orthodox and Communist: A History of a Christian Community in Mandate Palestine and Israel," *British Journal of*

This typology is well reflected in the transformations undergone by the Burdqush family, landowners from Jaffa who transformed into a medical household.[42] Dr. Jacob Salem (b. 1878) graduated from the AUB in 1904, and three of his brothers were trained there in pharmacy, graduating in the early 1900s. Two younger brothers graduated as a dentist (1920) and doctor (1922), respectively. Jacob was a central figure in the local and national political leadership. He was Jaffa's sole representative for the third Palestinian National Congress in 1920 and a member of the following conferences.[43] Elias was a candidate for Jaffa's mayorship and a central figure within the city's community.[44] When Elias died, his funeral was attended by a massive crowd, including consuls, notables, merchants, and Arab and Jewish doctors.[45]

Notable Christian families from villages and towns sought to integrate into this professional market. Daud Bulus from Kafr Yasif was the son of a tax collector under the Ottomans, who "succeeded in amassing a modest fortune."[46] Among Daud's brothers, there was a pharmacist, a qaymaqam, and the head of Kafr Yasif's local council. Daud's sons were sent to missionary schools, and three studied medicine at the AUB.[47]

Medical professions appealed to members of the Christian communities for interdenominational reasons as well. For the Greek Orthodox, climbing the patriarchy's hierarchical ladder was virtually impossible since Arabs were usually not appointed to high-ranking

Middle Eastern Studies 42 (2015): 338; Mayan Hilel, "Cultural Diplomacy in Mandatory Haifa: The Role of Christian Communities in the Cultural Transformation of the City," in *European Cultural Diplomacy and Arab Christians in Palestine, 1918–1948: Between Contention and Connection*, eds. Karène Sanchez Summerer and Sary Zananiri (Cham: Palgrave Macmillan, 2021), 130–31; Fawwaz ʿAwda al-Nuʿaimat, *Nasara al-Quds fi fatrat al-intidab al-Baritani (1917–1948)* (Beirut: Markaz dirasat al-wahda al-ʿArabiyya, 2016), 104–05.

42 Tahir Qalyoubi, *'A'ilat wa-shakhsiyat min Yafa' wa-qada'iha* (Beirut: al-Mu'assasah al-'Arabiyya li-l-dirasat wa-l-nashr, 2006), 55, 231–32.

43 Bayan Nuwayhid Al-Hut, *Al-Qiyadat wa-l-muʾassasat al-siyasiyya fi Filastin: 1917–1948* (Beirut: Muʾassasat al-dirasat al-Filastiniyya, 1981), 852–53, 859, 866.

44 "ʿAsim bek nivhar shuv le-ʿiryat Yafo," *Doʾar ha-Yom*, June 28, 1934, 1.

45 "Janaza hafila li-faqid Yafa wa-l-watan," *Filastin*, February 9, 1938, 4.

46 Nassib D. Bulos, *A Palestinian Landscape* (Beirut: Arab Institute for Research & Publishing, 1998), 19–20.

47 Ibid., 25, 30–33, 46; Rufaʾil Bulus, *Kafr Yasif bayna asalat al-madi wa-rawʿat al-hadir* (Kafr Yasif: R. B. Bulus, 2012), 229.

posts. This created a schism between some members of the Arab community and the Greek ecclesiastical administration.[48] Daud Bulus' family illustrates this schism. Daud's father-in-law, a fluent Greek-speaking priest in Kafr Yasif, and Daud's father converted to Protestantism after Acre's Greek bishop refused to increase the local school's funding, and the Anglican mission agreed to do so. Their affiliation with the Anglican mission enabled educational and social mobility through the connection to Anglican institutions. Similarly, the Itayim family converted to Protestantism; their sons became a doctor, a dentist, and a pharmacist.[49]

East of Kafr Yasif lies the village of Biʿna, which during the late nineteenth century saw the rise of Nimr Khazin, an Ottoman tithe inspector and wealthy landowner. Nimr donated one of his houses to Russian missionaries, where they established the first school in the village, where the Khazins received their elementary education, a stepping stone for higher education. It was only natural, then, that his son Adib (b. 1894) studied medicine at the University of Kyiv. His brothers were AUB-trained pharmacists.[50]

Strong ties with the Greek Orthodox Church were also conducive to professional mobility, and the Jerusalemite Tleel family is a good case in point. Brothers Daud and Futi Tleel were Greek Orthodox natives of Jerusalem who owned a souvenir shop in the Old City. Daud traveled to Istanbul and Moscow and spoke Russian, Greek, and Turkish.[51] He married a Greek woman from Istanbul, and his son Nicolas married a Greek woman who came to Jerusalem for eye treatment at the St. John Ophthalmic Hospital.[52] Nicolas practiced dentistry at the Ratisbonne Monastery in Jerusalem,[53] and his sons studied dentistry at St. Joseph in the 1940s. Futi's sons also practiced medicine: one became a surgeon, and another opened a pharmacy near the Jaffa Gate.

Salwa Khuri, the first Palestinian Arab woman doctor, was the daughter of an educator from Kafr Yasif, Habib Khuri (1879–1968).

48 Salim Tamari, *The Great War and the Remaking of Palestine* (Berkeley: University of California Press, 2017), 88–117.
49 Bulos, *A Palestinian*, 17; Bulus, *Kafr Yasif*, 20, 228.
50 ʿAql, *Muʿjam al-atibbaʾ*, 2: 149–51.
51 John N. Tleel, *I Am Jerusalem* (Jerusalem: J. N. Tleel, 2007), 51.
52 Ibid., 47–48; with a doctor, dentist, and pharmacist, the Saʿid family and its ties with the Greek Orthodox Patriarchate is another example; ibid., 55–56.
53 Ibid., 49, 75.

She was born in Gaza while he was working there as a school supervisor for the Anglican mission. Under the Mandate, Habib Khuri served in the Department of Education's senior positions. Upon graduating from the AUB in 1936, Salwa became the only female Arab doctor employed in the DoH.[54] Charlotte Saba was the second Palestinian-Arab woman to become a doctor after completing her training and internship in London and returning to Palestine in the mid 1940s. She was the daughter of Nicola Saba, another employee of the Mandate administration with firm ties to the CMS and Anglican institutions in Palestine.[55] Both women were the product of missionary connections and representative of the trajectories mentioned earlier.

Survivors of a National Trauma: Armenian Doctors in Palestine

Armenian doctors, numbering at least twenty-five during the late Ottoman and Mandate periods, were another distinctive group. For many, Palestine became a haven where they could rebuild their lives after the atrocities perpetrated against their communities during WWI. Arriving in Palestine, often with nothing but their trade, they settled where they could find employment. Many had studied at the SPC, which brought them closer to the region. Between 1885 and 1918, Armenian students constituted the largest non-Arab group at the SPC, and in 1907, they represented more than half of the student body. Several factors turned the SPC into an attractive destination for them: the closure of the Medical Department of Central Turkey College in Aintab in 1888; the opening of missionary hospitals in Anatolia – and hence more prospective employment opportunities for university-trained physicians; discounts, loans, and stipends for graduates of missionary schools and colleges; and the improvement of transportation routes between the Levant and Anatolia.[56] AUB's inclusive atmosphere and safe distance from persecution and discrimination were another source of attraction.

54 Nicola A. Ziadeh, *Ayyami: Sira dhatiyya*, vol. 2 (London: Hazar, 1992), 79; Farah, *wa-Kana sabah*, 75–76.

55 Ellen Fleischmann, *The Nation and Its "New" Women: The Palestinian Women's Movement, 1920–1948* (Berkeley: University of California Press, 2003), 56–58; Robson, *Colonialism and Christianity*, 155.

56 Hratch Kestenian, "Portrait of Armenian Student Life at the Syrian Protestant College, 1885–1920" (MA thesis, The American University of Beirut, 2015), 2–3, 6.

Samuel Donabedian was an Armenian from Hoghe near Harput, eastern Anatolia, whose parents had converted to Protestantism. His village healer mother sent him to the American Euphrates College, where he graduated and later taught. From Harput, he moved to continue his medical training at the SPC (1919), leaving his family behind. His daughters were killed during the Armenian Genocide while he was drafted into the Ottoman army. His wife survived the genocide, and Samuel graduated, ending up in Ramallah.[57]

Manouq Erdekian was born in Adana and completed his medical training in Istanbul. Like Donabedian, his family was murdered while he served in the Ottoman army, later defecting to the British army and reaching Palestine through Egypt. Erdekian married a Lebanese woman from a notable Catholic family and was able to bring his mother and his brother's family, who survived the massacre, to Palestine. He settled in Acre, served as its prison doctor, and continued to work there after the establishment of Israel.[58] Vahan Kalbian (1887–1968) was born in Diyarbakır and graduated from the SPC in 1914. Unlike Erdekian, he benefited from positive relations with Ottoman officials. He was posted at an American Red Cross Hospital in Auja al-Hafir on the Egypt-Palestine border, established for the treatment of Ottoman soldiers. Jamal Pasha visited the hospital and befriended Kalbian, later appointing him director of the Russian Hospital in Jerusalem with the rank of colonel.[59]

Coping with trauma and dispossession, medical training became a trajectory for the next generation of these Armenian refugees as well. Veronica Bacamijan (b. 1914) was still a baby when her parents escaped the genocide and started their long journey from Aintab to Lebanon. She graduated at age twenty-three and worked for almost a decade in Palestine before starting an academic and clinical career at

57 History of Health Services Research Project, Interview with Avedis Donabedian conducted by Edward Berkowitz, April 16, 1998, Ann Arbor, MI, www.nlm.nih.gov/hmd/nichsr/donabedian.html, accessed May 22, 2025.

58 Telephone interview with Dr. Leon Erdekian, August 5 and 8, 2021. Dr. Nazareth Yaghlian had a similar story. After graduating from the Istanbul Faculty, he was drafted to the Ottoman army, deserted to the British army, later entering Jerusalem with General Allenby; Arpine Khatchadourian, *David of Sassoun: An Introduction to the Study of the Armenian Epic* (Eugene: Wipf and Stock, 2016).

59 Vicken V. Kalbian, "The Field Hospital of Hafir-El-Auja and US-Ottoman Relations," *Jerusalem Quarterly* no. 63 (2015): 54–71.

the AUB and New York.[60] Samuel Donabedian's son Avedis was born in Beirut while his father completed his studies. He grew up in Ramallah, studied at the Quaker Friends College, graduated from the AUB in 1944, and became a doctor at the English Mission Hospital in Jerusalem.[61] Finally, Kalbian's sons also became doctors, and their brother became a pharmacist, all graduating in the late 1940s from the AUB.[62]

Primary Opportunities of Secondary Education

The available pool of medical students was a direct outcome of the expansion of modern primary and secondary education, both missionary and Ottoman. Education at these schools provided language skills and a curriculum that prepared students for future medical training. Missionary schools prepared students mainly for foreign medical faculties in Beirut and outside the Middle East; government schools prepared students mainly for the Ottoman faculties in Istanbul and Damascus.[63]

Language instruction played a meaningful role in professional career choices. Istanbul's medical faculties switched their language of instruction from French to Turkish in 1870, and similarly, Turkish was the Damascene faculty's language of instruction since its establishment.[64] This shift, meaningful as it was for the Empire, added a further barrier to Palestinian or Arab graduates of secondary schools, most of whom were educated in either French or English. Conversely, the entrance exams for Beirut's medical schools made them particularly accessible to graduates of missionary schools, although graduates of local and Ottoman schools did possess the required language skills as well.[65]

60 "Obituaries," *AMAA News* 37, no. 4 (2003): 18.

61 Interview with Avedis Donabedian.

62 "News of Alumni," *Al-Kulliyyah* 25, no. 6–7 (1950): IV.

63 Selim Deringil, *The Well-Protected Domains: Ideology and the Legitimation of Power in the Ottoman Empire, 1876–1909* (London: I. B. Tauris, 1999), 104–07; Benjamin C. Fortna, *Imperial Classroom: Islam, the State and Education in the Late Ottoman Empire* (Oxford: Oxford University Press, 2002), 44–60; Khaled Nashef, "Tawfiq Canaan: His Life and Works," *Jerusalem Quarterly* 16 (2002): 12–26.

64 Johann Strauss, *Language and Power in the Late Ottoman Empire* (Abingdon: Routledge, 2016), 122, 135–36.

65 Chantal Verdeil, "Naissance d'une nouvelle élite ottomane: Formation et trajectoires de médecins diplômés de Beyrouth à la fin du XIXe siècle," *Revue des mondes musulmans et de la Méditerranée* 121–122 (2008): 2.

Neighboring Lebanese cities and villages preceded the development process of secondary education in Palestine. As seen earlier, Lebanese doctors were integral to Palestine's professional community. From the mid nineteenth century onward, Mt. Lebanon and Beirut became educational battlegrounds between religious and national groups, including local communities, the Ottoman authorities, and American and European missionaries. The Ottomans sought to increase the cadre of educated youth to expand their administration and improve integration into the global economy, but they lacked the means to do so beyond the Ottoman center. The Empire outsourced education to private organizations, including Christian missions. These were not allowed to try to convert Muslims and initially taught only Christians, whom they hoped to convert to their respective denominations. Local students, however, were much more eager for scientific and practical education than for religious teaching. This combination of Ottoman, missionary, and communal interests resulted in the proliferation of education in Ottoman Mt. Lebanon.[66]

From the 1830s, the number of missionary, governmental, and communal schools grew significantly. Catholic schools, in particular, targeted the sons of well-off families for secondary and later university education.[67] Multiple schools were opened in urban centers and Mt. Lebanon's villages, which enjoyed dozens of schools by the early 1880s and hundreds by WWI.[68] The competition between different missionary groups, the Ottoman government, and local communities created the basis for a Lebanese medical community large enough to export

66 Ussama Makdisi, *Artillery of Heaven: American Missionaries and the Failed Conversion of the Middle East* (Ithaca, NY: Cornell University Press, 2007).

67 Edward Falk, "Lyon to Liban: Language, Nation and Faith in the Jesuit Schools of Ottoman Lebanon," in *Entangled Education: Foreign and Local Schools in Ottoman Syria and Mandate Lebanon (19–20th Centuries)*, eds. Julia Hauser, Christine Lindner, and Ester Möller (Beirut: Ergon Verlag Würzburg in Kommission, 2016), 166; Susanna Ferguson, "'A Fever for an Education': Pedagogical Thought and Social Transformation in Beirut and Mount Lebanon, 1861–1914," *Arab Studies Journal* 26 (2018): 58–83.

68 Shahin Makariyus, "al-Maʿarif fi Suriya," *al-Muqtataf* 7 (1883): 534–37; Muhammad Bahjat and Muhamad Tamimi, *Wilayat Bayrut* (Beirut: Mabaʿat al-iqbal, 1916), vol. 1, 143, 159; Hania Abou al-Shamat, "The Religious Educational Divide in Nineteenth Century Lebanon: Institutional Roots of Communal Educational Choices" (PhD diss., University of Southern California, 2008), 23.

graduates across the region. A similar process, albeit on a smaller scale, took place in Palestine.

Most Palestinian doctors whose place of secondary education is known studied at a mission school before proceeding to the SPC. The Jerusalemite missionary schools, mainly Protestant and Anglican, stand out as trainers of future doctors. The son of a Protestant preacher, prolific intellectual, and pioneering physician, Tawfiq Canaan (1882–1954), born in Beit Jala south of Jerusalem, graduated from the Teachers' Division (seminar, est. 1890) of the German Schneller School in Jerusalem.[69] Dr. ʿIzzat Tannous (b. 1886) mentions how natural it was for him to continue his education at the SPC after graduating from the Anglican St. George's School (est. 1899) since the language of instruction was English and the general ambiance felt familiar.[70]

Urban Muslims often preferred foreign secondary mission schools over Ottoman state schools. The former were considered more practical, preparing them for European university training. A famous example is the venerated religious scholar Sheikh Raghib al-Khalidi, a member of Jerusalem's Ottoman Education Department, who held Anglican education in the highest esteem. He sent three of his sons, future students of medicine, Hassan Shukri (1893–1966), Husayn Fakhri (1894–1962), and Ahmad Samih (1896–1951) to St. George's School.[71] Converting the symbolic capital of theology to medicine was an acknowledgment of a shifting zeitgeist.

This preference for missionary schools was not confined to Jerusalem. The sons of the ʿalim, Azhar student of Muhammad ʿAbdu and Jamal al-Din Afghani, qadi and mufti of the Fourth Ottoman Army, Asʿad al-Shuqayri, studied at the Anglican Bishop

[69] Nashef, "Tawfiq Canaan," 13.

[70] Izzat Tannous, *The Palestinians: A Detailed Documented Eyewitness History of Palestine under British Mandate* (New York: I. G. T. Co, 1988), 29.

[71] The two elder sons graduated as doctors. Ahmad Samih switched to pharmacy after vomiting on the sight of corpses as a medical student; interview of Walid Khalidi by Yoni Furas, Cambridge, MA, November 21, 2016. See also Johann Büssow, "Children of the Revolution: Youth in Palestinian Public Life, 1908–14," in *Late Ottoman Palestine: The Period of Young Turk Rule*, eds. Yuval Ben-Bassat and Eyal Ginio (London: I. B. Tauris, 2011), 55–78. On the Husayni family and St. George's School, see Samih Hammuda, *Sawt min al-Quds: al-Mujahid Dawud Salih al-Husayni min khilal mudhakkiratihi wa-awraqihi* (Ramallah: Manshurat maktabat sar al-fikr, 2015).

Gobat School (est. 1853) in Jerusalem. Anwar became a doctor, and Ahmad became a lawyer. Sheikh Hajj Khalil Taha, a wealthy landowner from Haifa, sent his son to study medicine in Geneva and later to an internship in Paris.[72]

Some future doctors, however, completed their education in Ottoman schools and continued medical training in Istanbul. Ottoman state schools attracted the sons, and sometimes daughters, of the rural and urban upper classes,[73] offering another venue for professional mobility and preparing students for higher state education and service in the growing Ottoman bureaucracy. Like the mission schools, they disconnected them from customary education patterns and their communities.[74] Dr. Muhammad Hathat (1881–1934) from Gaza, for example, completed his elementary education in local Ottoman state schools and proceeded to secondary education in the Ottoman Sultaniye High School (*Mekteb-i Sultani*) in Beirut. With his diploma from the Sultaniye, Hathat could enroll in Istanbul's Imperial School of Medicine. He later became a medical officer in the Ottoman army, defected, and then served as Sharif Husayn's personal doctor.[75]

The Ottoman demise reduced the incentive to study in Istanbul, and state education came under the British colonial Department of Education. A few secondary schools were established during the Mandate, and the ones that existed before the occupation expanded their student body and prepared their students for the government matriculation exams or other British A-level exams. Foreign missionary schools maintained their hegemonic role in secondary education, training most of Palestine's future doctors, dentists, and pharmacists. Aside from the Anglican schools mentioned earlier, these included the French Catholic Collège des Frères schools in Jerusalem, Jaffa, Haifa, Nazareth, and the Quaker Friends Boys School in Ramallah. To these institutions, one must

72 Yazbak, *Haifa*, 148–49; "al-Duktur Taha Khalil Taha," Ephemera collection, the National Library of Israel, www.nli.org.il/He/sheets/NNL_EPHEMERA997000724880405171/NLI#$FL4379521, accessed May 22, 2025.

73 Provence, *The Last*, 19–26.

74 Keith David Watenpaugh, *Being Modern in the Middle East: Revolution, Nationalism, Colonialism, and the Arab Middle Class* (Princeton, NJ; Woodstock: Princeton University Press, 2006), 52; Betty Anderson, *The American University of Beirut: Arab Nationalism and Liberal Education* (Austin: University of Texas Press, 2011), 9.

75 Ahmad Muhammad al-Sa'ati, *A'lam min Ghazza, 1876–1967* (Gaza: Matabi' markaz Rashshad al-Shawa al-thaqafi, 2005).

add the national schools sponsored by the Supreme Muslim Council and administered by local educators. The al-Najah College was one such institution, becoming a popular alternative to foreign schools. Available sources suggest that sixteen doctors, one dentist, and nine pharmacists studied there until the late 1930s. Government secondary schools operating under the colonial Department of Education were scarce and highly selective. During most of the Mandate period, the Jerusalem government Arab College (est. 1918) was the only one offering full secondary training. Haydar (b. 1919) and Mustafa (b. 1921) Abd al-Shafi from Gaza, for example, studied there during the late 1930s.

During the three decades of British rule, Palestine did not witness a dramatic change in the percentage of secondary school graduates. Although secondary education expanded steadily during the Mandate, it remained private, expensive, and confined almost exclusively to the upper and upper-middle classes. The increase in the number of students taking the first matriculation exam, from 20 in 1924 to 326 in 1947, is telling.[76] Alongside economic growth and urbanization, accessible secondary education enabled the expansion of the professional community during the Mandate and made the pursuit of higher education more relevant for larger sections of Palestinian-Arab society.

Studying Abroad, Becoming Global

Since the mid nineteenth century, university education has been crucial for the profession's formation, endowing our social actors with the training and skills for formal certification and professional and social networks.[77] It affected their worldview – connecting them to Arab and global intellectual and political thought and to regional and international professional networks. Palestine lacked a university or a medical school for its Arab population, and higher education, as professional training and a rite of passage, had to be gained abroad.

[76] To these numbers one can add the candidates of the London and Cambridge examinations; Yoni Furas, *Educating Palestine: Teaching and Learning History under the Mandate* (Oxford: Oxford University Press, 2020), 219.

[77] Michael Burrage, Konrad Jarausch, and Hannes Siegrist, "An Actor-Based Framework for the Study of the Professions," in *Professions in Theory and History: Rethinking the Study of the Professions*, eds. Michael Burrage and Rolf Torstendahl (London: Sage, 1990), 203–25.

Spending at least four intensive years far from home shaped the nature of the Palestinian medical community.[78] Palestine's doctors spent this period in Beirut or European urban centers. Beirut bore some resemblance to Jaffa or Haifa, but its cosmopolitan, urban, and cultural features were nothing like their previous lived experience. No other professional community bore these characteristics in the Palestinian community. University training turned them into an essential element in mediating between Palestine and the rest of the world.

Universities provide students with professional or academic training and the cultural and symbolic capital on which their status and practice depend. Academic education forms national and class group identities and bonds and provides a shared intensive experience, which creates *communitas*, a community of equals whose shared educational experience forges lifelong connections. In her study of Irish medical education, Laura Kelly argues that medical students' professional identity is cemented through shared educational and extracurricular experiences, a set of rites of passage into the profession, creating a shared language, and a close-knit social network. These processes make informal social interactions no less critical than classroom learning.[79]

Available data on medical training indicate that 230 (65.7 percent) of 350 Palestinian physicians whose place of education is known were AUB graduates, and 10.3 percent graduated from St. Joseph's. At least 28 (8 percent) graduated from Istanbul; the rest were trained in European and American institutions. Very few Palestinians studied in the medical schools of Cairo and Damascus. The Damascus faculty was considered inferior to its Beiruti counterparts, and its diploma was not recognized by the Mandate's authorities, contributing to its lack of popularity.[80] Beirut's American and French faculties of medicine were

[78] A fifth year was later added to medical training. Since 1925, AUB's diploma required five years, and later, medical students there were required to complete three college years prior to admission. Stephen Penrose, *That They May Have Life: The Story of the American University of Beirut 1866–1941* (Beirut: American University of Beirut, 1941), 223–24, 228.

[79] Laura Kelly, *Irish Medical Education and Student Culture, c. 1850–1950* (Liverpool: Liverpool University Press, 2017), 2–3, 10–11.

[80] See, for example, the case of Diya al-Din al-Khamash, in Sa'id Abdallah Al-Bishawi, *al-Doktor Ahmad "Mahmud 'Atallah" al-Sruri* (Ramallah, Amman: al-Ru'ah, jusur thakafiyyah li-l-nashr wa-l-tawzi', 2021), 66, fn 57; conversely, Sruji notes the ease with which AUB graduates obtained a DoH license, Ilyas Sruji, *Min muruj al-Jalil, Mudhakkirat tabib min al-Nasira* (Nazareth: Matba'at al-hakim, 2011), 142–43.

closer and more accessible for Palestinian students, while Palestine was a close-enough and attractive destination for Beirut's graduates.

In addition to schools in the region, some Palestinian doctors studied in Europe, particularly in the United Kingdom, France, and Switzerland, and the years they spent there had a lasting impact on their intellectual and political makeup. Several doctors of Greek origin graduated from Athens, three to four were trained in Edinburgh, Geneva, and Montpellier, and one to two graduated from around thirty other institutions. Colonized students who studied in European universities were connected to transnational networks of people, ideas, and political activism.[81] Some AUB graduates continued their studies in European universities: Vahan Kalbian completed an internship in London, Tawfiq Canaan in Berlin, and others in Rome, London, and Paris.[82]

The actual impact of studies in European universities on Palestinian doctors is difficult to trace. Ophthalmologist Khalil Budayri, for example, mentions meeting Lebanese author and political leader Shakib Arslan during his studies in Geneva as the latter was visiting the League of Nations and met Syrian and Lebanese medical and law students. He owed his Marxist education to these formative years.[83] Studying abroad often intensified their medical calling. After a year of internship at the Hospital for Sick Children, Tannous wrote, "London taught me to dedicate myself not only to my personal interests, but also to God and country."[84]

Zooming In on St. Joseph University

St. Joseph University, the second-largest training institution of Palestinian doctors, was founded in 1875 as a result of converging

81 For example, Marc Matera, *Black London: The Imperial Metropolis and Decolonization in the Twentieth Century* (Oakland: California University Press, 2015), 242–57; Michael Goebel, *Anti-Imperial Metropolis: Interwar Paris and the Seeds of Third World Nationalism* (New York: Cambridge University Press, 2015), 116–48; Götz Nordbruch, "Arab Students in Weimar Germany – Politics and Thought beyond Borders," *Journal of Contemporary History* 49 (2014): 275–95.

82 Tannous, *The Palestinians*, 143.

83 Khalil Budayri, *Sitta wa-sittun ʿaman maʿa al-harakah al-wataniyya al-Filastiniyya wa-fiha: Tarikh ma aghfalahu al-tarikh* (Al-Quds: Manshurat Salah al-Din, 1982), 44–45.

84 Tannous, *The Palestinians*, 143.

interests: the Jesuits needed religious and political legitimacy; the French needed this cultural and diplomatic stronghold in the Levant; and the Maronite elite needed a modern educational institution that would keep its youth away from American Protestant influence and within the community.[85] Like the university, its medical school (est. 1883) was designed for members of the Maronite community. Its admission exams required missionary training, and tuition and living expenses made the school accessible mainly to affluent families.[86]

Despite its relatively exclusive nature, the Faculty of Medicine boasted a diverse body of students "of all races and religions," a total of sixteen different religions or sects. In 1912, French physician Raphaël Blanchard noted that considering its inclusion of Turkish and Armenian students, "One might think that the Beirut Faculty would be the scene of daily horrific carnage. In our 29 years of existence, however, not a drop of blood had been spilled here ... They speak Turkish, Armenian, Hebrew, Greek, Arabic, and Persian. They all have one thing in common – their love of France, to whom they owe their education."[87] Blanchard's assertion regarding the shared love of France is disputable, but St. Joseph, like the AUB, indeed endowed students with a shared outlook and a professional ethos.

The new postwar borders, however, limited St. Joseph's cosmopolitan character. A 1924 report about students' origin noted that they were "more local in origin than those of the AUB."[88] A 1927 report estimated that its medical faculty students came "mainly from Syria."[89] St. Joseph's historical bias in favor of the sons of the

[85] Rafaël Herzstein, "The Foundation of the Saint-Joseph University of Beirut: The Teaching of the Maronites by the Second Jesuit Mission in the Levant," *Middle Eastern Studies* 43 (2007): 749–59.

[86] Chantal Verdeil, "L'empire, les communautés, la France: Les réseaux des médecins ottomans à la fin du xixe siècle," in *Hommes de l'entre-deux: Parcours individuels et portraits de groupes sur la frontière de la méditerranée xvie-xxe siècle*, eds. Bernard Heyberger and Chantal Verdeil (Paris: Les Indes savants, 2009), 133–50.

[87] Dr. Raphael Blanchard, "La Faculté de Médicine de Beyrouth," *Conférence faite au comité de l'Asie Française, 29.1.1912* (Paris: siège social du Comité de l'Asie Française, 1912), 7.

[88] Rockefeller Archive Center, RF, RG2, S1927/833A, FA, "French Faculty of medicine, Beirut, notes of the RMP based on visit of March 22, 192, supplementing report of director of the school."

[89] Rockefeller Archive Center, RF, RG2, S1927/833A, FA, Pierre R. P. L. Verney, Chancellor, and Pierre R. P. P. de Vregille, Vice Chancellor, "French Faculty of Medicine of Beirut," 3.

Maronite elite explains the disparity between the institutions. Moreover, the AUB strove to provide education for all, and its student population was always more diverse in class and religious affiliation. This diversity made AUB more attractive to students outside Beirut and Mt. Lebanon.

AUB: A Professional and Sociocultural Hub

Since the late Ottoman period, SPC has become the leading regional medical school.[90] The first class included eight students, trained by three men trained in the United States: Drs. John Wortabet, Cornelius Van Dyck, and George Edward Post. Devoted missionaries and well-read theologians, they were also prolific authors of books, dictionaries, and Arabic textbooks on various topics. Born in Sidon, Wortabet's father was a Protestant preacher of Armenian descent, while the other two were Americans, sons of doctors.[91]

The "Lewis Affair" (1882) marked a rupture in the school's history: a mention of Darwin in the graduation ceremony led to the dismissal of a professor, a students' strike, and a split among the faculty. Former professors resigned, and the newly appointed ones, all Americans, spoke no Arabic. This was probably the main reason why English became the language of instruction after fifteen years. Switching to English meant that the professional language and training of Arab doctors were detached from their language and culture. Since the mid 1880s, the school's new senior faculty remained strictly foreign, mostly Americans or Canadians.[92]

The Medical School has employed local graduates since the early 1900s as instructors and assistants, yet all full professorships were restricted to Americans while excluding local faculty employees from decision-making forums. This policy changed in the early 1920s when several local staff members were granted "permanent status" and equal institutional rights, including voting in the General Faculty.[93]

90 Nabil Muhi al-Din Kronfol, "The Migratory Flow of the Medical Graduates of the American University of Beirut" (PhD diss., Harvard University, 1979), 3.

91 Charles A. Webster, "The Development of the Medical School," *The Medical Society Gazette* 2, no. 3 (February 1929): 1–5; Penrose, *That They May Have Life*, 33–41.

92 Penrose, *That They May Have Life*, 61, 65–68.

93 Ibid., 122–23, 202; Anderson, *The American*, 48–50; Bayard Dodge, *The American University of Beirut: A Brief History of the University and the Lands Which It Serves* (Beirut: Khayyat's, 1958), 30, 66–67, 93.

Two pioneering Palestinian students, N'ima Nakhu (1878–1955) from Nazareth and Sami Ibrahim Haddad (1890–1957) from Jaffa, became professors at the medical school.[94] From the 1930s onward, local doctors gradually took more senior positions at the school.[95] This institutional mobility was a source of inspiration for the new generation of doctors. It enabled limited localization of the professional language, which remained English yet was reclaimed and taught by Arabs.

Students came from Beirut and its surroundings, the Levant, Anatolia, Egypt, Iraq, Iran, and the Balkans.[96] The transition from Arabic to English enabled the admission of Armenian, Greek, Persian, and Bosnian students. The class of 1948 included thirty doctors, almost four times the first cohort.[97] In the 1947–48 academic year, 148 students were enrolled in the School of Medicine, 92 in the School of Pharmacy (est. 1871), and 51 in the Nurses Training School (est. 1905).[98]

The foreign missions dominated secondary education for girls until the end of the Mandate, and continuing to a long university training abroad was a bold move for young women, including members of prominent Christian families. Furthermore, it was only in November 1920 that the AUB voted to admit female students to its professional schools under the condition that at least three women would be enrolled together. The first woman graduated from the School of Dentistry in 1925 and from the School of Medicine in 1931.[99]

94 Ghazi Zaatrai, *Pathology and Laboratory Medicine at the American University of Beirut 1866–2015* (Beirut: American University of Beirut, 2015), 11–14, 38–39.

95 "Dean Ward Meets Our Alumni in Egypt and Palestine," *Al-Kulliyyah* 16, no. 6 (April 1930): 152–54; "The Tenth Annual Conference of the Medical Alumni of the American University of Beirut," *Al-Kulliyyah* 21, no. 5 (May 1935): 167; "Alumni News and Publications," *Al-Kulliyyah* 22, no. 2 (March 1947): 24.

96 Verdeil, "Naissance," 217–37.

97 Alumni Association, *Directory of Alumni*, 393–96.

98 "Registration," *Al-Kulliyyah* 22, no. 8 (November 1947), 21.

99 Aleksandra Kobiljski, "Women Students at the American University of Beirut from the 1920s to the 1940s," in *Gender, Religion and Change in the Middle East: Two Hundred Years of History*, eds. Inger Marie Okkenhaug and Ingvild Flaskerud (Oxford: Berg, 2006), 69–70. Except for those professional schools, women who wanted to be admitted to the AUB had to graduate from the American Junior College for Girls (est. 1927). See: Ellen L. Fleischmann, "'Under an American Roof': The Beginnings of the American Junior College for Women in Beirut," *Arab Studies Journal* 17 (2009): 62–84.

The number of students and the quality of the professors and medical facilities turned AUB into the leading regional center of the medical professions. Mandate rule in Palestine made the AUB even more attractive for Palestinians. The colonial Department of Education formulated the Palestine Matriculation Examination according to AUB's requirements. The strong personal relations between the department's heads and the Anglophone-Protestant staff of the AUB and the fact that the department's leading local officials studied there only strengthened this connection.[100]

Educating hundreds of Palestinians throughout the Mandate period, the AUB thus became among the most influential institutes of Palestine's educated elite.[101] In the 1920–21 academic year, 97 Arabs and Jews from Palestine were enrolled. This was a small number compared to students from Beirut (348) but not compared to the students from Aleppo and northern Syria (48) or from Iraq (12).[102] In 1932–33, 240 students from Palestine studied at the AUB, including about 148 Jews,[103] and the total reached 417 students in 1939.[104] The percentage of Palestinians (presumably both Arab and Jewish) graduating from AUB's medical faculty between 1935 and 1949 was 17 percent, and that of Armenian doctors – many of whom ended up working in Palestine – was 15 percent.[105]

A few Jews studied in mission schools, yet Palestine's secondary education schools were mostly segregated. This turned the AUB and St. Joseph into major spaces of encounters between Palestine's Arab and Jewish students. A Zionist group of students from Palestine was active on campus – and Arab students thus encountered Zionism up

[100] Abdul Latif Tibawi, *Arab Education in Mandatory Palestine: A Study of Three Decades of British Administration* (London: Luzac, 1956), 111. See also the diary of Director of the Education Department Humphry Bowman, February 27, 1924, Bowman files, Middle East Centre Archive (MECA); Bowman's testimony before the Royal Commission, November 27, 1936, 2/2/33, BM, MECA.

[101] Verdeil, "Naissance"; Verdeil, "L'Empire," 133–50.

[102] "Registration 1920–21," *Al-Kulliyyah* 7, no. 1 (November 1920): 9.

[103] "Registration," *Al-Kulliyyah* 20, no. 2 (December 1933): 38–40. In 1931–32, 261 Palestinians and 162 Jews were registered, ibid., "Registration," *Al-Kulliyyah* 19, no. 3 (February 1933): 71–72.

[104] This number is taken from Penrose, *That They May Have Life*, 331–35. Other sources suggest lower numbers: Bowman's testimony; Tibawi, *Arab Education*, 111; "Geographical Distribution of the A.U.B. Alumni," *Al-Kulliyyah* 20, no. 3 (1934): 69.

[105] Kronfol, "Migration Flows," chapter 3, table 7, 45, 55.

close.[106] John Tleel, a St. Joseph dentistry student in the late 1940s, recalled his good relations with Sam Loya, a Jewish student in his faculty. Loya "was very helpful" in John's first year in Beirut. He was in his last year and reciprocated the help from John's brother, who had similarly helped him before graduation. John described the student community as "a cocktail of Muslim, Polish, Armenian, Jewish, Lebanese, Druze, Palestinian, Syrian, Egyptian and Christian students (of various denominations)." He studied with a Polish Jewish immigrant from Tel Aviv and befriended him. He recalled that the Jewish students of the 1948 class at the School of Dentistry were secretly allowed to take their test before the British departure.[107]

In and out of the classroom, students met peers from the entire region and formed personal, political, and professional networks. Their shared Arabness created a common ground within what historian Betty Anderson called an American conceptualization of modernity.[108] Historian Hilary Falb Kalisman further underlined the distinctive habitus created at the AUB, noting that social mobility was inseparable from the "achievement of educational capital." AUB students, she shows, viewed themselves as leaders for a better future. Indeed, many of its graduates occupied senior positions in their new states' administration, often employing fellow graduates. This was particularly true of senior officials of Palestine's Mandate administration, specifically the DoH.[109]

The intensive school days far from home turned AUB students into an intimate group and refined their political worldviews. Their clubs and extracurricular activities helped reinforce horizontal bonds along class lines, crossing religious and ethnic boundaries.[110] Theater productions such as the one presented in the opening and the university's popular sports club were among the venues it offered for networking and a novel definition of self. The SPC's administration saw these

[106] Caroline Kahlenberg, "The Star of David in a Cedar Tree: Jewish Students and Zionism at the American University of Beirut (1908–1948)," *Middle Eastern Studies* 55, no. 4 (2019): 570–89.

[107] Tleel, *I Am Jerusalem*, 23, 36–37.

[108] Anderson, *The American*, 20–22.

[109] Hilary Falb Kalisman, "Schooling the State: Educators in Iraq, Palestine and Transjordan: c. 1890–c. 1960" (PhD diss., University of California, Berkeley, 2015), chapter 3; Christoph Schumann, "The Generation of Broad Expectations: Nationalism, Education, and Autobiography in Syria and Lebanon, 1930–1958," *Die Welt des Islams* 41 (2001): 174–205.

[110] Watenpaugh, *Being Modern*, 52–53.

activities as a means for forging a "college spirit" that would weaken racial, national, and religious barriers between students.[111]

Being the second-largest national group on campus, during the early 1920s, a Palestinian Club was active in the university. Da'ud al-Husayni, a dentistry student, mentioned the establishment of an imaginary state after the dissolution of the Palestinian Club, where Palestinian students took "formal" positions. He and his roommate, future doctor Mahmud Tahir al-Dajani, were ministers, and Ra'fat Faris served as chief patriarch.[112] Saba ʿAzzar from Jaffa was captain of the hockey team in the 1920s,[113] and Elias Sruji from the class of 1944 recalled the activities of *al-Urwah al-Wuthqa* (the Firmest Bond Society), the most popular club in the AUB, where speeches and debates about Arab nationalism were often held. According to Sruji, Palestinian students were the most dominant group in the society.[114]

The influence and connections of the school did not end upon graduation. AUB's alumni associations were instrumental in opening career paths for their members – in both the public and private sectors.[115] The university remained a hub for many graduates, who kept visiting and remained in touch through its various alumni societies, conferences, and the journal *al-Kulliyyah*. Graduates established local branches in Palestine in the early 1920s.[116]

The university also had its own Medical Society.[117] Through its medical conferences that began before WWI, it became an active hub for doctors who discussed contemporary medical issues and organized lectures about medical research.[118] The university likewise hosted alumni reunions, with symposiums about various medical topics and

111 Kestenian, "Portrait," 66. 112 Hammuda, *Sawt min al-Quds*, 349–50.

113 Imtiyaz Diyyab, ʿ*Atr madinat Yafa* (Beirut: Dar al-fatah li-l-nashr wa-l-tawziʿ, 1991), 184

114 Sruji, *Min muruj*, 98, 104–05.

115 Esther Moller, "'We Do Not Learn for School, But For Life': Alumni Associations at French Schools in Lebanon in the 1930s and 1940s as Privileged Spaces of Sociability," in Hauser et al., eds., *Entangled Education*, 265–82.

116 Dr. Tawfiq Canaan, Dr. Ibrahim Itayim, and Dr. Munir Mishʿalani chaired the Jerusalem, Tulkarem, and Nazareth branches, respectively, "News from Jerusalem," *Al-Kulliyyah*, 7, no. 4 (1921): 62; C. B. Muammar, "Nazareth," *Al-Kulliyyah* 19, no. 5 (1933): 157; "Alumni News," *Al-Kulliyyah* 20, no. 2 (1933): 66; "Report of Progress: Medical Branch," *Al-Kulliyyah* 20, no. 3 (1934): 92–93.

117 A. Afghani, "The Medical Society," *Al-Kulliyyah*, 7, no. 8 (1921): 135–36; "Medical Branch," *Al-Kulliyyah* 19, no. 5 (1933): 156.

118 Dr. Ward, "Third Medical Alumni Conference," *Al-Kulliyyah* 7, no. 6 (1921): 94–97.

visits to clinics and hospitals.[119] The Jerusalem branch of the SPC's Alumni Association included fourteen members, of whom six were doctors and three pharmacists.[120] In the early years of the twentieth century, the YMCA and the SPC's alumni associations served as social centers for Palestinian medical professionals.[121] Within the emerging pre-WWI cultural and local medical scene, the American institute was highly influential for its graduates and the many students who aspired to study there.

The Medical Society was also a social clique. In one of its receptions in 1930, alongside formal faculty and students' speeches, a costume contest was held, and a jazz band "dressed as apache [sic]" entertained, with "hundreds of students from the School of Arts and Sciences peeping through the windows to see the costumes." The Society's journal conveyed a sense of camaraderie between the students and nonformal relationships with the faculty with its humoristic entries and amusing caricatures.[122] Editorial entries called for unity among medical students from different classes; one of them stated: "We are all here not to be turned out as Egyptian, Iraquian [sic] or Persian doctors but as Doctors, Graduates, of the Medical School."[123]

Conclusion

Within a few decades, Palestinians integrated into global academization and professionalization processes. The practice of medicine played a prestigious sociocultural role alongside the state bureaucracy, religious scholarship, and commerce. This manifested in the financial efforts that notable families from urban centers, towns, and even villages invested to send their sons to private secondary education and then to four long and expensive years abroad. Becoming a doctor was a realistic dream for those who could afford it and a lucrative

119 Almost a third of the participants in the 1932 doctors' reunion were Palestinian, "Report of Progress: Medical Alumni Reunion," *Al-Kulliyyah*, 19, no. 2 (1932): 56–60.

120 *Al-Kulliyyah* 5, no. 1 (November 1913): 23.

121 Philippe Bourmaud, "Epidemiology and the City: Communal vs. Intercommunal Health Policy-Making in Jerusalem from the Ottomans to the Mandate, 1908–1925," in Dalachanis and Lemire, eds., *Ordinary Jerusalem*, 450.

122 "The Annual Reception of the Medical Society," *The Medical Society Gazette* 2, no. 4–5 (June 1930): 25–26.

123 "Pleas," *The Medical Society Gazette* 1, no. 4 (June 1929): 25–26.

trajectory for those with fewer alternatives. In urban centers and towns, the Muslim notability and Christian communities were the main customers of missionary education, which enabled proceeding to academic training. Church connections eased the latter's acquaintance with the sociocultural and scholarly habitus of Beirut's faculties.

For Palestinians, becoming doctors also meant becoming global, living abroad, connecting with Armenian, Jewish, and Arab students from across the region, and gaining proficiency in a second or third language while studying under foreign professors. As a professional community, this made them a distinctive group within Palestinian society, an elite within the elite. The dominance of AUB's medical faculty was pivotal in characterizing this community. English finally claimed the throne of the scientific and professional lingua franca under British colonialism. The students were trained in American English and French and imbued with Western culture while forming professional networks and lifelong friendships with doctors from other parts of the Arab world. Local doctors' associations, conferences at the AUB, and regional medical conferences fostered a shared ethos of independent local empowerment, a joint effort in a national scientific civilizing mission.

Becoming a doctor was, to some degree, a class matter, but the professional features of the trade challenged its once impervious ranks. Palestinian doctors and those from Lebanon and Anatolia moved around the country, treating and marrying locals. This movement enhanced the connections between local notabilities from different localities and enabled the inclusion of new members. The practice of medicine was also a conduit through which those of less privileged backgrounds could relocate physically and socially through wit and effort. This movement within and into the expanding urban classes further enhanced the disintegration of previous class divisions and reshaped Palestine's social fabric.

Chapter 3 will take the group of men born, raised, and educated in this chapter to one of the main employers in the Mandate years – the DoH. Since the market for private practice was limited, government employment offered a reliable career trajectory, especially for the dozens of doctors who graduated during or around WWI. The DoH appreciated the ability to rely on local personnel educated in a European institution. Chapter 3 will examine the tensions and contradictions of this encounter.

3 Colonial Care: Understanding the Department of Health

On October 5, 1935, Dr. Sami Shihab appealed to his superiors in the colonial Department of Health (DoH) and requested to be transferred to a larger city:

> I beg to point out that the prevailant [sic.] local health conditions make it impossible for me to school my children in Hebron. Furthermore, I personally have had a number of break downs on account of the lumbago which I have contracted in Hebron and which neither the change of sites nor the houses has had any effect on me.

Shihab further noted that the absence of his young children, whom he had to send to their grandparents in Damascus for their education, "has been causing a lot of anxiety to the mother and constant worry to myself. This, coupled with certain inconveniences connected with the work is causing me extra mental strain and rendering my burden twice as heavy as it should be." The DoH consistently refused Shihab's requests.[1]

The current chapter concentrates on the DoH and its medical officers (MOs), with two goals in mind: to analyze the infrastructure of medical services in Mandate Palestine, and to situate Arab doctors within this grid. Shihab's is one of the only surviving personnel files of Arab physicians in the Israel State Archives. It sheds light on colonial modes of operation and reflects the experience of an Arab MO working in Palestine's periphery. Appointed to serve a population of over 80,000, Shihab usually met long queues of villagers to whom he could not possibly devote proper attention. Adding pain to injury, his Aleppo urbanite origins turned his experience in Palestine into one replete with cultural tensions and misunderstandings.

[1] Sami Shihab, "Application for Transfer," October 5, 1935; Sami Shihab, "Application for Transfer," February 1, 1938, in Shihab, Sami. Medical Officer of Health, 1st Jacket, M/4250/5, Israel State Archive (ISA).

The state, as noted earlier, is one of the main explanatory factors in analyzing the formation of the professions.[2] In the case of Palestine, as in other colonial settings, the fact that the state was an external actor entailed both complementary and conflictual relationships with the medical profession. On the one hand, the DoH was a significant employer: 25–35 percent of all Palestinian physicians worked there at any given time. On the other hand, they had minimal impact on decision-making: British MOs occupied the top administrative echelons, restricting local medical professionals' autonomy and career prospects.

Throughout the British Empire, medicine served the colonial project, initially by caring for the colonial military and administrative personnel, then by treating the local population to protect European enclaves from infectious diseases, and finally by providing healthcare to the colonized.[3] When the British occupied Palestine, they were already administering a decades-old colonial medical apparatus on a global scale. From Nigeria to Malaya, British colonial health services varied in structure, personnel, and outreach, mirroring the internal and external challenges they faced. Caught between the policy and vision of the Colonial Office and local realities, demands, and possibilities, colonial medicine involved maneuvering, negotiations, and leveraging. Moreover, despite a nearly total Anglo-Saxon supremacy in its institutional hierarchy since the late nineteenth century, the Empire's dependence on intermediaries and subordinates, local or non-European personnel, became a common feature. Indian doctors served in the colonial health services across India, Malaya, and Africa, and African auxiliary personnel became an indispensable part of hospitals, clinics, and dispensaries.[4]

[2] Michael Burrage, Konrad Jarausch, and Hannes Siegrist, "An Actor-Based Framework for the Study of the Professions," in *Professions in Theory and History: Rethinking the Study of the Professions*, eds. Michael Burrage and Rolf Torstendahl (London: Sage, 1990), 208.

[3] Shula Marks, "What Is Colonial about Colonial Medicine? And What Has Happened to Imperialism and Health?" *Social History of Medicine* 10 (1997): 205–19. Scholarship on colonial medicine is extensive. Examples include Luise White, *Speaking with Vampires: Rumor and History in Colonial Africa* (Berkeley: University of California Press, 2000); Shiyong Liu, *Prescribing Colonization: The Role of Medical Practices and Policies in Japan-Ruled Taiwan, 1895–1945* (Ann Arbor: Association for Asian Studies, 2009); Guillaume Lachenal, *The Lomidine Files: The Untold Story of a Medical Disaster in Colonial Africa* (Baltimore: Johns Hopkins University Press, 2017).

[4] Anna Khalid and Ryan Johnson, "Introduction," in *Public Health in the British Empire Intermediaries, Subordinates, and the Practice of Public Health,*

The Palestine DoH was yet another branch of this apparatus, and like all others, bore its own nuances. Unlike most other colonial possessions, in Palestine, British authorities met an existing medical infrastructure and university-trained Arab medical doctors. In addition, the state's approach to the Arab medical profession reflected the Mandate's dual role. The League of Nations Convention entrusted it with rendering the local communities "administrative advice and assistance [...] until such time as they are able to stand alone." At the same time, it required British authorities to promote the establishment of a Jewish "national home." This duality had concrete implications for local medical services. While the Jewish community started building a state-like medical infrastructure, the Arabs relied on the DoH's services. The outcome was inherent tension between the British imperial experience, the promise for self-rule, and the "national home" project.

The adjustment of imperial rule to Palestine's specific circumstances did not translate into a proto-state administrative structure – even when Palestinian society provided the necessary trained personnel. Local doctors were highly involved in health administration, but a process of statewide empowerment that would gradually enable medical self-rule never materialized. The Mandate authorities tried to balance their commitment to both communities, yet in terms of health services, it was limited to the bare minimum. Criticism by Palestinian urban and rural communities, the League of Nations' Permanent Mandate Commission, and the 1937 Peel Commission led to a measured increase in health services, particularly during the Arab Revolt (1936–39), and following World War II (1946–48).

This chapter charts the development of the DoH throughout the Mandate years and brings to the fore its relationship with this book's protagonists – Arab medical professionals and their communities. Its first section explores the transitionary stages of British control and its relationship with the Ottoman and voluntary medical infrastructures. It then maps the early British attempts to provide basic medical services and the measured increase in government investment in the 1930s and 1940s. Next, it examines the Palestinian physicians employed by the

1850–1960, eds. Anna Khalid and Ryan Johnson (New York: Routledge, 2012), 20; Ryan Johnson, "'An All-White Institution': Defending Private Practice and the Formation of the West African Medical Staff," *Medical History* 54 (2010): 237–54.

DoH, and proceeds to look at the patients and how they were represented by and made claims for improved medical services in the Palestinian press. The chapter concludes with attempts made by the DoH's last director to remedy its ills during the final two years of the British Mandate.

Transition

The Ottoman and missionary medical infrastructure described in Chapter 1 suffered a significant blow during World War I (WWI). Ottoman authorities hindered the operations of institutions belonging to British and French missionaries, limiting the medical assistance available to Palestine's inhabitants. Some of these establishments were ransacked and laid to waste, returning to service only months or years following the British occupation. In addition, missionary hospitals were in financial straits during the Mandate's early years and were forced to start charging fees or close down for several months a year.[5]

International charities such as the Ottoman Red Crescent and the American Red Cross partly filled the void created by the near paralysis of missionary services during the war and its immediate aftermath. Jerusalem's Pasteur Institute and Nathan Strauss' Health Station were among the Jewish institutions that did so. The Syria and Palestine Relief Society and the American Red Cross operated hospitals and clinics until voluntary hospitals gradually resumed their activities in mid 1919.

In the summer of 1919, when American Red Cross personnel left the country, they handed over their installations, equipment, and supplies to the British Health Service of the Occupied Enemy Territory Administration (OETA, active from 1917–20).[6] Operating under the OETA, the Health Service for Palestine started its activity in Jerusalem and Jaffa in December 1917, and extended its operation to Haifa,

[5] Muhammad Qaraqra, *al-Khidamat al-sihhiyya al-hukumiyya wa-l-ahliyya li-l-sha'b al-Filastini aban al-intidab, 1918–1948* (Shefa-ʿAmr: Jamaʿiyyat al-Jalil li-l-buhuth wa-l-khidamat al-sihhiyya, 2017), 247; *An Interim Report on the Civil Administration of Palestine during the Period 1st July 1920–30th June 1921* (London: HMSO, 1921), 4, 35 (henceforth: *An Interim Report, 1921*).

[6] *An Interim Report, 1921*, 1; Qaraqra, *al-Khidamat*, 61, 115; Nissim Levi, *Prakim be-toldot ha-refu'a be-Erets Yisra'el, 1799–1948* (Tel Aviv: ha-Kibbuts ha-Meuhad, 1998), 159–65.

Nablus, and the Galilee by the end of the war. The first steps taken included the obligatory notification of infectious diseases and the licensing of medical personnel. In May 1918, OETA issued a decree calling doctors and mukhtars to notify the authorities of all infectious diseases.[7] Another decree enabled the licensing of doctors holding a degree from recognized institutions to work in Palestine, laying the legal basis for medical practice under the Mandate.[8]

Initially, and to compensate for the lack of medical services, the OETA's Health Service established four- to eight-bed hospitals in Nazareth, Safad, Tiberias, Majdal, Bisan, and Jenin, and traveling hospitals on camels. During the first years of the Mandate, the authorities ran a mobile emergency clinic to deal with localized epidemic outbreaks and provide field hospital services. In 1919, it also initiated a traveling ophthalmic hospital for the countryside.[9]

Alongside medical doctors, missionary hospitals, and voluntary organizations' equipment, the DoH inherited from the Ottomans eleven governmental and municipal hospitals throughout Palestine.[10] In 1921, Mandate authorities noted that the Jerusalem, Haifa, Jaffa, Nablus, and Ramallah hospitals were "fairly well housed." In contrast, the hospital buildings of Ramleh, Tulkarem, Gaza, Acre, Hebron, and Beersheba were "entirely unsuitable," in ruinous condition. In some places, the Mandate's annual report asserted that work had begun on new buildings or the reconstruction and repair of existing ones.[11] Most of these initiatives were short-lived, and British authorities preferred missionary investment to funding health services themselves. Accordingly, they hastened to reopen the missionary hospitals and medical facilities that had closed down during the war but closed down government and municipal hospitals and clinics.[12]

7 Qaraqra, *al-Khidamat*, 294; *An Interim Report, 1921*, 27–28.

8 Mikhael Assaf, *ha-Yahasim ben Yehudim ve-ʿAravim be-Erets Yisraʾel, 1860–1948* (Tel Aviv: Tarbut ve-hinukh, 1970), 290; Philippe Bourmaud, "'Ya doktor': Devenir médecin et exercer son art en 'Terre sainte', une expérience du pluralisme médical dans l'Empire ottoman finissant (1871–1918)" (PhD diss., Aix-Marseille I, 2007), 748.

9 Qaraqra, *al-Khidamat*, 294; *An Interim Report, 1921*, 27–28.

10 Bourmaud, "'Ya doktor'," 504.

11 The DoH equipped hospitals with mattresses, blankets, sheets, clothing, English hospital beds, and new surgical instruments. *An Interim Report, 1921*, 33.

12 Frances S. Hasso, *Buried in the Red Dirt: Race, Reproduction, and Death in Modern Palestine* (Cambridge: Cambridge University Press, 2021), 83; Qaraqra, *al-Khidamat*, 63.

The Department of Health: Structure, Budget, and Institutions

After five years of tenure as Palestine's first High Commissioner, Herbert Samuel declared, "[n]owhere was there a more pressing need for action, and nowhere has greater progress been achieved than in the sphere of public health." Nevertheless, his report, which concluded the formative years that determined the Mandate's administrative modus operandi, reveals the British dependence on Zionist and missionary funding and capabilities in all fields of public health.[13] Despite expanding colonial services in the coming decades, they remained central players throughout the Mandate years.

The early 1920s marked the construction of the Department of Health and the laying of foundations for the country's public health infrastructure. Established in 1921, its initial goals were to treat British personnel, preserve the administration's political interests, and improve the population's health conditions, in that order. In 1945, 9.7 percent of the government hospital's beds were dedicated to British citizens and attended solely by British staff. In Jerusalem this was the case for 40.9 percent of the beds, and in Jaffa only 4.3 percent.[14] Additional goals included disease prevention through sanitation efforts, hospitalization, and isolation services for patients contaminated with infectious diseases and for the mentally ill. The DoH comprised five subdepartments: public health, hospitals, laboratory services, quarantine services, and logistics. The country was divided

[13] Herbert Samuel, *Palestine: Report of the High Commissioner on the Administration of Palestine, 1920–1925* (London: His Majesty's Stationery Office, 1925), 10–13; *A Survey of Palestine 1946* (Jerusalem: Government Printer, 1946–47), 610, 633–34; Muhammad Yunis al-Husayni, *al-Tatawwur al-ijtimaʿi wa-l-iqtisadi fi Filastin al-ʿArabiyya* (Jerusalem: Maktabat al-Tahir Ikhwan, 1947), 196–97; Nira Reiss, *Health Services to the Arab Population in Israel* (Tel Aviv: International Center for Peace in the Middle East, 1988), 17–18.

[14] As late as 1945, the government hospitals in Jerusalem, Haifa, and Jaffa, allocated 40 percent, 10 percent, and 4 percent of their beds, respectively, to British patients. Department of Health, *Annual Report for the Year 1945* (Jerusalem: Department of Health, 1946), 9 (henceforth: DoH, *Annual Report, 1946*); Nira Reiss, "British Public Health Policy in Palestine, 1918–1947," in *Health and Disease in the Holy Land: Studies in the History and Sociology of Medicine from Ancient Times to the Present*, eds. Samuel S. Kottek and Manfred Waserman (Lewiston, NY: Edwin Mellen Press, 1996), 302; Sandy Sufian, "Re-imagining Palestine: Scientific Knowledge and Malaria Control in Mandatory Palestine," *Dynamis* 25 (2005): 358.

into four districts, headed by a Senior MO, and eighteen subdistricts, headed by an MO and staffed by health inspectors, physicians, and nurses.[15]

The DoH's epidemic services included isolation wards in government hospitals, a quarantine department, epidemic disease hospitals, and government laboratories, which conducted blood tests and prepared vaccinations.[16] Hospitals for epidemic diseases and epidemic control stations were established in Nazareth, Safad, Tiberias, Majdal, Bisan, and Jenin. The DoH also supervised health regulations on food vendors and restaurants and enforced quarantine regulations.[17] With its expanding network of primary government schools in villages, the colonial Department of Education also served as a conduit for health regulation and health services. Students were vaccinated, examined by government physicians, and taught basic hygiene. This operation, however, was restricted to the localities in which a school operated, and thus only reached roughly a third of the school-age population by the end of the Mandate.[18]

Anat Mooreville showed that the DoH's ophthalmic service was designed to eradicate trachoma, the so-called scourge of the East.[19] Ophthalmic medicine also had the effect of "performative medicine," namely medical treatment intended to demonstrate the effectiveness of modern medicine and hence the benefits of colonial rule.[20] It was also highly cost-effective – eye drops were cheap, teachers and nurses could administer them to students, and a doctor would see eye patients weekly or biweekly. Most importantly, ophthalmic services reduced blindness, which burdened families and communities, with minimal

15 Qaraqra, *al-Khidamat*, 116–17.

16 Reiss, *Health Services*, 18–19; Sufian, "Re-imagining Palestine"; Zalman Greenberg and Rakefet Zalashik, "Masaʿ mishlahat hever ha-leʾummim le-hakirat ha-malariya be-Erets Yisraʾel bi-shnat 1925," *Cathedra* 134 (2010): 49–64. The Jewish National Fund and the Supreme Muslim Council also took part in swamp drainage, Assaf, *ha-Yahasim*, 180.

17 Aref Abu Rabia, "Bedouin Health Services in Mandate Palestine," *Middle Eastern Studies* 41 (2005): 421–22.

18 Reiss, "British Public," 307; Reiss, *Health Services*, 21.

19 Anat Mooreville, "Oculists in the Orient: A History of Trachoma, Zionism, and Global Health, 1882–1973" (PhD diss., UCLA, 2015), 113–19.

20 Robert Blecher, "Desert Medicine, Ethnography and Colonial Encounter in Mandatory Syria," in *The British and French Mandates in Comparative Perspectives*, eds. Nadine Meouchy and Peter Sluglett (Leiden: Brill, 2004), 249–68.

cost. During the Mandate's first summers, the DoH maintained traveling ophthalmic units in Nablus, Ramleh, and Hebron. In 1924, ophthalmic clinics were established in Gaza, Ramleh, Nablus, Beersheba, and Acre, alongside a traveling ophthalmic hospital in schools.[21]

In 1926, Mandate authorities operated fifteen public clinics, six ophthalmic dispensaries, and eight Infant Welfare Centers (IWCs). With relatively small financial investment, the latter two helped reduce two of the most significant health hazards: trachoma-induced blindness and infant mortality. The demand for modern healthcare in the rural periphery dramatically surpassed its supply.[22] In 1931, George Heron, the DoH Director since its foundation, observed that "wherever we have placed an Infant Welfare Center, the attendance has in a few months invariably out-numbered the capacity of the Center and the Nurse."[23]

In 1922, the DoH maintained that "the presence of the voluntary hospitals in Palestine very largely relieves the government from its responsibility for providing accommodation in its hospitals for the country's sick,"[24] and thus saw it as its duty to provide medical attention to British personnel and the very poor.[25] From 1930 onward, the DoH redefined its mission to providing medical services for the general population "where no provision or inadequate provision is made by voluntary organizations."[26] In 1933, medical services were to become available "where no private practitioner or other medical assistance is available." The change was not confined to colonial rhetoric. From this point on, there was an increase in government investment in public health, particularly in hospitalization services and ophthalmic and infant care.[27]

As for budget allocation, the beginning seemed promising. The first High Commissioner, Herbert Samuel, invested in infrastructure, for which he took loans and ran a deficit budget. From 1923 onward, however, the British Treasury and Colonial Office imposed a balanced budget policy in Palestine, despite Samuel's insistence that increasing social services would contribute to British popularity among the local

[21] Mooreville, "Oculists," 114–15. [22] DoH, *Annual Report, 1926*, 27–32.
[23] Letter from Heron to the Chief Secretary, Government Office, Jerusalem, "Report of the O'Donnell Commission," September 15, 1931, CO 733/208/9, NA, 10.
[24] *An Interim Report, 1921*, 35. [25] Hasso, *Buried in the Red Dirt*, 81.
[26] DoH, *Annual Report, 1930*, 42. [27] DoH, *Annual Report, 1933*, 44.

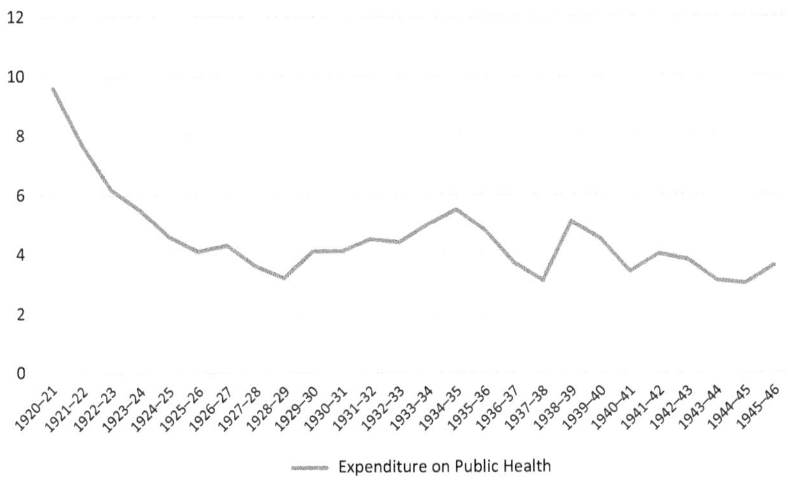

Figure 3.1 Annual expenditure on public health, percentage of the total budget.

population. The budget for the administration of Palestine was cut substantially, severely affecting the DoH.[28] The lion's share of the budget was spent on security and salaries, while only 4–5 percent was allotted to health.[29] Figure 3.1 shows these rates' fluctuations throughout the Mandate years.

One manifestation of this budgetary policy was the shutdown of government hospitals, whose number dropped to four in 1925. The DoH and the municipalities jointly maintained another four.[30] In 1923–24, the DoH transferred the responsibility for the Gaza, Tulkarem, Acre, and Jaffa government hospitals to their respective municipalities, leaving only the Jerusalem and Haifa hospitals under its responsibility. Clinics in villages and towns with missionary medical facilities were likewise closed.[31] From 1924 until the mid 1930s,

[28] Ya'kov Re'uveni, *Mimshal ha-mandat be-Erets Yisra'el, 1920–1948: Nittuah histori-medini* (Ramat Gan: Bar-Ilan University, 1993), 180.

[29] Hasso, *Buried in the Red Dirt*, 84–86; Nachum Gross, *The Economic Policy of the Mandatory Government in Palestine* (Jerusalem: Maurice Falk Institute for Economic Research in Israel, 1982), 5–8, 20; Jacob Norris, *Land of Progress: Palestine in the Age of Colonial Development, 1905–1948* (Oxford: Oxford University Press, 2013), 14, 116–17.

[30] *Reports of the Experts Submitted to the Joint Palestine Survey Commission, October 1st, 1928* (Boston: Daniels Printing, 1928), 635.

[31] Qaraqra, *al-Khidamat*, 122–24.

municipal hospitals were funded jointly by the respective municipal authority and the government. The Mandate authorities paid for the medical staff and medications, while the municipality paid for other hospital operations.[32] The government also covered half the cost of municipal hospitals, which allowed free treatment to government officers, police, prisoners, accident victims, and the poor.[33] In 1929, British authorities noted in retrospect that since the closing of the government hospitals in Tulkarem, Ramleh, Majdal, Ramallah, and Hebron, most of the Arab population had no adequate hospital facilities.[34] In 1932, the municipal hospitals of Beersheba and Acre also closed down.[35]

The budgetary policy also increased the MO's work overload, constantly yet unsuccessfully combating the absence of institutions and trained personnel. In cities and large towns, MOs and government hospitals were only a part of the local medical services, which included missionary hospitals, a small community of private practitioners, and a larger community of Jewish doctors. Smaller towns offered fewer alternatives, and MOs carried the weight of government policies. Since they served both the town and its surrounding villages, only a few days a week could be dedicated to the townspeople. For example, one MO was responsible for sixty-three villages around Ramallah, and another for the entire Naqab's Bedouin population.[36] In 1945, two government physicians in the Nablus District served a population of 94,000; in Hebron, two served 87,000; in Gaza, two served 105,400; and in Tulkarem, two served 72,000.[37] In clinics and weekly visits, their workload, daily routine, and interactions with patients reflected an inability to serve the population's needs.

Shihab's weekly schedule in Hebron (see Figure 3.2) attests to the consequences of MOs' responsibilities outside smaller urban centers

[32] "Note on the Central Emek Hospital," J1/4588, CZA.

[33] Heron to the Chief Secretary, "Report of the O'Donnell Commission," 7–8; Muhammad Qaraqra, "Maʿarekhet ha-briʾut ha-mandatorit ve-ha-voluntarit ve-ʿArviye Erets Yisraʾel, 1918–1948" (MA thesis, Haifa University, 1992), 64.

[34] *Report by His Majesty's Government in the United Kingdom of Great Britain and Northern Ireland to the Council of the League of Nations on the Administration of Palestine and Trans-Jordan for the Year 1929* (London: His Majesty's Stationery Office, 1930), 86 (henceforth: *Report to the LoN, year).*

[35] *Report to the LoN, 1933*, 138. [36] Qaraqra, "Maʿarekhet," 54.

[37] Yosef Washitz, *ha-ʿAravim be-Erets Yisraʾel* (Merhavia: al-Kibbuts ha-Artsi, 1947), 200; Qaraqra, "Maʿarekhet," 93; Reiss, "British Public," 308.

	1st Week	2nd Week	3rd Week	4th Week
Monday	Clinic at Hebron	Clinic at Hebron	Clinic at Hebron	Clinic at Hebron
Tuesday	Operations at Hebron	Operations at Hebron	Operations at Hebron	Operations at Hebron
Wednesday	DITTO	DITTO	DITTO	DITTO
Thursday	Targoumia and Area	Dewayma	Beit-Jibrin and Area	Ajjour and Area
Friday	OFF	OFF	OFF	OFF
Saturday	Operations At Beit-Jibrin	Operations At Beit-Jibrin	Operations At Beit-Jibrin	Operations At Beit-Jibrin
Sunday	Doura	Dahria	BeitOmmer and Area	Yatta and Area

Figure 3.2 Sami Shihab's weekly routine.[38]

and the limitations of government services, due to inadequate MO-patient ratios outside Palestine's larger cities. Based in Hebron, three of Shihab's working days were spent there, while the two other days were divided between al-Dawayima (24 km west of Hebron), Beit Ummar, Tarqumiya, Ajjur, and Beit Jibrin (11, 12, 21, and 24 km northwest of Hebron, respectively), Yatta and Dura (8 and 10 km south of Hebron, respectively), and al-Dhahiriya (22 km southwest of Hebron). These were eight relatively large villages, and Shihab's responsibility included their surrounding "area" as specified in Figure 3.2.

Similarly, Bertha Ma'luf, whose husband Mikha'il was Bethlehem's MO from 1930 until his murder in 1948, recounts that in addition to his regional duties, he was also in charge of Palestine's mental hospitals and served as a government expert in criminal cases. His daily routine started with three hours, from 8:30 to 11:30, at his Bethlehem clinic. He then drove his black Dodge to his other clinics in Deheisheh and Beit Jalla. His weekly routine included visits to Bethlehem's mental hospital and to villages and kibbutzim around town – the former to provide medical services and the latter only to inspect the Jewish ones. He also owned a horse for visiting remote villages inaccessible by car.[39] Such a routine left the town underserved and the MO exhausted.

[38] ISA, "Shihab, Dr. Sami. Medical Officer of Health, 1st Jacket," M/4250/5, Senior Medical Officer to District Health Office, Hebron, "Time-Table Dr. S. Shihab for Winter season 1937–8," December 23, 1937.

[39] Larry Collins Papers, GTM.Gamms315, Box 2, Folder 18, Interviews: Numbered Files, 4a, 1, 2, 6.

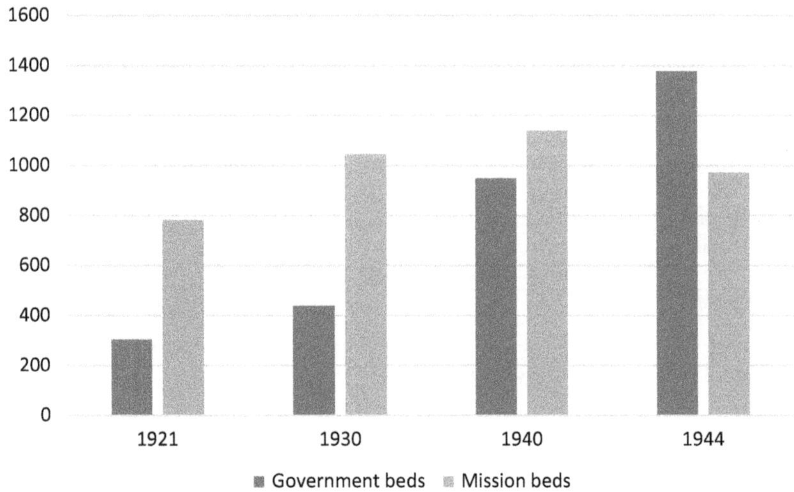

Figure 3.3 The total number of hospital beds.[40]

By the late 1930s, following increasing pressure by the local population and due to the repercussions of the Great Arab Revolt (1936–39), the DoH took greater responsibility for hospitalization services, and slightly increased its budget allocation (see Figure 3.1). While the size of missionary hospitals remained stable, government hospitals in Jerusalem and Haifa doubled in size. In addition, when community and municipal hospitals in Gaza, Jaffa, and Nablus struggled to survive during the Arab Revolt, the colonial authorities took them under their wings and expanded them (see Figures 3.3 and 3.4). A new hospital facility opened in Haifa in 1938, with installations and equipment "up to the standard of modern European hospitals." The same year, the government hospital in Jerusalem expanded to allow for additional beds for wives and families of British police and soldiers.[41] Overall, the percentage of government hospital beds went up from 14 percent in 1925 to 24 percent in 1935 and 33 percent in 1944.[42]

By 1939, trained medical orderlies managed ophthalmic services, which included a traveling ophthalmic unit, eight town clinics, twenty village first-aid units, whose personnel regularly visited neighboring villages, and thirty-nine IWCs (some of which were funded or co-

[40] *A Survey of Palestine 1946*, 615. [41] *Report to the LoN, … 1938*, 170.
[42] Gross, *The Economic Policy*, 50; *A Survey of Palestine 1946*, 610–11.

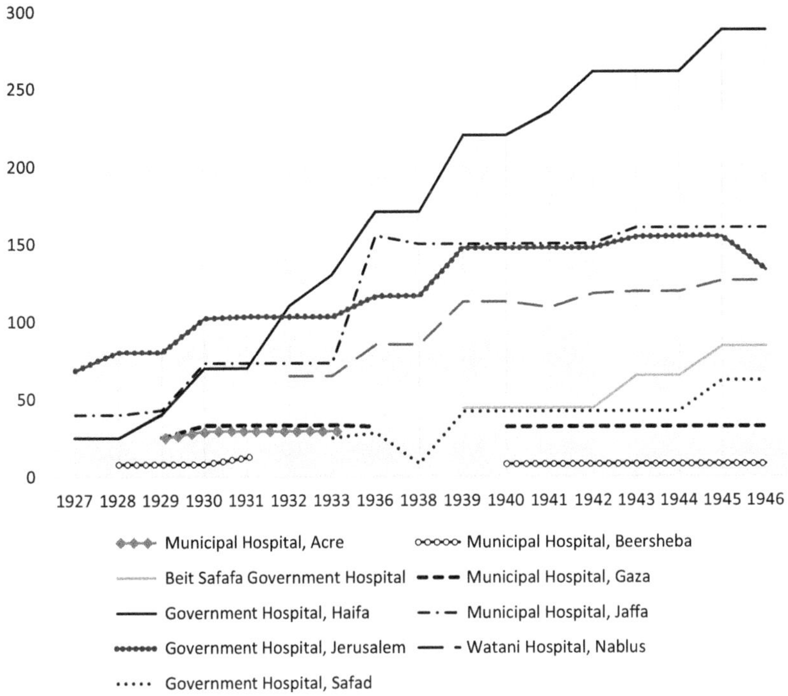

Figure 3.4 Bed strength of municipal and governmental hospitals.[43]

funded by municipalities and local voluntary associations) (see Figure 3.4).[44] The countrywide spread of government health facilities can be seen in Figure 3.5. By the mid 1940s, there were twenty-one outpatient clinics in cities and towns (see Figures 3.8 and 3.9), nineteen weekly village clinics, forty-one village ophthalmic clinics (see Figure 3.7), five gynecological stations, and thirty-eight IWCs. Local voluntary committees operated seven additional IWCs. Furthermore, government hospitals operated five hospital training centers for midwives and nurses. By the end of the Mandate period, there was one midwife for every 4,000 inhabitants.[45]

The impact of gradual expansion in public health services should be qualified, however, in view of the rapid demographic growth of the Arab population, which more than doubled between 1919 and 1948 –

[43] Based on DoH, *Annual Reports*, 1927–46.
[44] DoH, *Annual Report,* 1939, 52–53; Hasso, *Buried in the Red Dirt*, 89–90.
[45] Al-Husayni, *al-Tatawwur*, 176–77; Assaf, *ha-Yahasim*, 297.

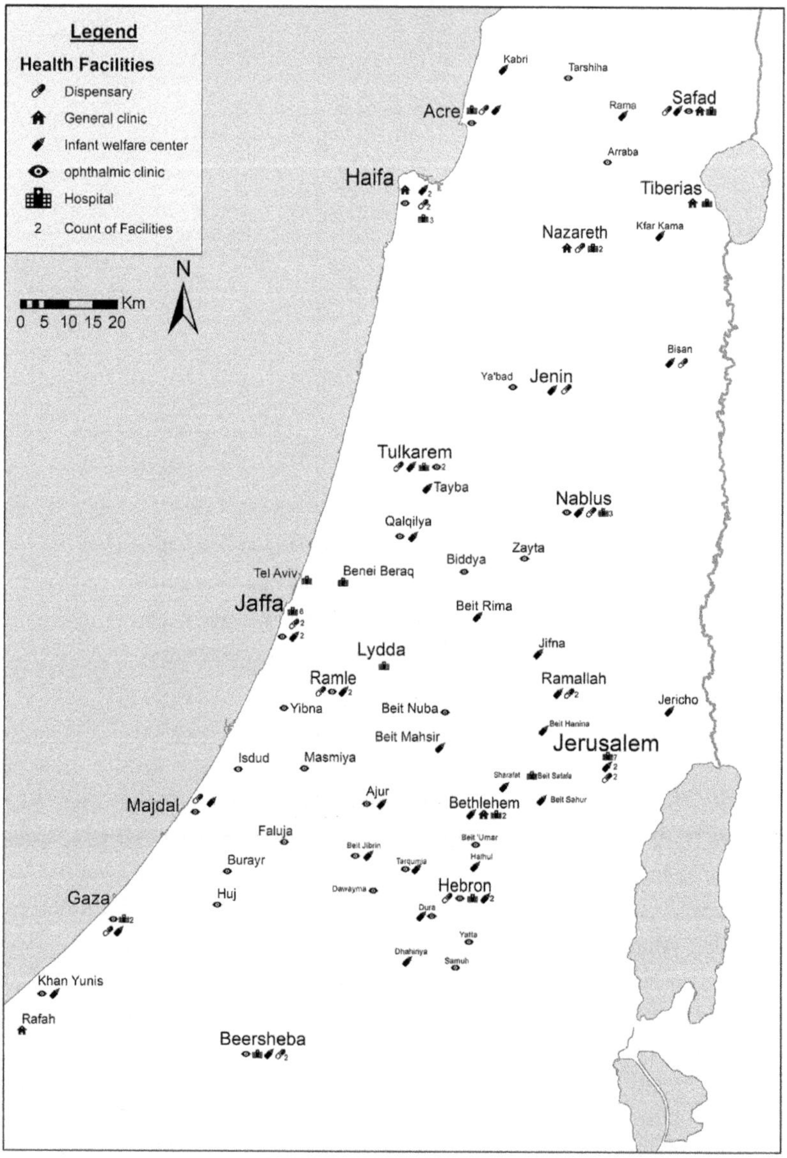

Figure 3.5 The countrywide spread of government health institutions, 1939.[46]

[46] DoH, *Annual Report, 1939*, 52–53.

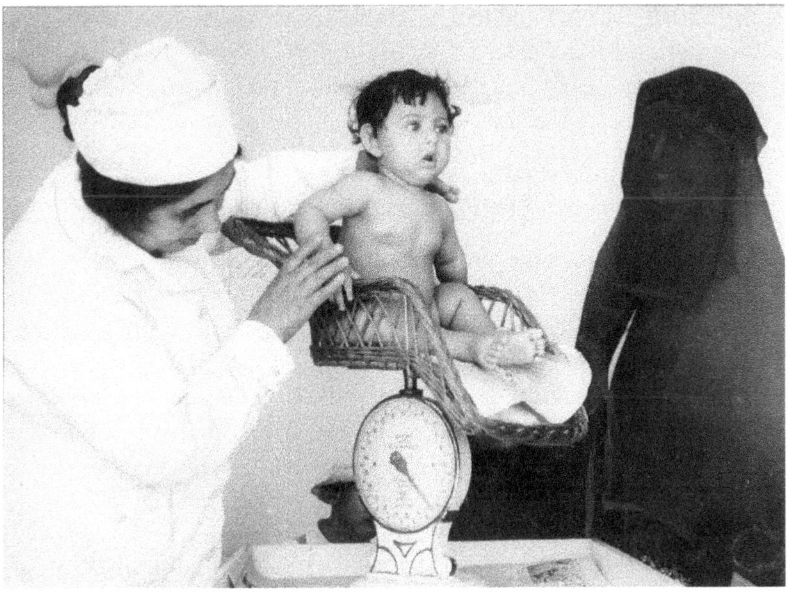

Figure 3.6 Nurse weighing a child at Haifa's government clinic.
TS-3024/60, Public Information Office Collection, ISA

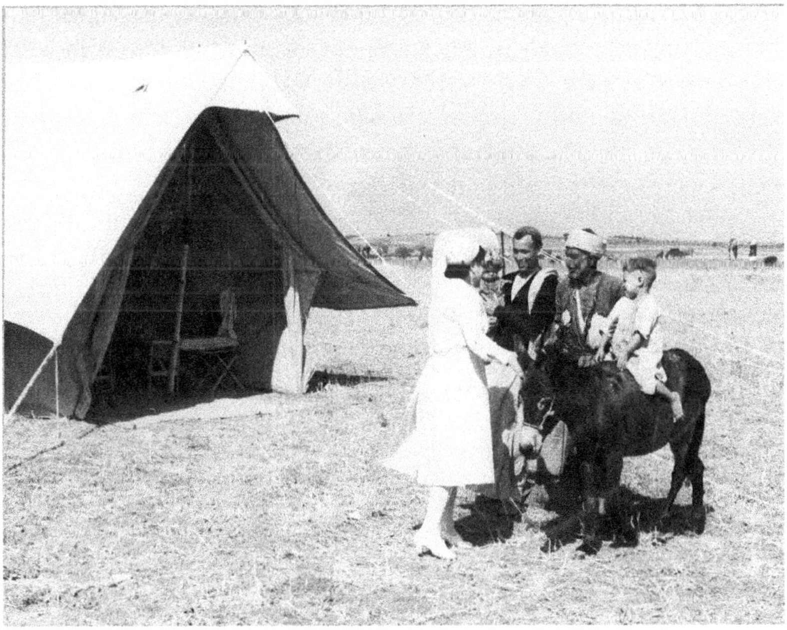

Figure 3.7 Field eye clinic receiving patients.
TS-3024/55, Public Information Office Collection, ISA

from 650,000 to 1.3 million. Nevertheless, between 1927 and 1942, infant mortality was reduced from 216 to 140 births per 1,000 (58 in the Jewish population).[47] In 1926–27, the life expectancy of Muslim men was 37–38, but by the end of the Mandate period, it reached 49–50.[48]

Satisfying No One: The PMC and the Colonial Office

The colonial budgetary policy and resulting restriction of medical services did not go unchallenged. In the field, British administrators were caught between demands to expand expenditure on social services by the League of Nations' Permanent Mandate Commission (PMC) and the local population,[49] and the Colonial Office's insistence to keep government expenditure to the bare minimum. With the Colonial Office having the upper hand, these conflicting pressures resulted in minor fluctuations in the DoH budget (see Figure 3.1) and expressed hopes that the cutbacks were only temporary.[50]

When the PMC questioned the British Mandate authorities about the budget decrease in 1926, Colonel Steward Symes, Chief Secretary to the Government of Palestine, explained that an apparent decrease in the DoH's budget represented the cost of services transferred to the local authorities. To justify the low budget allocations, he claimed that the DoH met the needs of the Arab population, while Jewish medical institutions met the needs of the Jewish one. The administration, he argued, treated both races on the same footing, but the Jews were "paying considerable sums in order to meet their own requirements, which were in excess of the requirements of the Arabs."[51]

Similarly, three years later, when the PMC questioned the British about the decrease from £146,000 in 1921 to £100,000 in 1929, Harry

[47] W. J. Vickers, *A Nutritional Economic Survey of Wartime Palestine, 1942–1943* (Jerusalem: Department of Health, 1944), 2.

[48] Al-Husayni, *al-Tatawwur*, 167–69, 193; Washitz, *ha-ʿAravim*, 198; Assaf, *ha-Yahasim*, 295–96.

[49] A critical survey of PMC's work in relation to Palestine Susan Pedersen, *The Guardians: The League of Nations and the Crisis of Empire* (Oxford: Oxford University Press, 2015).

[50] Permanent Mandate Commission (henceforth: PMC), *Minutes of the Seventh Session Held in Geneva from October 19th to October 30th 1925* (Geneva: The League of Nations, 1925), 120, 218.

[51] PMC, *Minutes of the Ninth Session Held in Geneva from June 8th to 25th, 1926* (Geneva: The League of Nations, 1926), 178.

Luke, Acting High Commissioner to Palestine in 1928, claimed that private and missionary hospitals compensated for this gap and that "it would be uneconomical for the Palestine Government to overlap with and duplicate work which was already being done by another institution." Luke further claimed that Palestine had sufficient medical personnel – one medical practitioner for every 1,500 inhabitants – a figure that did not consider the disparity between Palestine's Jewish and Arab populations.[52] In his testimony to the Peel Commission in November 1936, DoH Director Heron stated that the government health expenditure was around £180,000, whereas the Jewish organizations' medical expenses totaled around £318,000, for a much smaller population.

The British responses to the PMC reveal that as far as the Mandate administration was concerned, if missionary hospitals, municipalities, and Jewish medical institutions provided some health services, it was not obligated to provide them. The British administration resorted to cultural explanations to justify the neglect of Arab needs. In practice, whereas Palestine enjoyed multiple medical facilities and personnel, Jews and Arabs, urban centers and the rural periphery, were unevenly served.

Despite the PMC's criticism of British health services in Palestine, the O'Donnell Financial Commission, appointed by the Secretary of State for the Colonies to examine and report on the financial and general organization of the Palestine administration in 1931, recommended *further* budget cuts, including in the DoH.[53] The Commission believed that resource allocation in Palestine should be more in line with other parts of the British Empire, most notably India. These cuts included abolishing the post of the Inspector of Trade and Industry, responsible for licensing health-related trades and industries, as it was "trying to enforce standards not attainable save in the most advanced countries." The posts of epidemic MOs were also abolished, since the Commission maintained there were no major epidemics in Palestine. The Commission further suggested dividing the country into three, rather than four districts, which would save the costs of one British Senior MO. It saw the hands-on approach in Palestine as a waste of resources,

52 PMC, *Minutes of the Seventeenth (extraordinary) Session, Held in Geneva from June 3rd to 21st, 1930* (Geneva: League of Nations, 1930), 114–15.

53 Roza el-Eini, "Government Fiscal Policy in Mandatory Palestine in the 1930s," *Middle Eastern Studies* 33 (1997): 573–80.

as "larger staff are controlled in India by an Inspector General assisted by a junior officer." The Commission concluded that Palestinian MOs should not be promoted to Senior MOs for the time being.[54] Thus, from the colonial perspective, the point of comparison was not the British metropole or even the standard maintained by the Jewish community in Palestine, but rather health services in other colonial possessions.

Heron saw things differently. Before serving in Palestine, the colonel had served as an attaché to the British Public Health Department in Egypt. After a decade in Egypt and following the 1919 revolution, Heron came to Palestine in 1920. The Egypt he knew had an elaborate health system and growing local medical personnel.[55] In questions of medical policy, his colonial medical experience differed from that of most of his counterparts across the empire. The director's "strictly confidential" reply to the Committee's conclusions articulated inner colonial tensions and frustrations. Heron was very proud of his department's preventive health services in Palestine, and the comparison to India, he stated, was irrelevant, since disease prevention was not part of its medical services.[56] He insisted that the absence of major epidemics in Palestine was a tribute to health officers' success rather than their redundancy.[57]

Pointing to the proportional expenditure on health services in Kenya, Tanganyika, Ceylon, and the Straits Settlements (7–12.5 percent), Heron lamented that there "is no colony or Mandated territory that approaches" Palestine's "low figure" of 4.3 percent.[58] His resentment was overt, criticizing the Committee's recommendations to economize the "Department which is generally considered to have been starved, and has been reduced unmercifully on several previous occasions . . ."[59] If anything, he maintained, public health expenditure in the colonies should increase to save future expenses on medical

[54] Extract from the *O'Donnell Commission Report* (1931), 80, 82–84, CO 733/208/9, NA. During the Mandate's first nine months, DoH got 9.6 percent of the total budget, but it sunk to 4.1 percent in 1929–30 and to 3.7 percent in 1936–37, Qaraqra, *al-Khidamat*, 230.

[55] On the Egyptian medical system, see Amira Sonbol, *The Creation of a Medical Profession in Egypt, 1800–1922* (Syracuse, NY: Syracuse University Press, 1991), 106–32; Hibba Abugideiri, *Gender and the Making of Modern Medicine in Colonial Egypt* (London: Ashgate, 2010), 159–86.

[56] Heron to the Chief Secretary, "Report of the O'Donnell Commission," 14, 17.

[57] Ibid., 16. [58] Ibid., 12. [59] Ibid., 19.

services. Preventive medicine in Palestine was also to serve as a model for other colonies.[60] He concluded:

> In many of our colonies and dependencies, including such countries as Rhodesia, Kenya, and India, where the Medical Department has been in successful operation for a long time, the Health and Sanitary Service has only recently been considered. It is now a well-established fact that after the experience of the Sudan, Nigeria, Mauritius, Ceylon, etc., a Health and Sanitary Service, which deals with the prevention of disease, is just as important a factor as Medical service. The establishment of one, in fact, reduces the extent of the financial provision required for the other. With great respect, I venture to suggest that the commissioners did not fully realize this fact and were conversant with the old principle of purely medical service.[61]

Heron's apologetics was not only aimed at highlighting his own achievements. Based on his experience in Palestine, he envisioned a future health policy for the entire British Empire. His efforts notwithstanding, however, the tension between the men on the spot and the Colonial Office regarding social welfare budgets for areas such as health or education remained throughout the Mandate period.

Colonial Supply and Local Demand

Was Heron right? Or was the Mandate health budget sufficient to meet Arab needs? What exactly were they? In contrast to British claims, Palestine's Arabs did demand more medical services than the DoH was willing to provide. As early as 1921, the annual DoH report noted a surprise at the local demand. It was a "remarkable fact," it stated, "that people unused for centuries to sanitary reform has grasped with such readiness the essential fact that good sanitation means good health and health spells prosperity."[62]

The Palestinian daily press was a central stage for articulating public demands from the colonial government, including criticism of negligence and scarcity of services. Petitions to the government and stories in the Palestinian press demonstrate that residents in Ramleh, Lydda, and multiple other locations demanded the opening of a municipal hospital and improved or expanded healthcare.[63] In 1931, *Filastin*

[60] Ibid., 3–7. [61] Ibid., 2. [62] *An Interim Report, 1921*, 6.
[63] For example, "Mustashfa al-baladiya fi al-l-Ramleh," *Filastin*, March 10, 1933, 8.

demanded that the DoH open a hospital in Jenin, given that the peasants paid their taxes, which could be used for its construction. Jenin's MO, Dr. Khalil Abu Ghazalah, oversaw medical services in the town and its eighty-four surrounding villages. Like Shihab and other MOs, his office was constantly overflowing with patients. Peasants, *Filastin* lamented, sometimes traveled on foot for hours under the burning sun and waited four hours for their turn. In the absence of hospitalization services, patients in severe conditions had no choice but to return to their villages and await recovery or death.[64]

In addition to demanding expanded medical services, Arab communities protested the closure of existing ones. In March 1932, the inhabitants of Beersheba protested the closing of the municipal hospital and its conversion into a four-bed medical inspection room.[65] Later that month, the Muslim Brotherhood branch in Safad tried to collect donations for a local IWC but failed; the authorities opened one two years later.[66] In April, Tulkarem's inhabitants protested against the closure of the DoH's pharmacy, which also served neighboring villages and provided free medications to the poor.[67]

A 1934 report about a traffic accident in Haifa denounced the DoH for its staff's unavailability, which left the bleeding accident victim, who had no means to pay for a private physician, waiting long hours for a government doctor. Had he been British, the writer noted, he would have been treated with great care.[68] Similarly, in 1937 *al-Sirat al-Mustaqim* asserted that long lines formed daily in front of the DoH office in Jaffa, and suggested adding one more doctor or having all of Jaffa's doctors dedicate a daily hour to treating the poor.[69] Like other complaints, this had two targets: the government was to take action and the nation's physicians were to volunteer time and effort.

Dr. Shihab himself was also the target of such complaints. In a letter published in *al-Liwa'* in 1936, "Abu Hisham" from Hebron

64 "Hajat Jenin ila mustashfa," *Filastin*, July 29, 1931, 7.
65 "al-Mustashfa," *Filastin*, March 18, 1932, 4.
66 "Risalat Safad," *Filastin*, March 24, 1932, 4.
67 "Risalat Qalqilia," *Filastin*, April 23, 1932, 4.
68 "Ayna da'irat al-sihha wa-l-bulis fi Hayfa," *Mir'at al-Sharq*, September 5, 1934, 4.
69 "al-Marda wa-da'irat al-sihha," *al-Difa'*, July 6, 1937, 2; " 'Ala arsifa' da'irat al-sihha: mi'at al-marda yawmiyyan yantaziruna al-shifa'," *al-Sirat al-Mustaqim*, July 3, 1940, 4; "Manazir mu'lima fi da'irat al-sihha bi-Yafa," *al-Ittihad*, October 21, 1945, 3.

complained that the government employed only two doctors in town. Dr. Ahmad ʿAbd al-ʿAl was drowning in administrative work, whereas the other, Dr. Shihab, spent his days frequenting the nearby villages and only his weekly day off in Hebron. Hebronites thus demanded more physicians, nurses, and home visits.[70] While critical of the administration, the local population was highly appreciative of its physicians' hard work. In 1942, Hebron's *ulama*, *mukhtar*s, and notables petitioned against the decision to transfer ʿAbd al-ʿAl after twenty-five years in service: "A model of good character and good behavior ... honest and devoted to the health of the people ... he has now become one of the Hebronites, loves them, and they love him."[71]

From a countrywide perspective, a letter published in *al-Ittihad* in 1944 protested governmental neglect of rural areas. Doctors, the writer argued, should conduct more regular visits to the countryside and respond to urgent calls to visit the village. The government, the letter read, sent doctors for short and sporadic visits of limited effectiveness. Instead, it should establish fully equipped health centers in every village.[72]

In addition to understaffing, the local press also voiced protests against corruption. In 1945, *al-Ittihad* published a protest by the villagers of Isdud and its surroundings to the DoH, accusing an employee of selling them medications in exchange for sesame, eggs, vegetables, and chicken, instead of giving them for free.[73] The newspaper also harshly criticized the staff of Haifa's Government Hospital for favoritism. The writer lamented that only patients who had a written recommendation letter were allowed into the hospital, while the city's poor remained unattended.[74] In keeping with the pattern

70 Abu Hisham, "al-Sihha al-ʿamma fi al-Khalil," *al-Liwaʾ*, January 2, 1932, 6.

71 Petition of the ʿUlama, Mukhtars and People of Hebron to the District Commissioner, Jerusalem, through Assistant Director Commissioner, Hebron, November 29, 1942, ISA, M 853/10. See ibid. for a similar petition by the people of Jericho to District Commissioner, Jerusalem, through District Officer, Jerusalem Rural, November 30, 1942, regarding Dr. Shuqair's expected departure. The town's notables learned of his transfer from a newspaper ad.

72 "Ayna wasaʾil al-sihha fi qurana al-ʿArabiyya," *al-Ittihad*, July 30, 1944, 3.

73 "Yaʾkhudh min al-qarawiyyin bayd wa-dawajinu li-taqtir ʿuyunhum," *al-Ittihad*, September 23, 1945, 1; Washitz, *ha-ʿAravim*, 200.

74 Abu Ahmad, "Mustashfa al-hukuma bi-Hayfa," *al-Ittihad*, August 12, 1945, 3. *Al-Shaʿb* argued the hospital was releasing patients who had not fully recovered and subsequently died, "Mustashfa al-hukuma bi-Hayfa wa-ihmal al-marada," *al-Shaʿb*, November 7, 1947, 2; Washitz, *ha-ʿAravim*, 199.

already noted, notwithstanding this criticism, the writer praised the hospital and its staff.[75]

In the late 1930s, petitions from the local population, pressure by the PMC, the outbreak of the Arab Revolt, and the subsequent Peel Commission report all combined to cause the British authorities to expand infant care and ophthalmic services. Still, the uneven distribution of health services and limited promotion opportunities for Arab medical doctors remained painful issues within Palestinian-Arab society throughout the Mandate years.

Staffing a Colonial Service

High-ranking posts in the DoH remained in British hands, and English-speaking Arabs – Palestinian, Armenian, Syrian, and Lebanese graduates of missionary schools – occupied the lower ranks. Some low-ranking officials from the Ottoman period continued to hold the same ranks in the Mandatory administration.[76] The OETA's Health Services shared similar characteristics with other OETA departments. Its high-ranking British personnel were former military MOs, and its Arab and Armenian personnel were mostly young AUB graduates.[77] When the Mandate began, these men became the backbone of the DoH. Dr. Shihab joined a few years later, in the mid 1920s. A Syrian graduate of Montpellier's Faculty of Medicine, he received his Palestinian medical license after a short internship in Cairo.

The DoH was the largest Department in the British administration. In 1926, it included sixty-two administrators, compared to sixteen and forty-two in the Education and Judicial Departments, respectively.[78] By 1941, it almost doubled its staff, reaching 116 employees, including 34 midwives, nurses, and matrons.[79]

[75] "Mustashfa al-hukuma bi-Hayfa wa-ahmiyyatuhu," *al-Sirat al-Mustaqim*, December 31, 1942, 3.

[76] Abigail Jacobson, *From Empire to Empire: Jerusalem between Ottoman and British Rule* (Syracuse, NY: Syracuse University Press, 2011), 137.

[77] "Sir Joseph Harkness, C.M.G., O.B.E., M.B., Ch.B., B.Sc. D.P.H," *British Medical Journal*, no. 5237 (February 9, 1963), 407.

[78] *Staff List of the Government of Palestine Showing Appointments and Stations on 1st July 1926* (Jerusalem: Government Printing Press, 1926) (henceforth: *Staff List, Year*).

[79] *Staff List, 1941*, 11–15.

Of fifty Arab and Armenian doctors the DoH employed in 1941, twenty-nine had already been its employees in 1920–21, making them a tightly knit cohort. At least twenty-three had already worked at the OETA, twenty of whom after serving in the Ottoman army during WWI. As Abigail Jacobson demonstrates, General Edmund Allenby relied on Ottoman personnel for the British operation of the OETA. He respected their bureaucratic knowledge and familiarity with the land.[80] One of them, Dr. Munir Mishʿalani, started his career at the OETA, then served under the DoH, and after 1948 served as a health officer in the newly founded State of Israel.

The DoH's annual reports help reconstruct a collective biography of these longest-serving health officials. Most were born in the mid 1890s, and more than 80 percent graduated from the SPC during or around WWI. The Ottoman army and civil administration were starting points for many, and after the war, they were recruited to lay the department's foundations.[81] The DoH and this distinctive cohort had shared interests: the former needed young doctors with good medical training and acquaintance with the local population to establish the department at minimum cost, and the latter were in dire need of financial stability in the precarious postwar job market. Government employees earned less than established private practitioners did, but for the young doctors, this was exactly the opportunity they needed in the early stage of their careers.[82]

Beyond this specific cohort, MOs and assistant senior MOs were predominantly Arab and Armenian. Throughout the Mandate period, eighty-seven Arab and Armenian men and one Arab woman worked at the DoH. According to data available for seventy-eight employees, two thirds were born in Palestine, 20 percent in Lebanon, and the rest in present-day Turkey, Jordan, and Syria. The percentage of Lebanese recruited to the DoH dropped gradually throughout the Mandate years. The first twenty-five doctors recruited by 1921 included ten

80 "Sir Joseph Harkness."

81 Biographical data may be found in American University of Beirut, *Directory of Alumni, 1870–1952*; Government of Palestine, *Civil Service List: Revised to the 1st January 1931* (Alexandria: Whitehead Morris, 1931); Government of Palestine, *Civil Service List: Revised to the 1st January 1939* (Jerusalem: Government Printing Press, 1939).

82 See list of DoH doctors employed and income estimation of their private clinics in M/28/6601/3, ISA.

born in Lebanon, nine in Palestine, and three in southern Anatolia. The vast majority, 85 percent, graduated from the SPC/AUB, and the rest from Athens, Cairo, Edinburgh, Istanbul, and Montpellier.

The absence of women MOs presented a challenge to Arab women, who were reluctant to seek treatment from male doctors. From 1936, British women doctors and a Palestinian one – Salwa Khuri – provided gynecological services in government clinics in Jerusalem and Haifa. They offered weekly clinic hours in Ramleh, Jaffa, Nablus, and Acre.[83]

The British Imperial service only started relying on local medical personnel at the beginning of the twentieth century.[84] The reliance on Arab MOs, and more specifically, on SPC graduates, might have been inspired by the empire's experience in Anglo-Egyptian Sudan, whose medium-rank health administration was composed of SPC graduates from Greater Syria. In the 1910s, this empowerment and autonomy were an exception in the empire. The Indian Medical Service and East African Medical Service employed Indian doctors, and the West African Medical Service employed some African doctors. Unlike Sudan and later Palestine, however, these non-European doctors did not occupy the core of the medical service.[85]

At the beginning of the twentieth century, the colonial administration in Sudan employed more non-European doctors than did any other colonial administration in Africa south of the Sahara. It was only in the late 1920s, upon the graduation of the first cohorts of the Kitchener School of Medicine in Khartoum, that Sudanese doctors started replacing doctors from Greater Syria at the middle tiers of the administration.[86] For Palestinian doctors, experience in Sudan's colonial health administration meant a position within the British administration, which opened further possibilities in areas under British occupation. Raji Salim Nasr (b. 1895), for example, opened a private

83 *Report to the LoN, . . . 1936*, 183; Elise G. Young, *Gender and Nation Building in the Middle East: The Political Economy of Health from Mandate Palestine to Refugee Camps in Jordan* (London: I. B. Tauris, 2012), 62.

84 Sonbol, *The Creation*, 106–13; Mahmud al-Minawi, *Hukama' Qasr al-'Aini* (Cairo: Nahdat Masr, 1999), 25–26, 369–70.

85 Mark Harrison, *Public Health in British India, Anglo-Indian Preventive Medicine 1854–1914* (Cambridge: Cambridge University Press, 1994), 29–35; Anna Greenwood and Harshad Topiwala, *Indian Doctors in Kenya 1895–1940, the Forgotten History* (Basingstoke: Palgrave Macmillan, 2015), 87–88.

86 Heather Bell, *Frontiers of Medicine in the Anglo-Egyptian Sudan 1899–1940* (Oxford: Clarendon Press, 1999), 34–49.

clinic in Haifa after sixteen years of service in Sudan, and Sami Salim Bishara (b. 1902) joined the DoH after six years there.

Besides this continuity in reliance on SPC graduates, Palestine's health administration resembled its Sudanese counterpart also in the relationship between its British and Arab staff. As in other colonial health services, senior MOs of Sudanese provinces were British men seconded by the Royal Army Medical Corps. Their subordinates, however, were Syrian and Egyptian men who were often more experienced. They ran military and civilian hospitals under British supervision and, in remote posts, were much more independent and gained prestige and expertise.[87]

Unlike their Arab counterparts, only a few Jewish physicians served as MOs, and early recruits included Sephardi, Arabic-speaking Jews, native to Palestine. For example, Yeshuʿa Shami (1874–1944) was a native of Jerusalem whose father had immigrated from Istanbul. Dr. Shami graduated from the Imperial School of Medicine in Istanbul, served as a municipal doctor and in other official state positions under the Ottomans, and then joined the DoH. Other early recruits included Behor Benzion Franco (1894–1979) and Jacob Hassoun (1887–1967), sons of rabbis, who were born and raised in Hebron and were trained in St. Joseph. Some Jewish MOs immigrated to Palestine during the 1920s. Born in Balta (in today's Ukraine), Joseph Shapiro (1887–1978) immigrated to the United States in his teens, was trained in Colorado, and then immigrated to Palestine in 1919, before joining the DoH.[88]

The discrepancy between the number of Jewish doctors in Palestine and their ratio among DoH's employees was apparent throughout the Mandate years. As further discussed in Chapter 5, in 1925, Palestinians (Arabs, Armenians, and Greeks) represented 22.7 percent of all doctors, a rate that would drop dramatically to 10.5 percent in 1935 and 7.2 percent in 1947. In the DoH's last year, it employed 105 doctors, of whom 65 were Arabs, 26 Jews, and 14 British.[89]

Zionist criticism arose over the clear preference of Arab over Jewish doctors, failing to represent the much higher rate of Jewish doctors in

87 Ibid., 40–54; Heather Sharkey, *Living with Colonialism: Nationalism and Culture in the Anglo-Egyptian Sudan* (Berkeley: University of California Press, 2003), 75.

88 Nisim Levi and Yael Levi, *Rof'eha shel Erets-Israel 1948–1799* (Zikhron Yaʿakov: Itai Bahur, 2012), 221, 351, 418, 423

89 Levi, *Prakim*, 260–61.

the country. The Director of the American Zionist Medical Unit, Isaac Rabinow, complained already in 1922 that only about 10 percent of the physicians at the DoH were Jews: "Public health and sanitation in Palestine is entrusted by the government … to Syrians, Greek, and Armenian physicians, to anybody except Jews."[90] Similarly, in a memorandum submitted to the Royal Commission of Enquiry in 1937, the Jewish National Council protested this underrepresentation as a choice that "affects unfavorably the health services given by the government." The government, moreover, "has not taken advantage" of the influx of hundreds of doctors during the previous years, "many of them highly trained specialists."[91] Heron responded that the percentage of Jews at the DoH corresponded with their share of the population and that partial government funding of Jewish medical services in practice subsidized Jewish medical staff – thus favoring, rather than discriminating against, Jewish medical personnel. As for the employment of immigrant doctors, the response was that since the medical profession had already been overcrowded, the government was under no obligation to provide for their employment.[92]

Claims of underrepresentation in the colonial apparatus were not raised by the Yishuv alone. A series of articles in *Mir'at al-Sharq* in 1924 criticized the DoH for employing very few Palestinian Arabs, favoring Jews, British, Armenians, and Syrians instead. Palestinian Arabs at the DoH, critics claimed, held inferior ranks and were paid less than their British superiors.[93] Three years later, *Mir'at al-Sharq* called the DoH "the tower of Babylon," criticizing the overrepresentation of Armenians and Greeks, who "know nothing about this country

[90] Quoted in Philippe Bourmaud, "Epidemiology and the City: Communal vs. Intercommunal Health Policy-Making in Jerusalem from the Ottomans to the Mandate, 1908–1925," in *Ordinary Jerusalem, 1840–1940: Opening New Archives, Revisiting a Global City*, eds. Angelos Dalachanis and Vincent Lemire (Leiden: Brill, 2018), 454.

[91] "Medical and Health Services"; "Summary of the Grievances Contained in the Section on Health," 82, CO733/346/20, NA.

[92] Ibid., "Comments by Department of Health on pages 28–85 of Memorandum submitted by the Vaad Leumi to the Palestine Royal Commission on 'The Jewish Health System and the Government Policy,'" 15–16.

[93] "Da'irat al-sihha: 'Adad al-muwazafin fiha burhan 'ala al-israf," *Mir'at al-Sharq*, September 27, 1924, 1; "Da'irat al-sihha: al-Ghabn al-fahish 'ala al-Filastiniyyin al-wataniyyin – ayna nahnu?" *Mir'at al-Sharq*, October 1, 1924, 1; "Da'irat al-sihha: al-Muqabala bayna 'ahdayn – al-Filastiniyyin yamutuna wa-l-ghuraba' yahyuna," *Mir'at al-Sharq*, October 4, 1924, 1.

and could not care less." The editor reminded the British authorities that there were many Palestinian Arab doctors, no less capable than foreign ones.[94] There was truth in this criticism of disproportional representation. In 1926, out of the forty-four non-British employees of the DoH, less than half were Palestinian Arabs, nine were born in Lebanon, at least six were Armenian or Greek, and another seven were Jewish.[95]

There was some change of heart in *Mir'at al-Sharq* a few years later. In 1931, the newspaper rebuked those who had criticized the over-representation of Armenian doctors at the DoH. "Armenians have no homeland," an op-ed explained, "and they made Palestine into their home [...]. Unlike those foreigners who make their money here and spend it back in their homeland, the Armenians spend their salaries here. They are people who lost everything and saved themselves in our country."[96] When addressing the overrepresentation of Christians in the government, the newspaper argued that the Christians were Arabs just like the Muslims and were entitled to the same rights:[97] "If anything, it is not they who should be targeted, but the British who employ foreign employees, mostly British personnel with considerably higher salaries."[98] *Al-Sirat al-Mustaqim*'s criticism in 1932 was harsher in this respect, blaming Heron for his apparent disregard of the country's Muslim majority in the department's employment policy. The newspaper noted that Heron's "work is nothing but signing papers, and Palestine benefits nothing from his medical knowledge."[99]

This criticism reflected built-in discrimination in the colonial apparatus regarding personnel, salary, and benefits. A different salary scale for British and local personnel was also an administrative given. In 1931, for example, Heron earned a basic salary of 1,200 £P (Palestinian pound), and senior British staff made around 750–950 £P,

94 "Da'irat al-sihha," *Mir'at al-Sharq*, December 29, 1927, 4.
95 *Staff List, 1926*, 7–9.
96 "al-Atibba' al-Arman fi da'irat al-sihha," *Mir'at al-Sharq*, November 27, 1931, 5. See Lauren Banko, "Migrants, Residents, and the Cost of Illegal Home-Making in Mandate Palestine," *Jerusalem Quarterly* 84 (2020): 47–65.
97 "al-Waza'if fi dawa'ir al-hukuma tatahazimu 'ala al-'ubudiyya," *Mir'at al-Sharq*, September 28, 1932, 1, 6.
98 "Ayyuha al-shabb, la tatlub al-'ubudiyya, al-ingliz wa-l-ghuraba' hum aladhina ihtallu al-waza'if," *Mir'at al-Sharq*, October 1, 1932, 1.
99 "al-Hukuma wa-tansiq al-Muslimin," *Al-Sirat al-Mustaqim*, January 7, 1932, 2.

plus 100 in expatriation allowance. Non-British MDs earned 330–550 £P (the lowest paid were British matrons, whose salary ranged from 150–180 £P).[100] This disparity between British and non-European doctors was a common feature across the empire.[101]

Thus, both Jews and Arabs were frustrated with the DoH, which established its cohort of local MOs in the early years of British rule. The influx of Jewish doctors and the gradual growth in the Palestinian professional community made the demands for inclusion in the colonial apparatus an acute and, at times, urgent issue. While the Yishuv established its own occupational alternatives in the form of hospitals and National Health Fund clinics, the DoH remained a significant employer of the Palestinian-Arab professional community. Its failure or refusal to absorb young doctors had a dire effect on its institutionalization.

The British Personnel

The DoH, argued *Mir'at al-Sharq*'s editor in 1924, used Palestinian taxes to pay the high salaries of its employees rather than invest in the country's well-being. "The Englishman cannot work unless surrounded by an army of directors, hundreds of written papers, both useful and useless, dozens of typists clicking on their typewriters, and several guards standing at the door to prevent people from approaching his highness."[102] Service in the Empire allowed British doctors, sometimes of modest backgrounds, to combine adventure, professional promotion, and for some, social mobility that was unavailable at home. Several years of experience as house physicians or surgeons were required before serving in the colony. MO candidates were screened for their ability to run an independent post and earn the indigenous population's respect. Some were overworked, while others described a very relaxed experience, depending on both local conditions and their own initiatives. They often complained of exhaustion, low pay, and being overburdened with paperwork. At least in East

[100] See for example, Government of Palestine, *Civil Service List 1931*, 7, 77–107; *Staff List, 1941*, 11–15.

[101] Greenwood and Topiwala, *Indian Doctors*, 89–95.

[102] "Da'irat al-sihha: al-Muqabala bayna 'ahdayn – al-Filastiniyyin yamutuna wa-l-ghuraba' yahyuna," *Mir'at al-Sharq*, October 4, 1924, 1.

Africa and India, their relationship with the local population outside the clinic was mostly restricted to a master-servant relationship.[103]

The Senior MOs at the Palestine DoH were all British. Like their Arab and Armenian subordinates, members of the first cohort were born around 1890, served during the war, and arrived in Palestine right after graduation. Most had little civilian clinical experience. Some British senior MOs served elsewhere in the empire before coming to Palestine, or left for other colonial posts after serving there.

Senior personnel were of Scottish, Irish, and English descent.[104] Joseph Pottinger arrived in Palestine in 1933 after serving in the Ivory Coast and British Guinea. William John Wickers came to Palestine in 1938 after serving in Malaya.[105] Joseph Harkness (b. 1890, Glasgow) left Palestine in 1939, after nine years as Deputy Director of the Department, and from there, continued to the Gold Coast, Nigeria, and the West Indies.[106]

The British staff was superior to their native subordinates in power and service conditions, but their point of reference was other colonial officials and not their Palestinian colleagues. In 1937, four of Palestine's British senior MOs wrote the Secretary of State for the Colonies Malcolm McDonald to protest their lack of promotion prospects and inferior position compared to their counterparts in other colonial settings. Unlike British MOs in the Empire, they explained, their benefits did not include housing, they were barred from private practice, and they could not be promoted beyond the rank of senior MO. They demanded higher positions and suitable professional allowance. McDonald rejected their demand for a salary increase, noting that given former Palestine senior MOs' promotion to other posts in the British Empire, current senior MOs had little to complain about.[107] Nevertheless, upon his promotion to Director of the DoH in 1946, Dr. Hugh Lester stated that many of his better officers had left Palestine for these reasons.[108]

103 David Arnold, *Science, Technology, and Medicine in Colonial India* (Cambridge: Cambridge University Press, 2000), 52–91; Anna Crozier, *Practicing Colonial Medicine: The Colonial Medical Service in British East Africa* (London: I. B. Tauris, 2007).

104 As observed by Judge Kermack. See Kermack Collection, GB165-0169, MECA.

105 Nissim and Levi, *Rof'eha*, 327

106 "Sir Joseph Harkness."

107 "Conditions of Service: Department of Health," CO 733/362/7, NA.

108 Hugh Lester, The Department of Health Palestine, 1946–1948, "The Decline and Fall," CO 968/197, NA, p. 2.

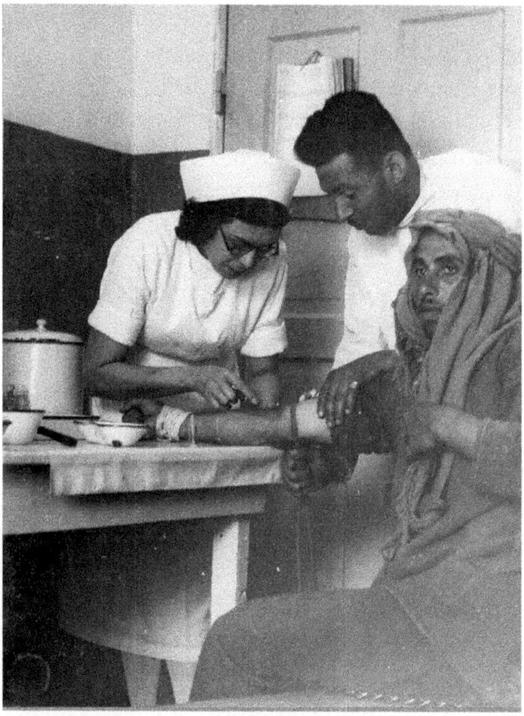

Figure 3.8 Prisoner receiving treatment, Tulkarem's government clinic
TS-3020/96, Public Information Office Collection, ISA

McDonald and Lester's observations once again highlight the difference between British and local personnel. Palestine was a branch of a global project, and London and other colonial health services were the points of reference. Non-British employees could be discriminated against mainly because they had no other alternatives, and little or no leverage against their employers.

The Pains and Pleasures of a Medical Officer

On September 24, 1936, Sami Shihab drove his car into a rebels' ambush and sought refuge in a ditch. Upon hearing that a British officer was shot, he bravely returned to his car, collected the wounded officer, and drove him back to Hebron under fire. Commendations for the MO's "gallant and humanitarian conduct" came from Roy Spicer,

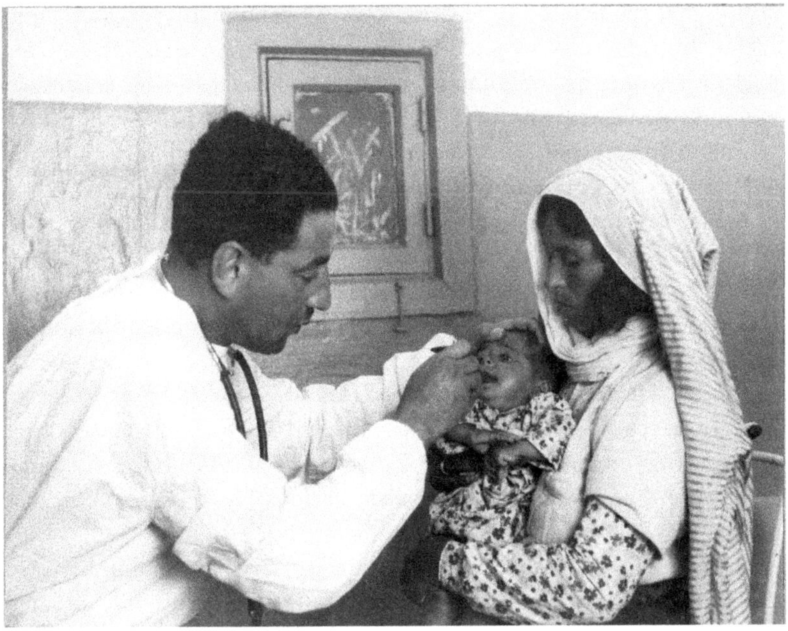

Figure 3.9 Government clinic at Tulkarem.
TS-3024/62, Public Information Office Collection, ISA

Inspector General of Police and Prisons, and the High Commissioner himself.[109] This incident illuminates the double obligation of the Arab employee to both his patients and his employers – at the expense, perhaps, of national loyalties. It also demonstrates adherence to the doctor's most basic calling: treating a person in need.

As shown in Figure 3.2, Shihab's weekly routine as Hebron's MO was demanding, and during the Great Arab Revolt, it also became risky. In August 1936, he requested permission to carry arms but was denied. "No hostility has been shown," Deputy DoH Director Harkness wrote Shihab, to "(o)fficers in the really disturbed areas of the country."[110] Previously, in July, Shihab was more optimistic,

[109] Roy Spicer to Director General of Medical Services, November 12, 1936, and John Shaw, Assistant Secretary to Director of Medical Services, December 23, 1936, Shihab, Dr. Sami. Medical Officer of Health, 1st Jacket," M/4250/5, ISA.

[110] Dr. Sami Shihab to Senior Medical Officer, Jerusalem, August 17, 1936; Joseph Harkness, Senior Medical Officer, Jerusalem to Dr. S. Shihab, Medical Officer, Hebron, August 24, 1936, M/4250/5, ISA.

noting that the fellahin in Hebron were "exceptionally peaceful," and asking his superiors to undertake all medical responsibilities in the villages beyond his ophthalmic duties. Another MO, he suggested, would be dedicated strictly to Hebron's medical needs.[111]

Shihab's correspondence with the DoH offers a glimpse into the MO's working conditions. A few years earlier, when he was transferred from Gaza to Tulkarem, Gaza's residents protested in *Mir'at al-Sharq* against the transfer of their beloved physician.[112] Public appreciation aside, Shihab wanted an upgrade to an urban center. Shihab refused to trust his children with the local town schools and preferred, as mentioned earlier, the distance over compromise in matters of education. He constantly begged the DoH to be transferred to a larger city so he could reunite with his family.[113] His experience raises questions about the relationship MOs forged in their different posts, given their frequent mobility between various Health Offices around the country.

Doctors such as Shihab were supposed to serve as the link between the Palestinian population and British authorities. This role situated them in an ambivalent position: as government representatives, they were often held accountable for government policies. During the political and violent turmoil of 1936–39, the inherent conflict between their formal responsibilities and national loyalties was accentuated. For better or worse, they were living manifestations of colonial control. Especially in the rural areas, they were "go-betweens," to borrow Anat Mooreville's terminology, between the medical administration and rural healthcare personnel.[114] For some, frequent transfers between duties hampered any connections and prestige they hoped to gain within the communities.[115]

As for social mobility, they were in-betweeners: they had the academic and professional accreditation that gave their claims relative leverage, but they were also entirely dependent on colonial goodwill

111 Shihab to Senior Medical Officer, Jerusalem, July 14, 1936, M/4250/5, ISA.
112 "Tabib al-mustashfa al-baladi fi Ghazza," *Mir'at al-Sharq*, June 15, 1932, 3.
113 Sami Shihab, "Application for transfer," October 5, 1935; Sami Shihab, "Application for Transfer," February 1, 1938, in Shihab, Sami. Medical Officer of Health, 1st Jacket, M/4250/5, ISA.
114 Mooreville, "Oculists," 86–89.
115 Ylana Miller, *Government and Society in Rural Palestine 1920–1948* (Austin: University of Texas Press, 1985), 45–53, 64, 66.

in their efforts to move up. This tension between the DoH's needs and local demand was not confined to MOs. Julia Shatz observes that nurses who staffed village clinics were embedded into intimate relationships with local populations that complicated the government's vision of fully standardized and interchangeable nursing staff. Village nurses became part of the community to such an extent that, as in the case of MOs, some communities petitioned against government intentions to transfer them.[116]

Only rarely did MOs spend all or even most of their career in one locale. Some moved around every three to four years, while others stayed even two decades in one post. Between 1928 and 1946, Shihab worked in Nablus, Beersheba, Gaza, Hebron, Majdal, and Acre. Originally from Marjayoun, Iskandar Hurani served over a decade in Gaza, moved to Ramallah in the early 1930s, and then to Safad in the late 1930s. Nasfat Nadim Kamal from Jenin graduated in 1937, worked in Amman, then at the DHO in Jerusalem, in 1940–41 in Beersheba, and later in Jenin.

MOs were forced to comply with this geographical mobility, mandated by the needs of the central authority. Having no other occupational alternative, most remained in government service throughout their career. In a few cases, however, MOs preferred to remain where they were initially posted and resigned when ordered to relocate. In 1931, when the British authorities decided to transfer a beloved physician from Jaffa's government hospital to Nablus, the people of Jaffa protested, and he resigned.[117] Two years later, this former government physician, Dr. Fu'ad Dajani, would establish the first Palestinian-Arab private hospital in the country. Dr. Ahmad al-Sururi, who headed the Watani Hospital in Nablus since 1934, had a similar story: upon the DoH's request that he leave Nablus in 1945, he quit, and opened a private clinic.[118]

Some MOs opened private clinics while in government employment. A 1945 government report noted that doctors favored their private

[116] Julia R. Shatz, "A Politics of Care: Local Nurses in Mandate Palestine," *International Journal of Middle East Studies* 50 (2018): 676–78.

[117] "Mustashfa Yafa al-baladi 'urida li-l-diya'," *al-Haya*, March 29, 1931, 2; "Sunduquki, ayyuha al-umma," *Filastin*, March 31, 1931, 1.

[118] Sa'id al-Bishawi, *al-Duktur Ahmad "Mahmud 'Atalla" al-Sururi: al-Tabib al-insan wa-l-idari al-bari' wa-l-siyasi wa-shahadat mu'assirihi, 1336–1408 H / 1908–1988* (Amman: Dar al-ru'a li-l-dirasat wa-l-nashr, 2021), 17, 22–23.

practice over their government post, undermining service quality.[119] More serious allegations were raised against doctors who used their government posts for personal profit. In July 1930, *al-Sirat al-Mustaqim* reported that Tulkarem's MO pressured patients to visit his private clinic and pay him for treatment after office hours. In addition, he allegedly demanded travel expenses by car, although Tulkarem's houses were close to each other.[120]

Shihab's file contains several complaints regarding his professional conduct. He was allegedly rude to the patients, and disrespectful of the elderly. In one case, he responded that the complainant was a shaykh who insisted on skipping the queue. Another complaint was, he argued, raised by a patient's brother he quarreled with after this man had insisted on whispering the eye chart figures in his sister's ears.[121] While the truth about these claims remains uncertain, they convey cultural expectations of appropriate patient – doctor relations regulated by a bureaucratic authority and underline the presence of a professional etiquette. Private practices of government employees flourished, but doctors were expected to remain committed to their patients' well-being rather than minding their bottom line.

Lester's "Decline and Fall"

Appointed in the summer of 1946, Dr. Hugh Lester arrived in Palestine after twenty years of service in Nigeria. He started as an MO, but his success in fighting the Tsetse Fly and Sleeping Sickness won him the promotion to Assistant Director of Medical Services.[122] Lester had no idea how short his tenure would be or that he would become the last DoH director. He did recognize in hindsight, albeit ironically, the historical importance of his role. He titled his

119 Chief Secretary to Director of Health Services, September 12, 1945 and Director of Health Services to Chief Secretary, September 20, 1945, M/28/6601/1–2, ISA.

120 The physician was Ibrahim Jiris Itayim. See "Tulkarem," *al-Sirat al-Mustaqim*, July 10, 1930, 2; a letter published eleven days later insisted allegations were false, "Tulkarem: Da'irat al-sihha," *al-Sirat al-Mustaqim*, July 21, 1930, 3.

121 ISA, "Shihab, Sami. Medical Officer of Health, 1st Jacket," M/4250/5, S. Shihab, District Health Office, Hebron, "Complaint – Jameel el-Sheriff," August 18, 1937.

122 "H.M.O. Lester," *British Medical Journal,* 4824 (1953): 1394.

fourteen-page eulogy of the department between 1946 and 1948 "The Decline and Fall."[123]

Upon his arrival, Lester was determined to revive the DoH, which had suffered significantly from the war. In his "Decline and Fall," he argued that when he started his position in 1946, the DoH, formerly regarded as "the only real Health Service in the Colonial Empire," was in a state of "genuine decline." Many of its British staff had been transferred to fill senior posts in other colonial medical services. The Palestinian staff, Lester added, "still acquired suitable prestige from the general public through belonging to the Department, but little from their fellow Department officials." He observed that Palestinian doctors' salaries in the service were "scandalously low," lower than private doctors' or other civil servants, and the medical staff's wages in his former post in Nigeria. The result was that Palestinian-Arab doctors were reluctant to take jobs at the DoH.[124]

To remedy this problem, he raised their salaries and opened promotion possibilities, thus reducing the incentive to supplement income with private practice.[125] He also promoted Palestinians to posts formerly occupied exclusively by British officials.[126] Under his leadership, the DoH had its first Arab senior MOs, who headed two of Palestine's four districts.[127] Lester also attempted to implement a small part of Acting High Commissioner John Valentine Wistar Shaw's 1945 plan for a rudimentary National Health Service in Palestine. This plan included the establishment of twenty-five rural health centers, that would include IWCs, antenatal care, health instruction, home visits, infectious disease centers, and health education classes for primary schoolchildren. In his funding application, Lester explained the need for rural health centers as one step toward closing the gap between the Jewish and Arab communities in Palestine. Work was to commence in 1948 and conclude in 1953. The Colonial Office canceled the plan in

123 Hugh Lester, "The Decline and Fall."

124 "Colonial Office and Commonwealth Office: Defense Department and successors: Original Correspondence. Palestine: report by Dr. H M O Lester on the Palestine Department of Health 1946–1948," 1–5, CO 968/197, NA.

125 Ibid.

126 Director of Medical Services (DMS) to Chief Secretary, September 9, 1946 and July 13, 1946; DMS to Acting Financial Secretary, Government of Palestine, January 25, 1947, M/28/6601, ISA.

127 Qaraqra, *al-Khidamat*, 161.

November 1947, estimating that there would be no time to implement it before the Mandate's conclusion.[128]

Lester's reform reflected long-term colonial learning processes and colonial acknowledgment of the greater need for local empowerment to strengthen the health system's sustainability. Lester was not alone in his visions of administrative reform and empowerment of Arabs in managing their own society. Bernard De-Bunsen, who initiated his directorship of the Department of Education at roughly the same time, reached similar conclusions. Both sought to remedy the decades-long barriers set by the colonial administration on empowerment, degrees of administrative autonomy, and promotion of local employees.[129] These ambitions were compromised by the tide of violence that ended British rule in Palestine.

Conclusion

The Palestine DoH is an example of the British Empire's reliance on local personnel to expand and improve its health services. The British were fortunate to find qualified local doctors, some of whom had already gained experience in the Ottoman administration or military. The colonial service employed dozens of doctors who constituted an interface between the British authorities and the local population. Doctors, newspaper editors, and local communities were overtly critical of the Mandate's resource allocation compared to Jewish institutions and of the neglect of the countryside. The physicians employed by the DoH were overworked. As Shihab's schedule shows, they traveled between villages outside their offices, chasing their own tail while trying (and failing) to attend to all patients. Government officials were supposed to showcase government concern for its subjects. In practice, their constant exhaustion manifested colonial incompetence.

[128] Hasso, *Buried in Red Dirt*, 92–94; "Application for a Clinical Development Fund Grant for Rural Health Centers in Palestine," M-4090/5, "Village Clinics," ISA; Director of Medical Services to Director of Public Works, "Rural Health Clinics," November 9, 1946, and Director of Public Works to Director of Medical Services, "Rural Health Centers," January 9, 1947, M-4090/5, "Village Clinics," ISA.

[129] Yoni Furas, *Educating Palestine: Teaching and Learning History under the Mandate* (Oxford: Oxford University Press, 2020), 44–45.

Reading the DoH's section in Palestine's government annual reports, it is possible to follow a narrative of colonial success. Each report includes subtle words of self-praise, depicting the gradual decrease in child mortality rates, successes in plague prevention, and the vaccination of thousands. It was a colonial narrative of development and progress. Within it, it carried the inherent contradiction of colonial burden: developments in healthcare (as in other government services) raised greater needs in the community, and subsequent demand for greater government aid. Men on the spot, such as Heron, Lester, and their subordinates, felt proud of their achievements using only a fraction of the total budget. The bigger their self-proclaimed achievements, the greater their appetite was for funding. The Colonial Office could or would not afford it. The roadmap to universal healthcare amplified the never-ending needs of the colonized for the better lives that the empire promised. More than any other colonial intervention, medicine underlined the Empire's inability and unwillingness to keep this promise.

4 *Medical Landscapes*

Doctor (Akram al-Sweidi): {After almost falling from his horse only to be saved by a fallah} I'm a doctor.

Fallah (Ahmad al-Sheikh Yunis): A doctor??? What brings a wise man [*hakim*, also doctor] to the peasantry [*ahl al-filh*]?

Doctor: We have a farm, an estate in the area.

Fallah: So you are . . .?

Doctor: Akram.

Fallah: You are Abu-Akram Sweidi's son?

Doctor: A doctor with a diploma from the American University. Three years in health and clinic [training], but still people know me through my father.

Fallah: . . . I wish we could all be doctors who can't ride a horse, right brother?

Doctor: Still, there are things in the *rif* [countryside] we are deprived of in the city.

Fallah: Oh sir [*ya sidi*], he who needs the *rif* for the green view, mountains, fresh air and water, can say what you've said.

Doctor: The *rif* for the fellah is not just the green [view] and the water.

Fallah: I didn't mean to . . .

Doctor: . . . I think all of us in the city know the fellah's situation, but here {points to his head}, in our minds, how we feel, that's another story.[1]

In this fictional encounter between a fellah and a doctor, taken from the popular 2004 Syrian TV series *al-Taghriba al-Filasiniyya* (The

[1] *al-Taghriba al-Filasiniyya*, chapter 2, 50: 42, https://bit.ly/4dYmyKy, accessed May 22, 2025.

Palestinian Exile), the two characters represent two completely different species of Palestinian society, separate essences.[2] Perhaps as a metaphor for the elite's inability or failure to control the fellahin, the doctor fails to rein in his horse and is ironically saved by them. With his effendi attire, language, and worldview, he is foreign to the land and its people, and the fellahin are surprised to see him there. The *hakim*, it is implied, has literally no business in the *rif*. Attempting to highlight the dramatic turning points in Palestinian history, the series, however, forefronts the doctor only as a signifier, an icon of Palestinian class, notability, and cultural capital during the Mandate period.

This chapter decodes this signifier and critically examines its sociocultural characteristics and location within Palestinian society. The chapter surveys Palestine's medical landscape, mapping the distribution of medical professionals across the country and the gap between the city and countryside. It concentrates on the spatial presence of Palestinian doctors – the communities they served and those they did not; spaces that enjoyed abundant medical services and those that had none. In short, this chapter places Palestine's doctors on the map and examines the social, spatial, and political entanglements of their positioning. It concentrates on the Mandate but, whenever relevant, backtracks to the late Ottoman backgrounds of the different localities.

In constructing a typology of Palestine's medical landscape, institutionally and professionally, we propose three analytic categories: villages, towns, and cities. The presence of medical services had different effects on residents of each category; and endowed the city and town with new roles, redefining their relationship with each other and with the countryside. This distinction thus outlines this chapter's structure. While neither of these categories represent complete homogeneity, they do share important characteristics shaping their respective medical landscapes.

Villages rarely had medical facilities or doctors. Peasants had to travel to the town or city for medical services and would otherwise rely on traditional practitioners. Akram, probably modeled after Acre doctor Anwar al-Shuqayri, may have been brought up in the countryside, but he opened his clinic in the city. Deprived of health services, yet gaining growing awareness of their benefits, peasants' demand for

[2] Mustafa Kabha, "The Palestinian Exile – Drama Shapes Memory," in *The War of 1948: Representations of Israeli and Palestinian Memories and Narratives*, eds. Avraham Sela and Alon Kadish (Bloomington: Indiana University Press, 2016), 194–202.

doctors was a constant reminder of the profession's shortcomings. Towns, the second category, include both coastal towns such as Acre and Gaza, and small urban centers in the hinterland like Nazareth and Nablus. What towns had in common was the presence of missionary medical facilities, a small community of doctors, some of whom were native to the town; one or two government medical facilities – a DHO (District Health Office), a government clinic, or a small hospital.

The third category includes three major cities – Jerusalem, Jaffa, and Haifa, and our main focus here will be on the latter two, as case studies. These urban centers were characterized by a relatively large professional community, a substantial Jewish presence (in Jaffa's case – in nearby Tel Aviv), a strong missionary presence that provided both educational and medical services, and a strong presence of the Mandate administration. Within urban centers, large concentrations of physicians did not necessarily mean medical services for all. The restricted investment in public medical services on both the municipal and government levels limited access to treatment to those who could afford private practitioners.

Medical services provided by university-trained and state-licensed doctors transformed the landscape. They created new links and routes between villages, towns, and cities, and supplemented existing relations between the village and the nearby city or town and accentuated sociocultural gaps. The town became the place a peasant would travel to for medical services; and the city – the hub of advanced medical care. The clinic, moreover, created new intimate spaces for encounter between the peasant and urban middle and upper class. For the new professional community, these encounters echoed existing tensions, as well as a new sense of responsibility for the peasants' welfare. Once modern medicine was available, moreover, it created demand in growing circles in Palestinian society.

Medical Landscapes: A Bird's-Eye View

Several factors affected the countrywide distribution of medical doctors. First, the preexistence of missionary facilities. These were attracted to cities of Christian significance (e.g., Jerusalem, Nazareth), to localities with relatively large Jewish communities, which they hoped to convert (e.g., Safad, Tiberias), and to ones with small Christian communities which they hoped to attract to their denomination (e.g., Haifa, Gaza). These hospitals employed the first Palestinian doctors. The second factor was governmental. Since the 1870s, Ottoman municipalities were supposed to employ a municipal doctor, and several localities also had a municipal or governmental hospital. The DoH's centers and British governmental hospitals, inspection rooms, and quarantine stations supplemented or at times replaced these facilities countrywide. Neither the Ottomans nor the British made any effort to force or encourage equitable distribution of medical services. A third factor was the existence of clientele – patients able to afford private practice – mainly the urban elite and upper-middle classes. Finally, the presence of Jewish urban population or proximity to a Jewish settlement affected patients' choices and doctors' professional competition.

Taken together, these factors made for an uneven distribution: concentration of health services in Jaffa, Jerusalem, and Haifa, with smaller clusters of medical doctors and clinics in Palestine's towns. Villagers' access to healthcare depended on their distance from urban centers, means of transportation, available income, and sporadic government initiatives.

Analysis of Palestinian doctors' workplace distribution indicates a growth in numbers, and a relatively constant countrywide spread. Palestinian urbanization, the cornerstone of the country's social trajectory during the Mandate period, fueled this spread throughout. Figure 4.1 illustrates the relative importance of each category throughout the Mandate years. More than half of the doctors were

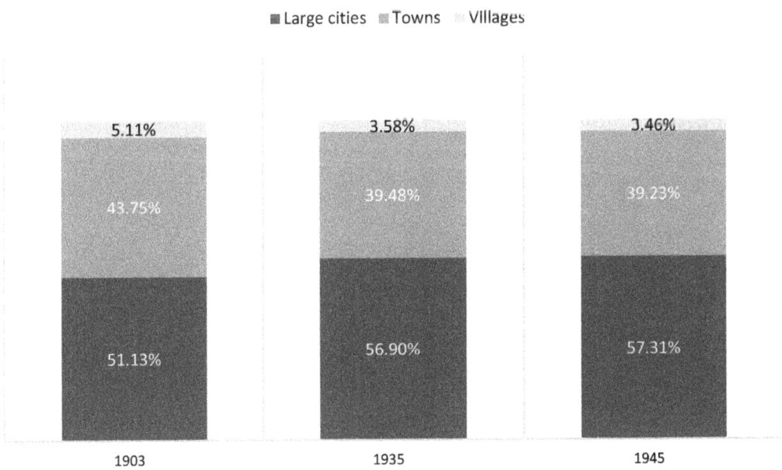

Figure 4.1 Palestinian doctors' distribution in cities, towns, and villages.

concentrated in Jerusalem, Jaffa, and Haifa. By 1946, they numbered about thirty to fifty in each city, representing 51 percent and 57 percent of Palestine's Arab medical community in 1930 and 1946, respectively. About 40 percent were distributed between about twenty towns, which had a constant presence of three to six doctors each, except for Nablus and Gaza, which enjoyed a larger medical community. Outside these locales, very few towns and villages had even a single doctor. Tiberias, Shefa-ʿAmr, Jaljulia, Bassa, Bidya, Tarshiha, Bisan, Kafr Kanna, Khan Yunis, Manshiat al-Hula, and Beit Jala housed one or two doctors for most of the period. Elsewhere, most Palestinians had no access to Palestinian Arab doctors.

The number of pharmacists increased steadily, and like doctors, they were concentrated mainly in Jerusalem, Jaffa, and Haifa – roughly 66–70 percent throughout the Mandate years. Other than that, in 1946, only Nablus had more than a handful. Palestine's roughly sixty Arab dentists practiced almost exclusively in cities, and their presence in towns was sporadic at best. Certified midwives were also

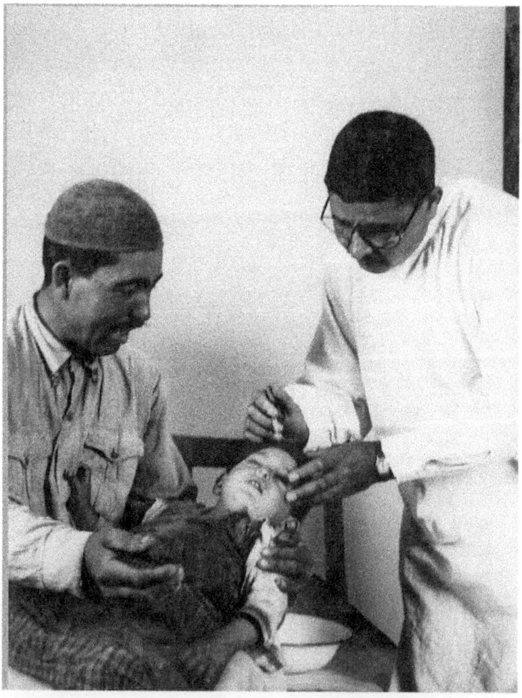

Figure 4.2 Eye treatment in Beit Nuba's government clinic.
TS-3024/41, Public Information Office Collection, ISA

concentrated in the cities, and to a smaller extent in towns. Their numbers also increased throughout the Mandate years, and they could be found in the countryside as well: beginning from the 1940s, they were located in dozens of villages countrywide.

Treating Rural Ills

In 1937, the inhabitants of Bir Zeit, then a small village north of Ramallah,[3] submitted an urgent petition to the DoH. Ella Hulbert was about to relocate to Kenya and leave the village without a qualified nurse. The villagers' request for a new nurse was denied, and Hulbert ended up staying in Bir Zeit for six more years.[4]

Most Palestinian villages had no medical personnel at all: a trained nurse, sometimes supplemented by weekly doctor visits, was a privilege few villages enjoyed. Some villagers had better access to hospitals than others: villagers from the Acre region, for example, went to Acre or Haifa, for more complicated procedures.[5] Jenin and Acre – homes to a small hospital or a small group of doctors – attracted patients from neighboring villages.[6] Villagers from the Bisan district went to Tiberias or Nazareth hospitals, or to the doctor in Bisan.[7]

3 Inhabited by 1,233 and 1,560 in 1931 and 1945, respectively, Eric Mills, *Census of Palestine 1931: Population of Villages, Towns and Administrative Areas* (Jerusalem: Greek Convent & Goldberg Press, 1932), 48; *Village Statistics, April 1945* (Jerusalem: Unknown publisher, 1945), 26.

4 Department of Health, Infant & Child Welfare, Bir Zeit, Government of Palestine, M/23/6572, ISA.

5 Muhammad ʿOmar Dheeb (b. 1931), al-Birwa, interviewed by Rakan Mahmoud, Shatila Camp, October 26, 2011, www.palestineremembered.com/Acre/al-Birwa/Story20811.html, accessed May 22, 2025; Faysal ʿAbdul ʿAziz al-Biqaʿi (b. 1934), al-Damun, interviewed by Rakan Mahmoud, Saadnayel, October 12, 2011, www.palestineremembered.com/Acre/al-Damun/Story26940.html, accessed November 28, 2022.

6 Ibrahim Jamil Mar'i and Salih 'Abd al-Jawad, *Qaryat Zar'in* (Bir Zayt: Jami'at Bir Zayt, markaz dirasat wa-tawthiq al-mujtama' al-Filastini, 1994); Sharif Kana'na, *al-Lajjun* (Bir Zayt: Jami'at Bir Zayt, markaz al-watha'iq wa-l-abhath, 1987), 49. For Acre, Muhammad Tawfiq Abu Raqabah (b. 1929), Acre, interviewed by Rakan Mahmoud, Beirut, December 2, 2010, www.palestineremembered.com/Acre/Acre/Story20810.html, accessed May 22, 2025.

7 Nimr Abu Hassouna (b. 1933), Bisan, interviewed by Fawwaz Salama, al-Mashariʿ, November 6, 2005, www.palestineremembered.com/Baysan/Baysan/Story1675.html, accessed May 22, 2025; Yousef al-Zinati (b. 1928), Bisan, interviewed by Fawwaz Salama, November 14, 2005, www.palestineremembered.com/Baysan/Baysan/Story1680.html, accessed May 22, 2025.

Villagers' testimonies also noted the role of Jewish doctors. The people of Dayr al-Qasi and al-Kabri mentioned Dr. Nathan Weill's clinic in Naharia.[8] This resonated in a memoir written by Dr. Max Krammer's wife, noting that his ophthalmic clinic in Naharia attracted hundreds of Arab patients from neighboring villages.[9] Bashit's inhabitants recalled a woman Jewish doctor nicknamed "Umm Yusuf" from Kvutzat Yavne;[10] and villagers from the Bisan and Nazareth districts frequented doctors in Afula.[11] The presence of Jewish doctors in the Palestinian-Arab countryside was sometimes criticized in the daily press, particularly in light of the gap between the Jewish settlements and Arab villages.[12] Arab doctors were also criticized for neglecting the countryside, thus creating a void, which Jewish doctors were only too happy to fill.[13]

It Takes a Town

Based on the criteria listed earlier – missionary presence, government investment, a paying clientele, and the presence of Jewish competition – we can characterize Palestinian towns as follows. Many had a missionary hospital, some of which went back to the late nineteenth century.

8 Subhi ʿAli al-Sadiq (b. 1929), Dayr al-Qasi, interviewed by Rakan Mahmoud; Niʿma Saleh al-Dibajeh (b. 1932), al-Kabri, interviewed by Rakan Mahmoud.

9 Jannie Krammer's memoire on her husband, Max Krammer's work in the villages around Nahariya, K13\167, CZA.

10 Iyad Shahin, *Hikayat qarya mudammara, Bashit* (Bir Zayt: Dar 'Allush li-l-nashr wa-l-tawziʿ, 2002), 20.

11 Ibrahim Muhammad al-Bawati (b. 1928), 'Arab al-Bawati, interviewed by Rakan Mahmoud, Waqqas, June 11, 2011, www.palestineremembered.com/Baysan/Arab-al-Bawati/Story20827.html, accessed November 28, 2022; Nasir al-Daʿoum (b. 1926), ʿArab al-Safa, interviewed by Fawwaz Salameh & Rakan Mahmoud, al-Husn, December 14, 2017, www.palestineremembered.com/Baysan/Arab-al-Safa/Story1678.html, accessed May 22, 2025; Rafiq al-Tahtamouni (b. 1937), Bisan, interviewed by Abdel Majeed Dandeis, al-Husn, June 22, 2004, www.palestineremembered.com/Baysan/Baysan/Story1264.html, accessed May 22, 2025; Lifta's inhabitants were treated in Jerusalem's Shaʿarei Tzedek, Sharif Kana'na, *Lifta* (Bir Zayt: Jamiʿat Bir Zayt, 1991), 23; ʿAin Hud's were treated in Atlit, Sharif Kana'na, *'Ayn Hawd* (Bir Zayt: Jami'at Bir Zayt, markaz al-watha'iq wa-l-abhath, 1987), 44–45.

12 Abu al-ʿAbd, "Fi sabil salamat al-fallah: Hajat al-qariya al-ʿArabiyya li-l-islah al-sihhi," *al-Difaʿ*, August 27, 1934, 7; Muharrir al-Difaʿ al-ziraʿi, "al-Islah al-sihhi wa-l-ijtimaʿi fi al-qariya al-ʿArabiyya," *al-Difaʿ*, February 26, 1937, 7.

13 "Atibbaʾ al-Yahud fi al-qura," *al-Kifah*, February 2, 1936, 3; "Kalimat al-ʿadad: Islah al-qariya al-ʿArabiyya," *al-Difaʿ*, August 17, 1944, 2.

As for governmental investment, towns became administrative district centers and housed several government institutions, including *shariʿa* courts, post offices, police stations, and DHOs. Most of their personnel were brought from outside the town, and were frequently replaced due to the government's changing administrative needs or their reluctance to remain for too long in a demanding job, away from the attractions of the city. All these towns had a small professional middle-class community in the Mandate years, able to afford medical treatment. As for Jewish competition, Palestinian-Arab towns were generally not a target of Jewish settlement. Some, such as Tiberias, Safad, and Hebron, had small Jewish communities, but these attracted little attention from Zionist medical services. Small Jewish settlements did, however, exist around some of these towns, increasing the availability of medical services to their hinterland.[14]

As Figures 4.3 through 4.5 demonstrate, towns, with populations ranging from several thousand to about 24,000, enjoyed a modest

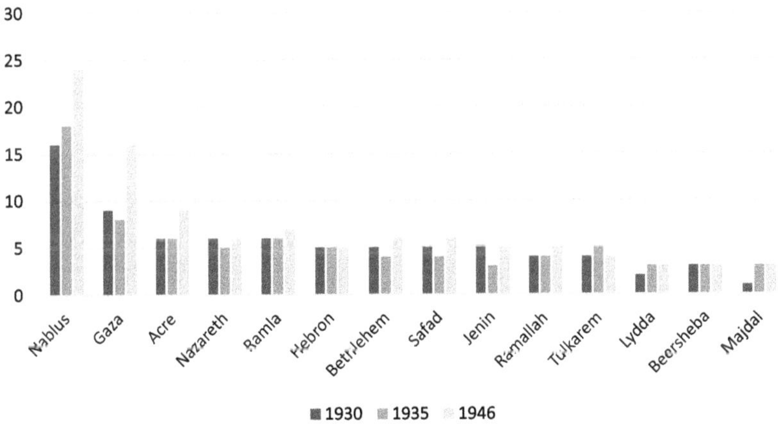

Figure 4.3 Numbers of doctors in Palestine's towns.[15]

[14] Mustafa Abbasi, "City of Farmers and Merchants: Beisan in the Palestine Mandate Period (1918–1948)," *Journal of Holy Land and Palestine Studies* 14 (2015): 206–09.

[15] Data is based on following publications, Government of Palestine, Department of Health, *List of Doctors, Pharmacists, Dentists and Midwives Who Have Been Licensed in Accordance with the Various Ordinances Regulating Their Professions* (Jerusalem, 1930), 22–23, 26–29; Government of Palestine, Department of Health, *List of Doctors, Dentists and Midwives Who Have Been*

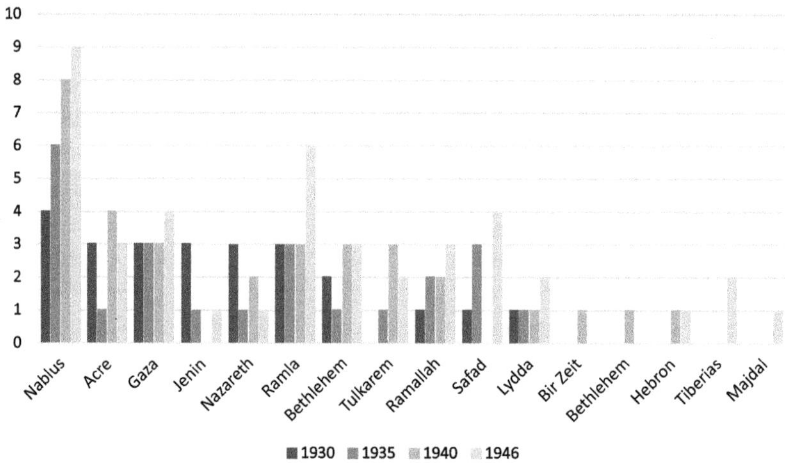

Figure 4.4 Numbers of pharmacists in Palestine's towns.[16]

medical community of about five doctors, three pharmacists, and five certified midwives. Usually, one or two of each profession worked for the DoH, and in some places, one or two worked for a missionary hospital or clinic. This left very little room for private practice, and indeed only a relatively small clientele could afford it.

During the Mandate years, Acre, Nazareth, Gaza, and Nablus were home to four out of nineteen DHOs. We focus on these towns for several reasons. All four boasted a relatively large medical community, thus providing richer material for discussion, and all had early medical presence, allowing longer-term analysis. These towns also supported a

Licensed in Accordance with the Various Ordinances Regulating Their Professions Including a Supplement of Licensed Veterinary Surgeons (Jerusalem, 1935), 6–49; Government of Palestine, Department of Health, *List of Medical Practitioners, Dentists, and Midwives Who Have Been Licensed in Accordance with the Various Ordinances Regulating Their Professions Including a Supplement of Licensed Veterinary Surgeons* (Jerusalem: Government Printing Press, 1940), 6–48; Government of Palestine, Department of Health, *List of Medical Practitioners, Dentists and Midwives Who Have Been Licensed in Accordance with the Various Ordinances Regulating Their Professions Including a Supplement of Licensed Veterinary Surgeons* (Jerusalem: Government Printing Press, 1946), 6–56 (henceforth: *List of Medical Practitioners, year*).

16 *List of Medical Practitioners, 1930*, 37–44; *List of Medical Practitioners, 1935*, 75–79; *List of Medical Practitioners, 1940*, 72–82; *List of Medical Practitioners, 1946*, 79–87.

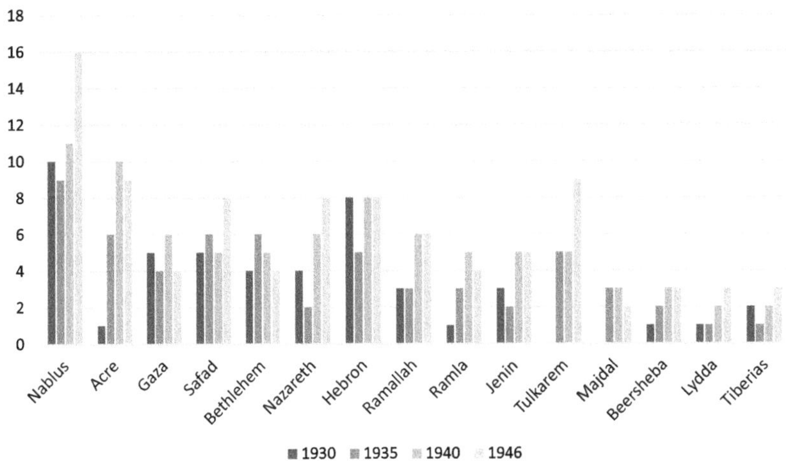

Figure 4.5 Numbers of midwives in Palestine's towns.[17]

large rural hinterland and underwent significant transformations during the later Ottoman and Mandate years. Finally, they offered a diversity of experiences – two coastal and two mountainside towns, one with a large Christian community and the others more homogeneously Muslim. Demographically, Acre and Nazareth both numbered around 10,000 inhabitants in the 1930s, while Gaza and Nablus were twice or thrice as large. In what follows, both similarities and differences are used to characterize the towns' positions in Palestine's medical landscape.

Acre

Acre's medical landscape is a microcosm of an East-Mediterranean town. Anwar Shuqayri, Ilyas Dib, and Manouq Erdekian's stories take us on fascinating tours within the old port city walls. The favorite son of an Azhar-educated scholar, Ottoman parliament member, and mufti of Jamal Pasha's army,[18] Asʿad Shuqayri sent his son Anwar to study in an Anglican missionary school in Jerusalem, and upon graduation,

[17] *List of Medical Practitioners, 1930*, 59–70; *List of Medical Practitioners, 1935*, 89–103; *List of Medical Practitioners, 1940*, 88–99; *List of Medical Practitioners, 1946*, 95–104.

[18] Mustafa Abbasi, "The Fall of Acre in the 1948 Palestine War," *Journal of Palestine Studies* 39 (2010): 6–7.

Anwar continued to the American University of Beirut (AUB). Ilyas Dib's father was a landowning olive grower from the village of Rama in the Galilee. His maternal grandfather was Iskandar Kazma, who studied in Moscow and was appointed by the Russian Tzar to establish and supervise the Russian missionary schools in the region.[19] Dib started his academic training in Beirut and gained his medical degree from the University of Geneva.[20] Born in Adana, Manouq Erdekian (b. 1890) was trained in Istanbul. After defecting from the Ottoman to the British army during World War I (WWI), he settled in Acre. He succeeded in bringing family members who survived the Armenian genocide to the city as well.[21]

In both biography and geography, the three doctors are representative of the greater regional medical landscape. Shuqayri was born in Acre. Erdekian was a DoH employee who decided to settle in town and quit his job when asked to relocate. Dib worked briefly in Jenin before settling in Acre and was one of the few Palestinian doctors of his generation hailing from the Palestinian countryside. Dib and Erdekian's descendants still live in Israel. Anwar, who was murdered in 1939 during the tide of intra-community violence of the Arab Revolt, left no descendants, but his older brother Ahmad was the first chair of the PLO. Their origins, choices, and circumstances are reflective of diverse doctors' biographies.[22]

In the late eighteenth century, the Ottoman district (Liwa) town gained regional administrative and economic prominence. Acre also gained religious importance with the construction of al-Jazzar Mosque and Ahmadiyya madrasa and library, and since the mid nineteenth century, the settlement of shaykh ʿAli Nur al-Din al-Yashruti and the Shadhaliyya sufi order, as well as a small Bahai community.[23]

[19] Hanna Kildani, *Modern Christianity in the Holy Land: Development of the Structure of Churches and the Growth of Christian Institutions in Jordan and Palestine* (Bloomington: AuthorHouse, 2010), 141–42.

[20] Interview with Dr. Ziad Dib, son of Ilyas by Yoni Furas and Liat Kozma, June 11, 2018.

[21] Telephone interview with Dr. Leon Erdekian by Yoni Furas, August 8, 2021, 5.

[22] Another Acre-based physician was Naʿim Qutran, Sherene Seikaly, "The Matter of Time," *American Historical Review* 124 (2019): 1681–88; and Sherene Seikaly, "How I Met My Great-Grandfather: Archives and the Writing of History," *Comparative Studies of South Asia, Africa, and the Middle East* 38 (2018): 6–20.

[23] Zuhayr Ghanayim, *Liwa ʿAkka fi ʿahd al-tanzimat al-ʿUthmaniyya,* 1281–1337 H / 1864–1918M (Beirut: Muʾassasat al-dirasat al-Filastiniyya, 1999), 19–43;

Nevertheless, the town's nineteenth-century history was marked by political and economic decline. The steamship made Acre's shallow-water port obsolete, contributing to the subsequent rise of Haifa's port. The Ottoman employment of Acre as a garrison town and the presence of soldiers in town made it even less attractive to merchants, who started relocating to Haifa, to which merchandise was increasingly imported directly. The connection of Haifa to the extension of the Hejaz Railway, inaugurated in 1905, further marginalized Acre, and the British decision to turn Haifa's port into a Mediterranean hub and pipeline station accelerated the process.[24] In 1908, the Ottoman ban on building outside the town walls was lifted, enabling gradual growth, attracting Lebanese merchants, Sufi followers, Bahais, and Jewish immigrants, but mostly migrants from neighboring villages. In the Mandate years, Acre grew from 6,420 in 1922 to 8,165 in 1931 and 13,560 in 1946.[25]

Around 1930, a DHO, a dispensary, an Infant Welfare Centre (IWC), and an ophthalmic clinic operated in Acre (see Figure 4.6). It also had a small municipal hospital, roughly thirty-bed strong, which was closed in 1933, leaving Haifa, about 25 kilometers to the south, as the location of the nearest hospital. The DHO in town was left with an MO, a pharmacist, two female nurses, and one male nurse specializing in ophthalmology.[26] This meant that most of the city's medical services were left to private practitioners. Still, with Acre's DHO and private clinics, it became the medical center of its rural periphery. Under the British, it came to serve as the administrative, political, and economic center of sixty-three villages inhabited by 55,970 people in 1944.

Mustafa Abbasi, "Mishpahot ha-nikhbadim ha-ʿArviyot be-ʿAko be-shalhei ha shilton ha-ʿOthmani u-bi-tkufat ha-mandat: Hemshekh o tmura," *Cathedra* 130 (2008): 54–61.

24 Ghanaym, *Liwa ʿAkka*, 104–05; Yuval Ben-Bassat and Yossi Ben-Artzi, "Cartographical Evidence of Efforts to Develop Acre during the Last Decades of Ottoman Rule: Did the Ottomans Neglect the City?" *Mediterranean Historical Review* 31 (2016): 65–70.

25 In 1931, e.g., 7,303 of its inhabitants were Muslims, 1,525 Christians, 231 Jews, 86 Bahai, and 10 Druze, Anat Kidron and Shuli Yarkoni, "Hityashvut Yehudim be-ʿarim meʿoravot bi-tkufat ha-mandat: ha-Mikre shel ʿAko," *Israel* 27–28 (2021): 119–22.

26 Department of Health, *Annual Report for the Year 1933* (Jerusalem: Department of Health, 1934), 38; "Risalat ʿAkka: Ikfal al-mustashfa," *Filastin*, May 3, 1933, 7; "Limadha alghat al-hukuma mustashfa ʿAkka?" *al-Jamiʿa al-ʿArabiyya*, December 26, 1933, 1.

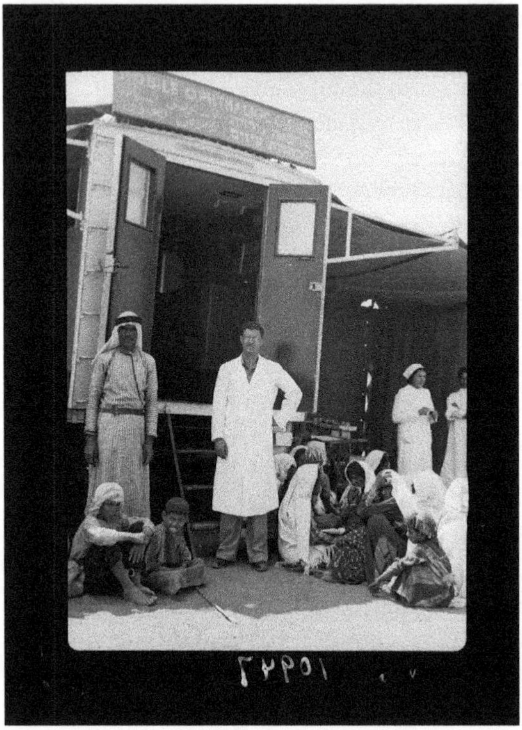

Figure 4.6 The Department of Health, Mobile Ophthalmic Clinic. Operating in Arab Villages of the South Country, N.E. of Gaza. Looking into the ophthalmic van, showing local Doctor Shukeir, photos taken outside Nejd [i.e., Najd] Village, August 1939. G. Eric and Edith Matson Photograph Collection, Library of Congress, Prints & Photographs Division.

Villagers now came to town for services such as education and health. In 1934, Dr. Anwar Shuqayri's request to establish a five-bed maternity unit in town that would serve the Acre subdistrict was denied by the DoH.[27]

Zooming into the city's medical community, we find four private practitioners in the 1920s and ten in the 1940s. Acre was also served by six midwives in the 1930s and ten in the 1940s; three to four pharmacists and one to three dentists. Like in the case of Drs. Shuqayri, Dib, and Erdekian, among them there were natives of Acre

27 "Medical Institutions – Voluntary & Private – Maternity Home – Dr Anwar Shukayri, Acre," December 24, 1934, M/11/610, ISA.

(including a descendant of Shaykh Yashruti) and medical professionals born in neighboring villages such as Biʿna, Kafr Yasif, and Rama. Others came from different parts of the Ottoman Empire such as Istanbul and Marash (Anatolia) or present-day Lebanon, including the brothers Naji and ʿAsim Baydun, a doctor and a pharmacist, from a Beiruti merchant family.

To conclude, Acre's medical landscape and professional medical community were a mosaic of regional possibilities and developments of a small late Ottoman coastal town. The life stories of this community's members – the son of a notable Ottoman *ʿalim*, an Armenian refugee, and migrants from neighboring villages, and members of the Christian rural notability in the Galilee – illustrate the diversity of this mosaic. Its proximity to Haifa was to its own detriment, nonetheless, its medical services allowed it to serve its own inhabitants, as well as the villages of the western Galilee.

Gaza

Let us now journey south to Gaza, another coastal town on the Mediterranean with its own distinctive story. Like Acre, Gaza's medical landscape reflected its importance and gradual marginalization. Located on the historical border between Egypt and the Ottoman Empire, and after WWI, Mandate Palestine, it was a frontier town. The 1869 inauguration of the Suez Canal dramatically transformed Gaza's position as a caravan waystation. Maritime trade and hajj routes replaced the desert transport, and Gaza's economic and political importance declined. Its position as the capital of an Ottoman subdistrict somewhat diminished with the foundation of Beersheba in 1900 and its declaration as a parallel subdistrict. Despite this decline, with a population of around 40,000 at the eve of WWI, it was Palestine's third most populated city.

WWI left Gaza in ruins. In early 1917, the Ottomans evacuated it in anticipation of British forces in order to spare their army the burden of protecting civilians. Its inhabitants escaped with little of their belongings, and as the British approached, the Ottomans deliberately demolished large parts of the town.[28] Many Gazans chose not to return after

[28] Dotan Halevy, "The Rear Side of the Front: Gaza and Its People in World War I," *Journal of Levantine Studies* 5 (2015): 44–49.

the war, and in the 1922 British census, a population of 17,480 was documented, less than half the pre-war number. The city's population reached 37,820 in 1946.[29]

Unlike Acre, Gaza had a missionary medical facility and benefited from limited state investment in medical infrastructure already in the late Ottoman period. The Church Mission Society (CMS) started providing basic medical services in 1882. A British doctor joined the mission in 1886, and an inpatient clinic and dispensary were established later. In the early 1900s, the CMS started constructing its own hospital, while the Ottoman authorities began building a municipal one. The CMS managed to work closely with the local Greek Orthodox community and Muslim elite. Its staff studied Arabic and helped train local nurses. The relationship the mission managed to forge in town led to the establishment of a new CMS medical facility in 1908, funded by Gaza's own community.[30] The CMS hospital employed Arab doctors since the 1890s and throughout the Mandate years.

The construction of Gaza's municipal hospital lagged. The Ottoman authorities used it as a pretext to levy a new port tax, against which foreign traders and consuls were quick to protest. The completion of the CMS hospital, they argued, obviated the need for a municipal one. The hospital was eventually opened under the British in 1924.[31] The DoH's 1927 annual report documented an eighteen-bed municipal hospital in Gaza, and sixty-three beds in the CMS hospital. The municipal hospital would grow to a thirty-three-bed hospital by 1930 and become a government hospital in 1937, maintaining the same bed-strength until 1948.[32] In addition, Gaza had a DHO, which included a dispensary and an IWC.

There was one attempt to establish an independent Palestinian-Arab hospital in Gaza. In early 1945, ʿA'isha Abu Khadra and her daughter donated 44,000 pounds for the foundation of a voluntary Islamic fifty-bed hospital and dedicated a waqf of the family's lands to its maintenance.

[29] Mustafa Murad al-Dabbagh, *Biladuna Filastin* (Beirut: Mu'assasat al-dirasat al-Filastiniyya, 2016), vol. 1, no. 2, 106–07.

[30] Philippe Bourmaud, "Discipline et familiarisation à travers la médecine: Une mission médicale à Gaza (1878–1914)," *Histoire et missions chrétiennes* 21 (2012): 81–102.

[31] *Political Diaries of the Arab World: Palestine & Jordan* (Slough: Archive Editions, 2001), 2: 48.

[32] Al-Dabbagh, *Biladuna Filastin*, vol. 1, no. 2, 123.

They requested that the DoH pay for the plans, and its Director supported the request, yet there is no evidence of further developments.[33]

Gaza had a very small community of medical professionals relative to its population: nine medical doctors in 1930 and sixteen in 1946, one and later two dentists, three to four pharmacists, and four to six midwives. Their origins were highly diverse, and only three of its doctors throughout the period were native to the town. Except for Dr. Hathat, who had been trained prior to WWI, only five others were born in Gaza and trained in the 1940s. One, Jirair Arsenian, was the son of an Armenian pharmacist, a refugee from Anatolia. Arsenian graduated from the AUB in 1947. Unlike Acre, which relied on its neighboring villages, here medical professionals originated from Jerusalem, Haifa, and Lebanese villages.

Gaza's Medical Officers visited the larger neighboring villages on a regular basis. Dr. Hurani, for example, had a regular clinic which he operated in Khan Yunis on Thursdays.[34] Some private practitioners did so as well. The ʿAbd al-Shafi brothers, who graduated from the AUB four years apart, Haydar in 1942 and Mustafa in 1946, opened clinics in Gaza and Khan Yunis.

The distance from Gaza's medical facilities determined the medical solutions available to its hinterland. The people of Najd, a small village 14 kilometers to the northeast, traveled to town for medical treatment mostly in severe cases, otherwise relying on local healers.[35] During the late 1940s, Najd and neighboring Simsim resorted to Kibbutz Gvarʿam's clinic.[36] Located 30 kilometers northeast of Gaza, Faluja had its own clinic with a male nurse and a government doctor who made weekly visits. For hospital treatment, they traveled to Gaza or Jaffa.[37]

33 "Proposed Voluntary Hospital in Gaza," M-325/38, ISA; "Mustashfa Ghazza al-khayri: Hadith hamm maʿ sahibatay al-mashruʿ," *al-Sirat*, July 25, 1943, 2.

34 "Kabir sihhat al-Qadaʾ," *Filastin*, June 9, 1932, 7.

35 Mansour al-Kurdi (1934), Najd, interviewed by Rakan Mahmoud, Jordan, October 16, 2008, www.palestineremembered.com/Gaza/Najd/Story12147.html, accessed November 28, 2022; Khatima al-Qiram (1918) and her son Fayez Abu Farda (1958), interviewed by Rakan Mahmoud, December 5, 2005.

36 Avraham S., "Bikur be-Gvarʿam," *Haaretz*, February 20, 1948, 6; Jamal Abu ʿAwn (1934), Simsim, interviewed by Rakan Mahmoud, Khittin Camp, April 2, 2008, www.palestineremembered.com/Gaza/Simsim/Story9469.html.

37 Muhammad Abu Sirdaneh (1924), al-Faluja, interviewed by Said ʿAjjawi, June 17, 2007, www.palestineremembered.com/Gaza/al-Faluja/Story3984.html, accessed May 22, 2025; www.youtube.com/watch?v=w1R23sayH60, accessed May 22, 2025.

Both Gaza and Acre were coastal towns, both marginalized by war and changing maritime routes. Their differences lie, first, in their proximity to other medical hubs. Acre had nearby Haifa, while Gaza had none. Gaza's hinterland, which included a huge Bedouin population, did not experience the social developments that transformed Acre's surroundings. This rural population relied on Gaza's medical services and did not contribute to the expansion of its medical community. Second, the good relationship between the missionaries and the city enabled Gaza's inhabitants to enjoy a missionary hospital alongside a municipal one throughout the Mandate period.

Nazareth

During the late Ottoman period, Nazareth belonged to Acre's subdistrict, part of *Wilayat* Beirut. Under the British Mandate, Nazareth was the administrative center for the Nazareth subdistrict and the headquarters for the Galilee district. In the 1922 census, 7,424 inhabitants were documented, 8,756 in 1931, and around 12,000 in 1946, most of whom were members of the Greek Orthodox and Latin denominations.[38] Due to its religious importance and its sizable Christian population, Nazareth became a site for missionary settlement already in the mid nineteenth century. As in Jerusalem and Jaffa, this presence enhanced inter-denominational and imperial competition between British Protestants, French Franciscans, and Russian Presbyterians, which involved the establishment of monasteries, churches, schools, and clinics.[39] Nazareth's early introduction to missionary schools and hospitals explains the number of medical professionals born in the city, and the number of medical professionals who worked there – much exceeding other towns of similar size. Indeed, during the last Ottoman decades, the city's missionary schools, churches, and hospitals also attracted Lebanese and rural immigration for education and employment.[40]

[38] In 1922, Nazareth's population was 33 percent Muslim and 66 percent Christian (28 percent Greek Orthodox, 16 percent Roman Catholic, 13 percent Greek Catholic, and the rest belonging to nine other denominations).

[39] Siham Fahoum Ghunaym, *Tahaddiyyat taghayyurat wa-tahawulat fi ta'rikh al-Nasira* (Nazareth: Matba'at al-nahda, 2003), 79–84, 110–11; As'ad Mansur, *Ta'rikh al-Nasira min aqdam azmaniha ila ayamina al-hadira* (Cairo: Matba'at al-Hilal, 1924), 82–87, 101.

[40] Ghunaym, *Tahadiyyat*, 113–15.

Several developments changed Nazareth's economy during this period. The growing trade with Europe benefited Nazareth's Christian merchants. Some of them would accumulate wealth that enabled them to purchase land in and around Nazareth. At the beginning of the twentieth century, the Darʿa-Haifa branch of the Hejaz Railway diverted some of this trade and diminished Nazareth's involvement in it. Changing Ottoman land laws enabled the wealthy Beiruti Sursuq family to purchase many of the agricultural lands around Nazareth and in the nearby Ibn ʿAmir Valley. They would start selling this land to Jewish settlers already in the 1880s – turning the hinterland of Nazareth into the first and most affected by Zionist endeavors of all the towns discussed in this chapter.

Dr. Kaloost Vartan, an Ottoman Armenian from Istanbul, reached Nazareth in the 1860s and inaugurated the Edinburgh Medical Mission Society (EMMS) clinic, which would later become a hospital. This was a unique missionary endeavor, by a non-European who joined the British army in the Crimean War and then trained in Edinburgh.[41] An Austrian hospital was opened in the city in 1884, located east of the town, and a dispensary operated at its center.[42] These hospitals were joined by the French Sœurs de Charité in 1898 who opened a clinic which later became a hospital.[43]

During WWI, Ottoman and German army camps were located in Nazareth, taking their toll on the population, which was depleted of its resources. The town's hospitals were closed as enemy institutions, or used for military purposes, while olive trees around Nazareth were cut down for firewood. Missionary hospitals gradually resumed their activities in the early years of the Mandate. The subsequent British decision to turn Nazareth into an administrative center changed its position once again, attracting both administrative employees and migrant laborers.[44]

During the Mandate years, Nazareth also housed a government medical inspection room. The EMMS Hospital grew from forty beds in 1926 to seventy beds in 1936. In the early Mandate period, the French hospital started with fifty-six beds, growing to ninety by the

[41] Nakhla Bishara, *Irus Vartani: Sippuro shel bet ha-holim Natseret* (Zikhron Yaʿakov: Itay Bakhur, 2001), 18–29.

[42] Kildani, *Modern Christianity*, 409.

[43] Mansur, *Taʾrikh al-Nasira*, 156.

[44] Ibid., 119–26; Mansur, *Taʾrikh al-Nasira*, 97–98, 106–107.

mid 1940s. These numbers underline the dominant role of missionary facilities in Nazareth's medical landscape.

About six doctors, two to four pharmacists, one to two dentists, and four to eight certified midwives worked in Nazareth at any given time. The dentist ʿArif Bulus Qaʿwar worked in Nazareth throughout the Mandate years, shortly after his graduation from the Faculty of Medicine of the newly founded Damascus University in 1920.

Serving as an educational center already from the late nineteenth century, Nazareth produced eighteen physicians, most of whom did not return there upon graduation. Born in 1878, the first Nazareth-born physician was Niʿma Nakhu, who worked as the city's municipal physician during the early years of the century and later settled in Lebanon to become the director of a sanatorium. Amin ʿAwda studied at the Russian Seminary in Nazareth and after graduating from the AUB, proceeded to his residency at Kiev University. His personal story also exemplifies the role of the foreign mission in enabling social and occupational mobility.

The Nazareth subdistrict included 22,681 inhabitants in 1922, of whom 700 were Jews, who had their autonomous medical services. In 1945, the subdistrict numbered 46,100, including 7,600 Jews. The town's hospitals served the population of both Nazareth and Bisan subdistricts. These villagers also resorted to HaEmek hospital founded in the Jewish settlement of Afula, south of Nazareth, in 1927. The uniqueness of Nazareth's hinterland in comparison to other towns discussed here lies also in the presence of monasteries and doctors in Jewish settlements, both serving the local Palestinian-Arab population. The people of Safuriyya, Mujaydal, and Kafr Kanna, for example, were treated by local nuns who lived in nearby monasteries.[45] In Shefa-ʿAmr, there was a clinic operated by a CMS nurse, weekly visited by a Nazareth doctor.[46]

[45] ʿAli Nijim (1918), Safuriyya, interviewed by Abdelmajeed Dandeis, Jordan, June 4, 2004, www.palestineremembered.com/Nazareth/Saffuriyya/Story1280.html, accessed May 4, 2021; Abdulmajeed Kanʿan (1929), Safuriyya, interviewed by Rakan Mahmud, Damascus, February 16, 2009, www.palestineremembered.com/Nazareth/Saffuriyya/Story13968.html, accessed May 22, 2025.

[46] Muhammad Qaraqra, "Maʿarekhet ha-briʾut ha-mandatorit ve-ha-voluntarit ve-ʿArviye Erets Yisraʾel, 1918–1948" (Master's thesis, Haifa University, 1992), 161.

Administratively, and in most demographic characteristics, Nazareth was similar to neighboring Acre, yet the contours of its medical landscape were determined by its religious importance, which attracted multiple missionary endeavors at an early stage, accounting for the relatively large number of Nazareth-born physicians. At the same time, local doctors who practiced in Nazareth had to compete with missionary and foreign doctors, which might explain their migration to other localities. The Jewish presence in the Ibn ʿAmir Valley with its expanding medical facilities, virtually nonexistent around the Gaza and Nablus hinterlands, competed with Nazareth in treating nearby villagers.

Nablus

Until the mid nineteenth century, Nablus and its surroundings were the most populated and productive region in Palestine. Nablus had one of the first municipal councils in the Ottoman Empire, established in 1868, and its activity reflected the town's economic power and relative autonomy. Surrounded by olive groves, it became a regional capital of soap production, exporting its products regionally and globally. This industry's reliance on agricultural products also entailed close ties to the rural hinterland. Like Gaza, the city had an overwhelming Muslim majority and its remoteness from the Mediterranean meant lesser interaction with outsiders. As economic hegemony was shifting toward the coast in the later decades of the nineteenth century, Nablus lost some of its socioeconomic centrality.[47] As for its population, the 1922 census recorded 15,947 inhabitants, 17,498 in 1931, and 23,250 in 1945.[48]

Nablus owes its relatively high number of native doctors to two factors: the early arrival of modern education and the presence of several families known for their role in the apprentice-based medical

[47] Beshara Doumani, *Rediscovering Palestine: Merchants and Peasants in Jabal Nablus, 1700–1900* (Berkeley: University of California Press, 1995); Salim Tamari, *Mountain against the Sea: Essays on Palestinian Society and Culture* (Berkeley: University of California Press, 2009), 22–35; Baruch Kimmerling and Joel S. Migdal, *The Palestinian People: A History* (Cambridge, MA: Harvard University Press, 2003), 41–46; Mahmoud Yazbak, "The Municipality of a Muslim Town: Nablus 1868–1914," *Archív Orientální* 67 (1999): 339–60.

[48] Al-Dabbagh, *Biladuna Filastin*, vol. 1, no. 2, 208–09.

landscape before the introduction of modern medical education. Some families maintained their role in the local medical scene by adaptation to university-based education and accreditation. Its first state primary school was founded in 1879, and more advanced education was available since 1889. Missionary schools were likewise founded in the 1870s, providing multiple educational opportunities and preparing Nabulsians for studies in Istanbul or Beirut.[49]

Although a short-lived endeavor, the first hospital in Nablus was a two-room municipal institute founded in 1888 and funded by Hajj Salih Kharim, subsequently bearing his name.[50] The arrival of the Anglican mission marked a turning point in the town's medical history. Unlike in Gaza, the relationship between the missionaries and the local community in Nablus was marked by ongoing conflict. Already in 1891, a few days after the opening of the CMS dispensary, the local governor ordered its shutdown for employing an unlicensed pharmacist. The CMS managed to reopen its hospital in 1901 only by appealing directly to the Ottoman authorities in Beirut while circumventing local opposition. Moreover, the Nablus CMS missionaries were unapologetic about their conversion efforts and even managed to antagonize the local Protestant community.[51] According to Ottoman officials Muhammad Bahjat and Rafiq al-Tamimi, writing in 1915, the hospital did attract patients but yielded only one convert in all its years of operation. Patients had to hear a daily sermon, and if they died at the hospital, receive a Christian funeral before being handed over to their families.[52]

The missionaries found themselves in direct professional conflict with local physicians and pharmacists. During the Mandate period, this conflict may have subsided, as at least two Palestinian-Arab physicians worked in the CMS hospital from the 1930s onward. Like in Jerusalem, the presence of foreign medical institutions encouraged the pursuit of university training. Indeed, the Abu Ghazalah, Jabbur, and

[49] Ibid., vol. 1, no. 2, 213–21.

[50] Ihsan Nimr, *Taʾrikh jabal Nablus wa-l-Balqaʾ* (Nablus: Jamaʿiyyat ʿummal al-matabiʿ al-taʿawwuniyya, 1975), 3: 78–81.

[51] Philippe Bourmaud, "Public Space and Private Spheres: The Foundation of St. Luke's Hospital of Nablus by the CMS," in *New Faith in Ancient Lands: Western Missions in the Middle East in the Nineteenth and Early Twentieth Centuries*, ed. Heleen Murre-van den Berg (Leiden: Brill, 2006), 133–50.

[52] Muhammad Bahjat and Muhamad Tamimi, *Wilayat Bayrut* (Beirut: Matbaʿat al-iqbal, 1916), 1: 95–96; Moshe Schalit, *bi-Ntivot hayyay* (Tel Aviv: Y. Golan, 2000), 271–72.

Tuqan families, who for generations practiced apprentice-based medicine and pharmacy, now sent their sons to Beirut's medical schools.

This ongoing tension between the local population and the mission was the background for the 1908 establishment of Nablus' Watani Hospital. Its establishing committee was composed of members of the city's notable families who raised the required funds,[53] and its operation was funded by new taxes levied on the town's slaughterhouses.[54] It was directed by Dr. Nur al-Din al-Karidi, a graduate of Istanbul's Imperial Medical School, who worked there until his death in 1920.[55] An infant welfare center and ophthalmic clinic were added later. This sixty-bed-strong medical facility, as well as the doctors themselves, served the city and the surrounding villages. In the mid 1930s, the Mandate authorities took over the hospital's administration, and it became a government hospital. By that time, it had expanded to eighty-five beds, and to 126 by the end of the Mandate.

During the Mandate period, Nablus became the center of a subdistrict and thus home to a DHO and an adjacent IWC, a dispensary, and an ophthalmic clinic. It hosted the largest medical community outside the cities: sixteen to twenty-four doctors, six to nine pharmacists, and ten to sixteen midwives in 1930–46, and a dentist or two throughout the period.

Bahjat and Tamimi's report on Nablus concluded that the town had nothing to offer to Nabulsis who had graduated from Istanbul, Beirut, or European universities. After acquiring a taste for the larger cities, they argued, these graduates would refuse to return to the damp alleyways, heavy food, and monotonous routine of Nablus. Al-Tamimi, a native of Nablus, did not return, but many others did. Unlike other towns discussed in this chapter, the list of longest-serving doctors in Nablus is dominated by its natives. George Daʿdas was one of the first Arab doctors in Palestine. He was first recorded in Nablus at the beginning of the century and worked there throughout his life. His

53 Philippe Bourmaud, "'Ya doktor': Devenir médecin et exercer son art en 'Terre sainte', une expérience du pluralisme médical dans l'Empire ottoman finissant (1871–1918)" (PhD diss., Aix-Marseille 1, 2007), 713–14.

54 Bashshar Saʿid al-Tamam, *Baladiyyat Nablus fi al-ʿahd al-ʿUthmani, 1868–1918* (Nablus: Maktabat baladiyyat Nablus al-ʿama, 2012), 86–89; Nimr, *Taʾrikh jabal Nablus*, 3: 78–81.

55 Bahjat and Tamimi, *Wilayat Bayrut*, 1: 95–96.

son, Fu'ad, graduated from the AUB in 1930 and returned to his hometown as well.

Among the doctors and pharmacists working in Nablus during the Mandate period, we find sons of the city's notable families. Wasif ʿAbd al-Hadi was trained in Istanbul in parallel to Tamimi. He graduated in 1911, and in 1918 he settled in Nablus where he opened a private clinic, remaining there at least until the end of the Mandate. Ashraf Abd al-Hadi studied dentistry in Nancy and returned. The ʿArafat family provided the city with both pharmacists and doctors. Four members of the Abu-Ghazaleh family returned to town after their training and worked in local pharmacies, while four others worked elsewhere in Palestine.

As far as its medical community is concerned, Nablus was almost a category of its own. Like Gaza and its hinterland, Nablus was characterized by religious homogeneity. Unlike the coastal border town, it maintained its economic, cultural, and political importance during the Mandate, which enabled the expansion of its medical community. Slightly larger than Nazareth and Acre, it had a much larger medical community. We see a group of men from notable families, some of whom were traditional healers, who returned home to Nablus and established their clinics and pharmacies there. Unlike Nazareth, which also had a similar output of doctors, they faced little competition back home, which made their return easier, as the missionary presence was smaller than in Nazareth. The lack of competition with Jewish doctors and the close economic relations Nablus enjoyed with its hinterland helped turn it into an exclusive regional service provider.

Urban Centers as Medical Centers

The evolution of medical communities in Palestine's largest urban centers (illustrated in Figures 4.7–4.9) was tightly connected to several intertwined processes: an expanding market economy leading to rapid urbanization, the presence of foreigners who took advantage of this development, an expanding network of foreign and local schools, and several wealthy families able to afford quality education. The urbanization of Jaffa, Haifa, and Jerusalem also went hand in hand with the growing Jewish presence. Since we discussed Jerusalem extensively in Chapter 1, we dedicate the remainder of this chapter to Haifa and Jaffa.

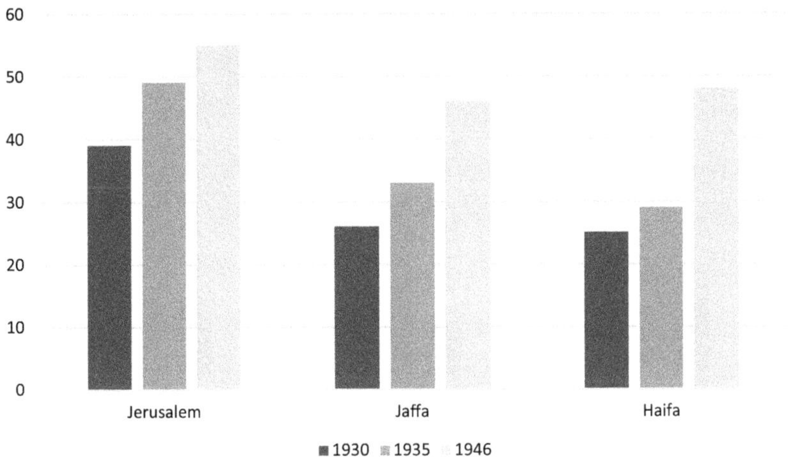

Figure 4.7 Number of doctors in Palestine's largest cities.[56]

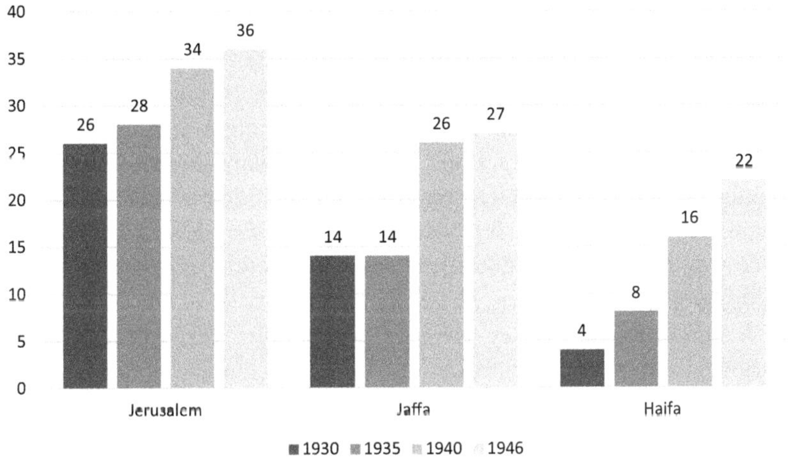

Figure 4.8 Number of pharmacists in Palestine's largest cities.[57]

Haifa and Jaffa's rebirth in the late eighteenth and early nineteenth centuries is commonly attributed to two men. Dahir al-ʿUmar rebuilt and fortified Haifa in 1761 and built its port, which would – a century

[56] *List of Medical Practitioners, 1930*, 11–16, 23–25; *List of Medical Practitioners, 1935*, 6–49; *List of Medical Practitioners, 1946*, 6–56.
[57] Ibid.

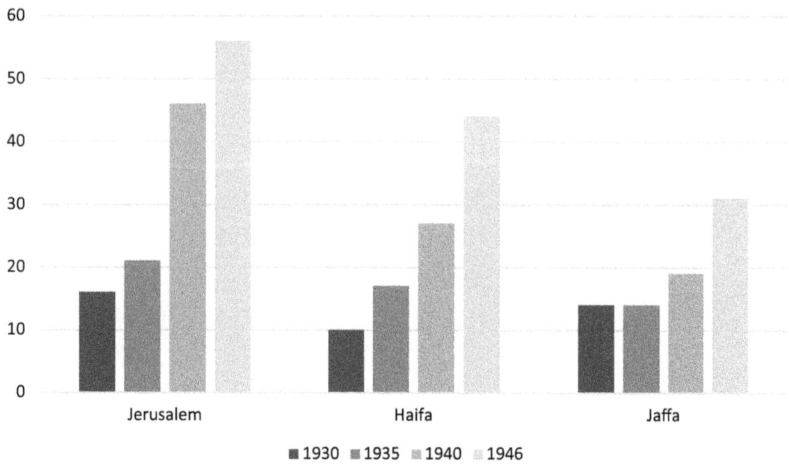

Figure 4.9 Number of midwives in Palestine's largest cities.[58]

later – replace Acre's as the main port of northern Palestine.[59] Similarly, Muhammad Agha al-Shami, Jaffa's governor from 1807 to 1818, reconstructed the city from its ruins after Napoleon's invasion, rebuilding the city's walls and port and opening a customs station. Another late Ottoman development was the establishment of a municipality in the 1870s, which meant a municipal doctor and municipal regulation of and responsibility over the city's cleanliness, hygiene, and quarantine post. Jaffa's municipal council was first recorded in 1872, and Haifa's in 1873.[60]

A significant missionary presence also entailed early medical institutions – and indeed, both cities were home to a number of hospitals by WWI. Jaffa and Haifa's position as Palestine's port cities made them the first entry points of epidemics; accordingly, they housed two of Palestine's quarantine stations. Both coastal cities were severely affected by the 1865 and 1902–3 cholera epidemics. Jaffa was spared the 1911–12 cholera contagion, while half of Haifa's inhabitants fled

58 Ibid.

59 Mahmoud Yazbak, *Haifa in the Late Ottoman Period 1860–1914: A Muslim Town in Transition* (Leiden: Brill, 1998), 13–15.

60 Ibid., 76–80; Ruth Kark, *Yafo: Tsmihata shel 'ir, 1799–1917* (Jerusalem: Yad Itzhak Ben Tsvi, 1984), 180–83; 'Ali Hasan Al-Bawwab, *Mawsu'at Yafa al-jamila* (Beirut: al-Muasasa al-'Aarabiya lil-dirasat wa-l-nashr, 2003), 2: 1029–31, 1047.

the city, and many died.[61] Smallpox entered through Jaffa and the plague through Haifa in 1924 and 1942, respectively. In both cases, an effective response from the British authorities prevented an outbreak outside the cities.

Both Haifa and Jaffa became capitals of administrative districts and housed district administration – including a Senior MO, a DHO, and relatively large government hospitals. Haifa was also home to a large British community, mediating between the British imperial project, Arabs, and Jews. Numbering about 1,200, the large community of British personnel was second only to Jerusalem and also affected the city's government medical services. In 1945, 10 percent of the government hospital beds were dedicated to British citizens and attended solely by British staff.[62]

In these urban centers, private clinics, pharmacies, and hospitals were in proximity to each other. This centralized proliferation of medical services amplified gaps within the city itself. Clinics and hospitals could not be found outside the well-off neighborhoods, turning them into intimate spaces of interclass encounters. These encounters underlined doctors' responsibility for their urban poor and their inability to equally serve them. Both cities had a vibrant civil society and a proliferation of clubs, associations, and newspapers, which catered to the metropolitan appetite of urban doctors and their class members.[63]

The development of Jaffa and Haifa was defined by the interaction with the Jewish immigrants much more than in any other locale discussed in this chapter. Due to middle- and working-class immigration, Haifa's Jewish population grew from a couple of thousand at the beginning of the Mandate to more than 74,000 by 1948. Jaffa's Jewish neighborhoods also grew at a steady pace, but it was neighboring Tel

[61] Another outbreak struck Jaffa in 1916; Dan Barel, *Ruah ra'a: Magefot ha-kolera ve-hitpathut ha-refu'a be-Erets Yisra'el be-shalhe ha-tkufa ha-'Othmanit* (Jerusalem: Bialik Institute, 2010), 36–38, 88, 99–100, 162–69, 223–25.

[62] Department of Health, *Annual Report for the Year 1945* (Jerusalem: Department of Health, 1946), 9.

[63] Maayan Hillel, "Constructing Modern Identity – New Patterns of Leisure and Recreation in Mandatory Palestine," *Contemporary Levant* 4 (2019): 75–90; Naama Ben Zeev, "Civil Associations in Mandatory Haifa: A New Perspective on Palestinian-Arab Political Life," *Middle Eastern Studies* 49 (2013): 958–72; Johny Mansur, *al-Madina al-Filastiniyya fi fatrat al-intidab al-Baritani: Tatawwurat wa-tahawwulat ijtima'iyya wa-iqtisadiyya wa-thaqafiyya, Hayfa namudhajan* (Ramallah: Al-Ru'at li-l-dirasat wa-l-nashr, 2009).

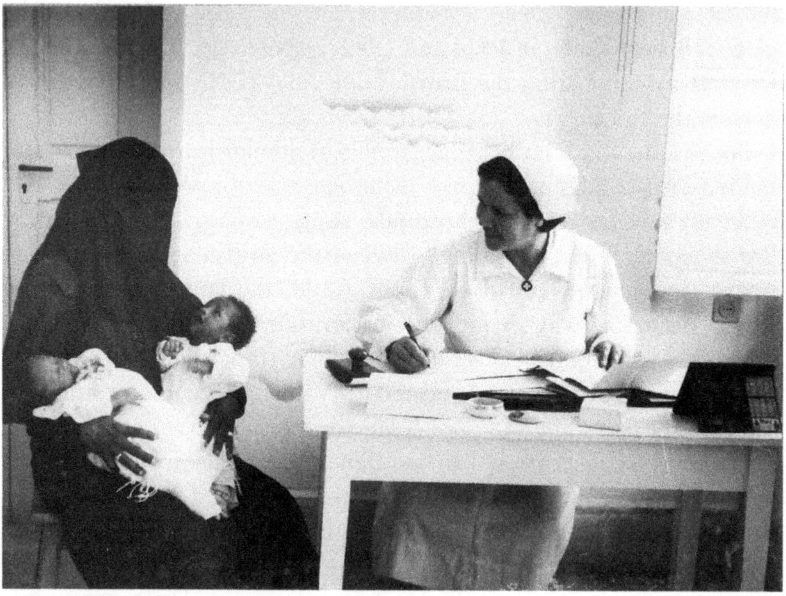

Figure 4.10 Mother with twins at Haifa's IWC.
TS-3024/48, Public Information Office Collection, ISA

Aviv that figured most largely in Jaffa's interaction with Jewish society – home, by 1948, for 200,000 Jews, one-third of Palestine's Jewish population. This proximity had a direct impact on the medical realm as well. Palestine's Arab medical professionals in Jaffa and Haifa had to compete with a much larger Jewish medical community and a superior institutional infrastructure – a competition that was hardly felt in the more homogenous towns. Arab patients, particularly the more affluent, had access to Jewish medical professionals and institutions. Jewish doctors from Tel Aviv and Haifa advertised their private clinics and hospitals in the Arab press.[64] Some operated their clinics in downtown, mostly Arab, Haifa.[65] While Jewish doctors, dentists, and pharmacists opened private clinics in Arab neighborhoods, the opposite phenomenon was nonexistent.

[64] See the ads for Dr. Itzko Freid's private hospital in Tel Aviv, in *Filastin*, February 17, 1928, 3; Nina Berlin Shlush, Clinic in Tel Aviv, *Filastin*, March 6, 1928, 8.

[65] *Filastin*, January 16, 1932, 6; October 8, 1932, 8; August 22, 1941, 3; August 6, 1944, 3.

Haifa

With an estimated population of 3,500–4,000 in the 1870s, Haifa's gradual transformation into an urban center began toward the turn of the twentieth century. Under the British occupation, Haifa became the educational, cultural, and economic center of northern Palestine.[66] The city's economic development attracted rural immigrants who worked in the railway and harbor, merchants from neighboring Mediterranean port cities, Jewish immigrants, Ottoman officials, and professionals from Mt. Lebanon and beyond.[67] These developments fueled growth – sixfold by the end of the Ottoman era. For the growing Jewish community in Palestine, Haifa became a distribution center for agricultural products and a home for heavy industries. It likewise attracted Egyptian, Lebanese, and British migration, seeking employment in its expanding industries.[68] Several factories were established by Palestinian entrepreneurs as well.[69] Its estimated 15,000 inhabitants after WWI grew to 24,634 in 1922, including 9,377 Muslims, 8,863 Christians, and 6,230 Jews.[70] Within a decade, it doubled its size and maintained a clear Arab majority of roughly 60 percent. Toward the end of the Mandate, however, Jews represented over half of its population of around 150,000.[71]

The relatively large community of Palestinian Arab doctors in Haifa can be attributed, in part, to its educational infrastructure. Greek Orthodox and Protestants were educated in missionary schools and joined the class of lawyers, doctors, and pharmacists.[72] The community's size can also be attributed to the presence of foreign medical institutions. The establishment of three hospitals preceded the British occupation: the Deutsche Spital, the Anglican St. Luke's (1899–1928), and the Italian Hospital (1907). Haifa's government hospital was

[66] May Seikaly, *Haifa: Transformation of a Palestinian Arab Society, 1918–1939* (London: I. B. Tauris, 1995), 22–23; Alex Carmel, *Ottoman Haifa: A History of Four Centuries under Turkish Rule* (London: I. B. Tauris, 2011); 79–80; Mansur, *al-Madina*, 30–34.

[67] Ghanaym, *Liwa ʿAkka*, 98–100.

[68] Seikaly, *Haifa*, 5–6.

[69] Amir Kulick, "Manhigut," 60; Shimon Shtern, "Hitpathut ha-maʿarakh ha-ʿironi shel Hefa ba-shanim 1918–1947" (PhD diss., the Hebrew University, 1974), 13–16.

[70] Carmel, *Ottoman Haifa,* 142–43.

[71] Shtern, "Hitpathut," 17–18.

[72] Seikaly, *Haifa*, 32.

established shortly after the war.[73] One of the city's IWCs can be seen in Figure 4.10.

Some of Haifa's doctors were born there. These were members of the more affluent families that were able to send their children to private missionary education and later to the medical faculties abroad. Such was the case with Drs. Maurice and Anthony Sahyun, sons of a rich merchant of European education and member of the municipal council.[74] Yet most of the city's Arab doctors migrated into the expanding city, attracted by the employment opportunities it provided. Families such as Nassar, Tabari, Musallam, and Zuʿrub from Nazareth, Jdeide, Ain Aanoub, and Tyre respectively, opened clinics and pharmacies all over the city. Poet and writer Dr. Qaisar Khuri (1893), a Maronite from the village of Bkassine near Jezzine, served as an Ottoman army doctor and settled in Haifa after the war, where he remained until the Mandate's end.[75] Born in Bisan in 1913, Dr. Omar al-Khalil arrived in Haifa in 1937 and opened a private clinic, making a name for himself not only for treating the poor but also as a workers' leader and publicist.[76]

Other notable doctors included Dr. Rushdi Tamimi from Nablus and Dr. Naif Hamzeh from Abey, Mount Lebanon. The Government Hospital was popularly known as the Hamzeh hospital, after Dr. Hamzeh, who directed its native ward. Tamimi headed the Muslim Polyclinic (*al-Mustawsif al-Tibbi al-Islami*, est. 1929), in a building designed for this purpose near the Istiqlal Mosque. The clinic was established by Haifa's Islamic Association and the Muslim Young Men Association in Haifa, which were affiliated with the mosque and headed, for some years, by popular leader ʿIzz al-Din al-Qassam.[77] The clinic was funded by donations and offered treatment and medication

73 Nissim Levi, *Prakim be-toldot ha-refuʾa be-Erets Yisraʾel, 1799–1948* (Tel Aviv: ha-Kibbuts ha-Meuhad, 1998), 361–64.

74 Kulick, "Manhigut," 133, n. 536.

75 "Dr Qaysar al-Khuri," Shai Files, Truman Archive, Hebrew University, Series 2, File no. 2, 224.

76 "Dr ʿOmar al-Khalil," February 19, 1948, Shai Files, Truman Archive, Hebrew University, Series 2, File no. 2, 218.

77 Naama Ben Zeev, "Ben ha-kfar la-ʿir: Hayye mehagrim kafriyyim Falestinim be-Hefa bi-tkufat ha-mandat" (PhD diss., Ben-Gurion University of the Negev, 2010), 117–21.

to the city's poor at affordable rates or free of charge.[78] In the summer of 1935, donations were collected by the Islamic Teaching and Guidance Association (*Jama'iyyat al-ta'lim wa-l-irshad al-Islami*) for the foundation of a surgical clinic, to be established above the Arab Workers' Union's building.[79]

Haifa's clinics were concentrated within a one-mile radius, around Stanton (today, Shivat Zion) and Allenby Streets. As noted earlier, clinics and pharmacies were built next to each other, sometimes by members of the same family. The location of the old Government Hospital, the English and the German hospitals (both closed in the late 1920s), and the Italian Hospital, explained the location of some of these clinics. Dr. Anthony Sahyun's clinic was on Mountain Road (today, Ha-Tzionut Ave.) and his brother's pharmacy on Allenby Square. Dr. Isbir and pharmacist Rashid Nassar's clinic and pharmacy could be found in Khamra Square next to Dr. Fu'ad and dentist Rafiq Tabari's clinic in the Carmelite Building, in the same square. Omar al-Khalil's clinic, with another doctor and two midwives, was at 52 Stanton Street, alongside ten other clinics, a few minutes' walk from the central square. Tamimi's Muslim Polyclinic was further down Stanton Street.

As the city's Arab inhabitants turned from a large majority to slightly less than half its population, the disparity in the medical sphere became much more dramatic. Already in 1930, most physicians in Haifa were Jewish – only about twenty (26 percent) of the city's seventy-six doctors were Arabs, as were only four of its twenty-two pharmacists and two of its twenty-five dentists. In August 1936, *Haaretz* noted that there were 240 Jewish doctors compared to

78 "al-Mustawsif al-Islami," *Yarmuq*, September 14, 1928, 2; "al-Mustawsif al-tibbi al-Islami bi-Hayfa," *Filastin*, January 21, 1931, 6. The Supreme Muslim Council was not involved in the Muslim clinics in Haifa or Jaffa. It operated clinics with an annex pharmacy in Jerusalem and Hebron established in 1924 and 1928, respectively. See Uri Kupferschmidt, *The Supreme Muslim Council: Islam under the British Mandate for Palestine* (Leiden: Brill, 1987), 144–45; *Bayan al-majlis al-Islami al-a'la li-sana 1349–1350 hijriyya wafq 1931* (Jerusalem: Matba'at dar al-aytam, 1932), 11. In later years, it operated other clinics, but exact details are not specified. *Bayan al-majlis al-shar'i al-Islami 'an al-sanawat 1358, 1359, 1360 al-muwafaqa l-sani 1939, 1940, 1941* (Jerusalem: Matba'at dar al-aytam, 1932), 12.

79 "al-Mustawsif al-jirahi bi-Hayfa wa-furu'uhu," *Al-Sirat al-Mustaqim*, June 3, 1935, 3; "al-Mustawsif al-jirahi wa-furu'uhu bi-Hayfa," *Al-Difa'*, June 5, 1935, 7.

30 Arab doctors in Haifa,[80] and by 1946, the gap widened. The city then had 330 doctors, 30 (9 percent) of whom were Arabs; 107 dentists, 9 (8 percent) of whom were Arabs; and 68 pharmacists, 18 (28 percent) of whom were Arabs.[81] Pharmacy was, therefore, the only realm in which Arab professionals were somewhat closing the gap. These numbers partly explain the nature and politics of Arab doctors' unionization in the city, as early as 1928, preceding similar developments elsewhere in the country. Arab medical professionals were overwhelmed by their Jewish counterparts, driving them to unionize.

More striking perhaps is the way in which these professionals' geographical distribution mirrored Haifa's inner segregation. Even if in other realms,[82] Jews and Arabs worked together, Arab and Jewish medical professionals worked in different institutions located in different parts of the city. The only exception was the Government Hospital, which would become a site of conflict in the winter of 1948. Most Jewish medical professionals who worked in the Arab neighborhoods in the 1930s moved to the Jewish neighborhoods or left the city by 1946: thirteen doctors, seven pharmacists, and seven dentists worked in the Arab neighborhoods in 1930, and few remained by 1946. The violent clashes in the city during the Arab Revolt enhanced this process.[83]

Whereas the smaller towns discussed earlier served as medical centers for nearby villages, Haifa constituted the main medical center of northern Palestine. It had the best surgical unit in the region, several hospitals, and many physicians. When Dr. Anwar Shuqayri bled to death after having been shot in his native Acre in June 1939, for example, his father's driver rushed him to the Italian Hospital in Haifa – the nearest hospital capable of saving his life – to

[80] B. Economicus, "ba-Miktsoʿot ha-hofshiyyim," *Haaretz*, August 16, 1936; Haifa's Jewish community 1938 census mentions much higher numbers: 408 doctors, 356 pharmacists and chemists, and 246 nurses, ʿOvadia Eizanberg, *Mifkad ha-okhlusiya ha-Yehudit be-Hefa – trts"h (5698)* (Haifa: M. Shoham press, 1940), 10.

[81] *List of Medical Practitioners, 1946*, 6–56.

[82] Deborah S. Bernstein, *Constructing Boundaries: Jewish and Arab Workers in Mandatory Palestine* (Albany: SUNY Press, 2000); Zachary Lockman, "Railway Workers and Relational History: Arabs and Jews in British-Ruled Palestine," *Comparative Studies in Society and History* 35 (1993): 601–27.

[83] Tamir Goren, "The Judaization of Haifa at the Time of the Arab Revolt," *Middle East Studies* 40 (2004): 135–52.

no avail.[84] Villagers from Wadi ʿAra would travel to nearby Tulkarem, where they could catch a taxi or bus to Haifa's Government Hospital.[85]

Haifa's ascendance into a regional medical hub was a mandatory development. Its importance was determined by colonial interests, the rapid expansion of a professional urban class, and a Jewish demographic boom. These elements turned its medical community into the second largest in the country and the home of Palestine's largest government hospital. Rising and expanding as a result of migration, Haifa's Arab medical community was composed of immigrants. It was a diverse and dynamic community that bordered a ten-times-larger Jewish one, turning Haifa's medical landscape into a space of cooperation as well as friction. Whereas the distribution of medical doctors in Palestine privileged its larger cities, within Haifa itself, the Arab doctors concentrated in specific streets downtown. This uneven distribution also meant that residents of Haifa's poorer districts had to travel or walk downtown for medical attention, if they could afford it.

Jaffa

"I returned to Jaffa," Dr. Saba ʿAzzar recalled, "and opened a clinic in ʿAjami Road. Next door was Burdqush's Pharmacy, which Yusuf Abu Daba later bought from him … and then next to me there were Dr. Saʿid al-Hajj, a dentist, and Dr. Ilyas Baghruth, also a dentist."[86] Close by, in one of the alleys adjacent to Howard Street, Dr. Wahbi Jabji opened an ophthalmological clinic neighboring many local clinics and pharmacies. "I equipped it with modern equipment," he noted, and "the people of Jaffa started saying – we now have an eye clinic that rivals [the famous Jewish] Dr Ticho's clinic in Jerusalem."[87] Although doctors left little evidence about the medical landscapes in which they operated, ʿAzzar and Jabji's recollections offer a glimpse into Jaffa's vibrant medical market in the 1930s.

[84] "The murder of an Arab doctor named Anwar Asʿad al-Shuqayri in Acre by Arab terrorists," P-176/56, ISA.

[85] Ahmad Mahmoud, "al-Sihha wa-l-sihha al-ʿamma fi taʾrikh Hayfa khilal fatrat al-intidab al-Baritani, 1920–1934" (MA thesis, Hebrew University, 2019).

[86] Saba ʿAzzar in ed. Imtiyaz Diyyab, *ʿAtr madinat Yafa* (Beirut: dar al-fata al-ʿArabi, 1991), 184.

[87] Wahbi Jabji in Diyyab, *ʿAtr madinat Yafa*, 196.

From the turn of the nineteenth century to 1948, Jaffa underwent a consistent process of demographic expansion and urban development. From a small urban center of 35,000 at the end of the nineteenth century, it grew to number 51,866 inhabitants in 1931, and 70,760 by the end of the Mandate.[88] During the Mandate, two of Jaffa's neighborhoods were Jewish, and their inhabitants had closer ties with neighboring Tel Aviv than with their Arab neighbors.[89]

Unlike Haifa's industrial port, Jaffa's port was based mainly on passenger traffic, and agricultural import and export.[90] Jaffa's Mediterranean port was the country's main point of exit and entry for goods and people, turning it into Palestine's quintessential cosmopolitan, modern, urban center. After the British occupation, Jaffa became the administrative center of the Lydda district, and the British administrative offices concentrated there. The city flourished, its population grew, and its port expanded.[91]

Several hospitals operated in Jaffa since the late Ottoman period. A maristan had already existed at the beginning of the nineteenth century and a quarantine hospital was established in 1836, during the Egyptian occupation of the city. Several Christian denominations operated small quarantine posts for their pilgrims, who landed in Jaffa on their way to Jerusalem and Bethlehem. Several hospitals operated in the late 1800s: a German hospital in the Templar colony (1869), a French hospital, St. Louis (1880), a CMS hospital (1882), and the Jewish Shaʿar Zion Hospital (1891). The last relocated to Tel Aviv in 1920. Jaffa's shariʿa court records mention about a dozen foreign and local doctors, who worked in the city's various hospitals, quarantine, and municipality.[92] The French Hospital employed mainly French

[88] Al-Dabbagh, *Biladuna Filastin*, vol. 4, no. 2, 216–19.

[89] Tamir Goren, "The Jews of Jaffa at the Time of the Arab Revolt: The Emergence of the Demand for Annexation," *Journal of Modern Jewish Studies* 15 (2016): 267–81; Tamir Goren, "The Jewish Neighbourhoods of Jaffa and the Question of Annexation to Tel Aviv at the End of the British Mandate," *Middle Eastern Studies* 52 (2016): 917–37; Tamir Goren, "Annexation or Separation? The Municipal Status of the Jewish Neighborhoods of Jaffa 1940–1944," *Israel Studies* 21 (2016): 77–101.

[90] Hanna ʿIsa Malak, *al-Judhur al-Yafiyya* (Jerusalem: Matbaʿat al-sharq al-ʿArabiyya, 1996), 53.

[91] Tamir Goren, "Tel Aviv and the Question of Separation from Jaffa 1921–1936," *Middle Eastern Studies* 52 (2016): 473–87.

[92] Malak, *al-Judhur*, 100; Levi, *Prakim*, 434–37; Al-Dabbagh, *Biladuna Filastin*, vol. 4, no. 2, 238–39; Al-Bawwab, *Mawsuʿat Yafa al-jamila*, 1025–33.

physicians, and an Arab doctor or two. According to ʿAzzar, the hospital conducted no medical research, and sent samples to the government laboratory in Jerusalem or to Jewish laboratories in Tel Aviv for analysis.[93]

Jaffa's CMS hospital caused much controversy. Similarly to the Nablus hospital, the Palestinian press accused its Jaffa counterpart of forcing its patients to attend morning preaching sessions, and at least on one occasion, of converting a minor patient against her family's wishes.[94] It also ascribed the pre-war construction of the municipal hospital to an effort to create an alternative to the aggressive missionary tactics at the CMS.[95] In 1946, the hospital closed down, as its physician left Jaffa to replace the Nablus CMS doctor and its nurses left for England. *Filastin* urged the DoH and Jaffa's municipality to find a solution that would enable its reopening. This eventually happened very briefly during the 1948 war.[96]

The Ottoman Municipal Hospital in ʿAjami continued to operate in the same building throughout the Mandate years, changing its name in 1935 to the Government Hospital.[97] The Government Hospital operated outpatient clinics, an IWC at Jaffa's center, and conducted small-scale medical research. Jaffa's MO regularly inspected the city's schoolchildren for signs of trachoma.[98] In the early 1930s, the Hospital became a bone of contention when the British authorities demanded participation in the hospital's administration. The demands included the employment of Jewish staff and the reservation of twenty beds at the new infectious disease ward for Jewish patients. The Palestinian press reminded the British authorities that the hospital was built before the war and funded by municipal taxes, and that Jewish patients had their own hospitalization option in Tel Aviv.[99]

93 Diyyab, *ʿAtr madinat Yafa*, 184.

94 "al-Mustashfa al-Inglizi wakr wasiʿ li-l-tabshir," *al-Jamiʿa al-Islamiyya*, January 9, 1933, 4.

95 "Mustashfa Yafa al-baladi ʿurida li-l-diyaʿ," *al-Haya,* March 29, 1931, 2.

96 "Ila al-masʾulin fi al-baladiyya wa-l-hukuma: Hawwalu dun ighlaq al-mustashfa al-Inglizi bi-Yafa," *Filastin*, May 28, 1946, 2.

97 Muhammad ʿAql, *Muʿjam al-atibbaʾ wa-l-sayadila al-Filastiniyyin (1758–1948)*, vol. 1 (Arara: Self-published, 2021), 313–14.

98 Thabit al-Dabbagh in Diyyab, *ʿAtr madinat Yafa*, 187.

99 "Mustashfa Yafa al-baladi ʿurida li-l-diyaʿ," *al-Haya*, March 29, 1931, 2; "Sunduquki, ayyuha al-umma," *Filastin*, March 31, 1931, 1.

One of the British demands went too far but yielded a project that was one of its kind. They demanded the removal of admired hospital doctor Fu'ad Dajani to the DHO in Nablus.[100] The outcome was Dajani's resignation from the DoH and his embarkment on his life project, the establishment of Jaffa's most famous health institution. Established in 1933, the Dajani Hospital was built on the Dajani family's land, in Nuzha neighborhood. In 1939, Dr. Dajani asked the British authorities for tax exemption. He protested what he described as discrimination against his institution, compared to Christian missionary and the Hadassah hospitals. The British authorities denied his request: hospitals could be eligible for tax exemption only if they were nonprofit institutions and owned and operated by a religious or charitable organization. He was advised to render his hospital eligible for exemption by converting it into a charitable trust. In his correspondence with the DoH, Dajani presented his enterprise as the first Palestinian competition to foreign institutions, a model for other Palestinian cities. His full-time work at the hospital as well as part-time work by two of his colleagues, he explained, were voluntary, and he dedicated his private funds to the hospital's establishment and operation. Hospital charges were lower than those of missionary or Jewish equivalents, and the poor were treated for free. He stated that both the Muslim Council and the Awqaf (religious endowments) considered donating to the hospital, but also bemoaned his community's reluctance to donate to the hospital. British taxes, he argued, further crippled his initiative and hence Arab society's ability to create an alternative medical infrastructure.[101] Like Haifa, Jaffa had a clinic funded by the Young Muslim Men Association. In 1939, the Islamic aid clinic (Mustawsif al-muwasah al-Islami) was founded in Bustrus Street, where some of the city's leading physicians offered free treatment several hours a week.[102]

Limited healthcare for the city's poor produced public debates and action. In an opinion piece from July 1937, *Filastin* urged the Supreme Muslim Council (SMC) to take responsibility for the poor's medical care. The Dajani Hospital, it argued, received patients free of charge,

[100] Ibid.

[101] "Colonial Office: Palestine Original Correspondence. Petitions. Dr Dajani," 1939, CO 733/390/15, NA.

[102] "Mustawsif al-mu'asa al-Islami bi-Yafa yaftahu ghadan li-mu'alaja al-marda," *Al-Difa'*, March 5, 1940, 2.

referred to it by the municipality. The hospital agreed to receive a limited number of patients, a number that did not meet the city's needs, and it was impossible to require the private hospital to subsidize medication.[103] SMC took upon itself to subsidize the hospitalization of destitute patients in Dajani Hospital and in one of the city's clinics.[104] In 1944, *al-Difa'* urged the Mandate authorities and Jaffa municipality to increase the number of beds in Jaffa's hospitals allotted to poor patients.[105] In October 1947, the construction of al-Maqasid Hospital, an Islamic benevolent initiative in the Abu-Kabir neighborhood, was inaugurated. The timing did not enable the completion of the work.[106]

A substantial number of Jaffa's doctors were native to the city. Of the sixty-five doctors out of ninety-two who worked at some point in Jaffa, about whom we have that information, twenty-six were born in Jaffa. This stands in contrast to Haifa, whose community of doctors was composed largely of immigrants.[107] Jaffa's branch of the Dajani family was a local notability with a lineage of ulama, dating back at least to the late eighteenth century. From the turn of the twentieth century, its offspring became doctors and pharmacists. Muhammad Zuhdi Dajani directed the Dajani Hospital after Fu'ad's death in 1940. Rashid Munib Dajani and Ishaq Shihada Dajani operated the Grand Pharmacy in Bustrus Street since 1930. Similarly, the Halabi family included two brothers, Iskandar Nikula and 'Isa Nikula, and the latter's two sons, Suhayl and Sami, who operated the Halabi Pharmacy with him. All were Jaffa-born, all studied at the AUB, and all spent their entire career in the city.[108]

As in Haifa, the Arab medical community grew in proximity to a much larger Jewish community of doctors and well-structured medical

103 "Masa'il al-yawm: Mustashfa al-Dajani wa-baladiyyat Yafa wa-l-awqaf," *Filastin*, July 1, 1937, 1.
104 Kupferschmidt, *The Supreme*, 144; *Bayan al-Majlis*, 12.
105 "Hajat Yafa ila mustashfa shabh majani li-fuqara' al-madina," *al-Difa'*, December 27, 1944, 2.
106 "Mustashfa al-maqasid al-khayriyya," *Filastin*, September 30, 1947; "Mustashfa jama'iyyat al-maqasid al-Islamiyya," *Al-Sha'b*, November 12, 1947, 2.
107 Rustum Shafiq Dawud Abu-Ghazala (1878–1957), in Tahir Adib Qalyubi, *'A'ilat wa-shahsiyat min Yafa wa-wada'iha* (Beirut: al-Mu'asasa al-'Arabiyya li-l-dirasat wa-l-nashr, 2006), 214, 251.
108 Qalyubi, *'A'ilat*, 254.

institutions. In 1934, for example, the hospital bed distribution was as follows: Jaffa had a total of 240 hospital beds at the CMS (57), St. Louis (90), German (20), and Municipal (73) hospitals. This was while neighboring Tel Aviv had 500 hospital beds.[109] Tahir al-Qalyubi, a native of Jaffa and one of its famous historians, mentioned his mother's treatment at Tel Aviv's Assuta Hospital by Dr. Marcus and more generally, the treatment of severe cases by Jewish doctors.[110]

Jaffa's medical landscape was even more segregated than Haifa's. In 1930, six out of Jaffa's thirty doctors were Jewish, as were six of its nineteen pharmacists and nine of its thirteen dentists. By 1946 – except a few doctors in its Jewish neighborhoods–no Jewish doctors, pharmacists, or dentists worked in the city. Those who had worked there in 1930 were not registered in 1946, or registered as working elsewhere.

Jaffa's medical landscape is personified in Fuʾad Dajani's story. A talented Palestinian, educated abroad, returning to his homeland for government service, resigning upon the DoH's attempts to transfer him, and ending up establishing the first and only private Arab hospital in Palestine. This is a story of an urban elite, which, as in Nablus and Acre, integrates its sons into the profession, who then become part of the urban social landscape. This is also a story of national commitment – but one which builds on family capital and is located at the heart of Jaffa's orchards. Dajani's initiative was a personal attempt to fill the gap between growing demand for and stagnant supply of medical services. Despite being a brave and unique intervention in the city's medical landscape, the hospital symbolizes the ongoing disparity between Jaffa's medical services and its demographic growth.

Jaffa's medical community, however, was more than Dajani's hospital. It included a plethora of medical services and an urban

109 300 at the Municipal Hospital, 100 at the private Assuta Hospital, and 100 in smaller private hospitals. Levi, *Prakim*, 444.

110 Professor Max Markus (1892–1983) headed the surgical ward at Hadassah and was among the founders of Assuta Hospital, Nisim Levi, *Rofʾeha shel Erets Yisraʾel*, 3rd ed. (Zikhron Yaʿakov: Itay Bakhur, 2012), 294; Tahir al-Qalyubi (b. 1929), interviewed by Said ʿAjjawi, Amman, November 3, 2007, www.youtube.com/watch?v=OWbo-hEBzgQ, accessed May 22, 2025. See also Ahmad Abu Taha (b. 1930), interviewed by Abd al-Majid Dandeis, Amman, May 22, 2005, https://bit.ly/3NFf0lk, accessed May 22, 2025.

middle class which created demand for them. Like in Haifa, their clinics could be traced on the cityscape – doctors and pharmacists offered their services along Bustrus, Howard, Nuzha, and Ajami streets – and like in Haifa, very few opened clinics in the poorer parts of the city. They were part and parcel of Palestine's vibrant economic and cultural capital.

Conclusion

Looking at the map of Palestine through medical lenses, what we trace are contours of class formation, migration, and changing forms of capital. On this map, the countryside is virtually invisible, except for its lifelines to the city. The towns tell a story of transitions in the local elite's investment, the changing economic status of different localities, and their different ability to attract and maintain educated elites. Jaffa and Haifa bring in the professional and the national tensions with the Jewish medical community, further discussed in Chapter 5.

This chapter mapped Palestine's landscape by looking at densities of medical services and personnel. It differentiated between larger urban centers characterized by clusters of doctors, towns that enjoyed a smaller medical community, and villages that had very limited access to medical services. This mapping situated the book's protagonists within the communities in which they worked and for which they cared. It showed how in both Haifa and Jaffa, medical professionals were connected directly to the urban commercial arteries and the upper middle classes.

The four smaller urban centers, or towns, reflected four different historical trajectories. Taken together, they also reflected developments that took place in towns of similar size elsewhere in Palestine. Fifteen other towns served as subdistrict offices, which meant a permanent presence of a medical officer, who served both the town and the surrounding villages. Some of these also had a missionary hospital or a small municipal or governmental one. The accessibility and quality of medical care depended on proximity to the larger urban centers of Jaffa, Haifa, and Jerusalem, which had the larger and better-equipped hospitals.

Finally, Palestinian doctors did not live in the villages, and very few villages enjoyed regular doctors' visits. The expanding medical community, especially in the cities but also in towns, enabled greater movement of doctors into the countryside and from it into the cities and towns. This movement only made the deprivation of sustainable and regular healthcare more apparent for the fellahin. They knew of and had great esteem for doctors, but the sight of one such as Dr. Akram Sweidi in their natural habitat was akin to an apparition, a present absentee.

5 Conflicting Medicines and the Politicization of Health

Flies were an inter-city story between Tel Aviv and Jaffa: Tel Aviv's mayor used to complain to the district's governor that flies arrive in Tel Aviv from Jaffa, despite Tel Aviv's efforts to combat them. He asked the governor, before my tenure as mayor, to charge Jaffa's municipality with cleaning the city. When the flies were eliminated from Jaffa, they started coming from Tel Aviv. I turned to the governor and asked him to ask Tel Aviv municipality to clean their city to prevent its flies from coming to Jaffa.[1]

The previous chapters examined the social and spatial attributes of the Palestinian doctors' community and its multifaceted links with the colonial Department of Health (DoH). This chapter adds a further layer to this analysis by examining this community's encounter with its Jewish counterparts. Relations between Arab and Jewish doctors, it argues, were a reflection of Arab-Jewish relations more broadly, but also had unique aspects and variations across space and time.

The relational analytical framework for studying Palestine's social history is useful for this end. While considering the myriad forms of separation and segregation between Arabs and Jews, this approach stresses the determinative effects of intercommunal segregations, encounters, and interactions on the social, economic, and cultural evolution of both professional communities.[2] The relationship between Jewish and Arab medical doctors lends itself to such an analysis. The two professional communities operated and were organized separately, and mixed healthcare services were provided at their margins.

1 Yusuf Haykal, in Imtiyaz Diyyab, *'Atr madinat Yafa* (Beirut: Dar al-Fata al-'Arabi, 1991), 30.

2 Zachary Lockman, "Railway Workers and Relational History: Arabs and Jews in British-Ruled Palestine," *Comparative Studies in Society and History* 35 (1993): 604; Baruch Kimmerling, "A Model of Analysis of Reciprocal Relations between the Jewish and Arab Communities in Mandatory Palestine," *Plural Societies* 14 (1983): 46–47; Deborah Bernstein, *Constructing Boundaries: Jewish and Arab Workers in Mandatory Palestine* (Albany, NY: SUNY Press, 2000), 6–10.

Palestinian doctors, specifically, operated within a complex professional network composed of Arab and Jewish doctors, the DoH, and Arab patients. This chapter situates the Arab medical community within this relational matrix by examining Jewish doctors' and Zionist healthcare institutions' medical and other contacts with the Arab population and Palestinian doctors. Such an analysis is instrumental in understanding Arab doctors' political and professional predicament and, more broadly, the formative role of these interactions for the Palestinians and the Yishuv.

Historical works on colonial medicine offer a useful analytical framework as well. As in other colonial contexts, Jewish medical services were designed to serve, first and foremost, the settlement project: Jewish doctors treated Jews and were instrumental in making Palestine more inhabitable for Zionist immigration and settlement. Colonial doctors in other contexts treated native populations in order to protect their own personnel and civilian populations from disease and to justify the colonial project to both the metropole and the colonized. In the Zionist case, by contrast, institutional medical assistance to Palestine's Arabs was limited and varied according to place and time. According to Sandy Sufian, Zionist planners, epidemiologists, and physicians were interested in "healing the land" by combating malaria – but not as much in healing Palestine's Arab inhabitants.[3]

Conversely, treatment by Jewish doctors and in Zionist institutions was the lived reality across Palestine throughout the late Ottoman and Mandate periods. Moreover, the high number of Jewish doctors compared to both the Jewish and overall Palestinian populations had no parallels in other colonial cases. From the late nineteenth century until the Arab Revolt, Jewish doctors even settled for several years in Arab towns and cities, operated clinics, and provided healthcare; many settled in mixed cities, offering treatment to their non-Jewish populations as well. Most of them were immigrants, but many were natives of Palestine and members of prominent Old Yishuv families. Arab patients provided them with livelihoods, much needed in an oversaturated medical market. For some doctors, treating patients regardless of creed or ethnicity meant following their professional calling. Whether treating the Jerusalemite elite who could afford treatment, or the poor *fellahin* of

[3] Sandy Sufian, "Re-imagining Palestine: Scientific Knowledge and Malaria Control in Mandatory Palestine," *Dynamis* 25 (2005): 358.

the Hula Valley who could not, the presence of Jewish doctors in Palestinian lives complicated their relationship with Palestinian doctors.

Arab and Jewish doctors had much more in common than other middle-class men and women: they shared professional knowledge, a vocation, and, in some cases, the same training. They worked together in government institutions, shared clinics, consulted one another, and fought common enemies of morbidity and mortality on the same land. Whereas in many other realms, Jews and Arabs could operate along parallel or separate lines, shared health challenges created ad hoc collaborations. Furthermore, whereas Arabs could boycott Jewish goods, life-saving health services were too precious to be abandoned.

Dr. Haykal's opening quote exemplifies the way in which health challenges crossed political boundaries far more than many other aspects of life in Palestine. As Jaffa's last Arab mayor in the late 1940s, he positioned the city in relation to neighboring Tel Aviv: Jaffa's cleanliness was a precondition for Tel Aviv's health and hygiene, and vice versa. The two cities in this anecdote communicated through the mediation of British authorities as well as through flies, which did not care about municipal or ethnic boundaries.

This chapter is organized as follows. It begins with some data on the relative size of both medical communities. It continues with a close reading of Hebrew texts about Arab doctors, followed by Arab texts about Jewish doctors. It then focuses on waves of violence, particularly the Great Arab Revolt, and the ways in which they affected health-related interactions between the communities. The chapter ends by presenting a few attempts at Arab-Jewish cooperation in healthcare.

The Politics of Licensing

Medicine and health were realms of continuity and rupture whose periodization and modes of operation were different from those of other political or economic relations. In late Ottoman Palestine, Jewish doctors represented an essential part of a growing decentralized medical community, which operated under different missions, municipalities, or the private sector. Upon the outbreak of World War I (WWI), there were sixty-three Jewish doctors in Palestine,[4] four times as many as their Arab counterparts.

[4] Nissim Levi, *Rof'eha shel Eretz Yisra'el, 1799–1948*, 3rd ed. (Zikhron Ya'akov: Itai Bachur, 2012), 33.

This numerical gap widened under the British. In 1921, there were 274 licensed doctors, of whom 109 (38.78 percent) were Jewish – a fairly high ratio for a population of 752,000, of whom only 11 percent were Jews. The rest were Europeans and Arabs.[5] In 1928, an expert commission noted a surplus of medical personnel – 600 physicians, 400 of whom were Jewish.[6] The Simpson Report (1930), drafted by the British Commission of Inquiry into the 1929 Disturbances, noted the negative influence of the growing number of Jewish doctors on Arab employment and added that Jewish families rarely consulted Arab doctors, while Arab patients had no problem consulting Jewish doctors.[7]

The year 1933 stands out as a watershed in the conflict and the medical profession in particular. Massive waves of Jewish immigrants fleeing Nazi Germany dramatically changed Palestine's demography. These included hundreds of highly skilled German-Jewish doctors shifting the numerical imbalance between Jewish and Arab medical communities further in favor of the former. From the turn of the twentieth century, Jews were overrepresented in Central European medical schools. This trend reflected their overrepresentation in higher education more broadly, quota policies in Eastern Europe that pushed Jews to German and Austrian universities, and antisemitic employment restrictions that made medicine one of their only routes for upward mobility.[8] These processes explain the disproportionate number of doctors among European Jewish immigrants. Between 1933 and 1935, Jewish German doctors who had lost their livelihoods immigrated to Palestine, increasing the number of licensed Jewish doctors in the country from 658 at the end of 1932 to 2,082 at the end of 1935.

[5] Ibid., 34–35.

[6] *Reports of the Experts Submitted to the Joint Palestine Survey Commission, October 1st, 1928* (Boston: Press of Daniels Printing Co., 1928), 732.

[7] John Hope Simpson, *Palestine: Report on Immigration, Land Settlement and Development, Presented by the Secretary of State for the Colonies to Parliament by Command of His Majesty, October 1930* (London: H.M.S.O, 1930), 23–26. An anonymous Jewish physician challenged Simpson's arguments, writing about superior education of Jewish doctors and their contributions to medicine in Palestine. "Hashkafotav shel Heron ve-maskanotav shel Simpson," *Davar*, November 24, 1930, 2.

[8] John Efron, *Medicine and the German Jews: A History* (New Haven, CT: Yale University Press, 2008), 234–38.

Consequently, the ratio of doctors rose by 1937 to 1:176 in the Jewish community compared to 1:3,779 in the Arab community.

As a result, legislation to control the overcrowding of the medical profession by limiting the number of new licenses came into effect in late 1935. The publication of the draft law that year led to massive immigration of Jewish doctors in the following months and a subsequent decline in the following years.[9] The number of applicants for medical, dental, and pharmaceutical licenses remained high, but the number of new medical licenses dropped from 596 in 1935 to 68 in 1939.[10] In 1946, there were 2,257 licensed Jewish doctors in Palestine, out of a total of 2,520. This meant that the ratio of Jewish to Arab doctors was 9:1. From one doctor per 1,300 inhabitants in 1930, the ratio shifted to one per 650 in 1946.[11]

The influx of Jewish doctors also affected the quality of medical care. Unlike Arab and Jewish doctors working in Palestine up to that point, who were mostly general practitioners, the German immigrant doctors had a wide variety of specializations.[12] By the mid 1940s, almost half of Palestine's Jews enjoyed medical insurance through the Histadrut's Sick Fund (Kupat Holim), which served as a virtual monopoly in the Jewish medical market, operating 2 hospitals, 274 clinics, and numerous additional stations. Its physicians and nurses worked in 50

[9] *Report by His Majesty's Government in the United Kingdom of Great Britain and Northern Ireland to the Council of the League of Nations on the Administration of Palestine and Trans-Jordan for the Year 1936* (London: His Majesty's Stationery Office, 1937), 176; Doron Niederland, "Hashpa'at harof'im ha-'olim mi-Germaniya 'al hiptathut ha-refu'a be-Erets Yisra'el, 1933–1948," *Catedra* 30 (1984): 119–20, 124.

[10] Philippe Bourmaud, "Ya Doktor! Devenir médecin et exercer son art en 'Terre Sainte', une expérience du pluralisme médical dans l'Empire ottoman finissant (1871–1918)" (PhD dissertation, Aix-Marseille 1 University, 2007): 752; Department of Health, *Annual Report for the Year 1936* (Jerusalem: Government Printing Press, 1936), 53; Department of Health, *Annual Report for the Year 1937* (Jerusalem: Government Printing Press, 1937), 70; Department of Health, *Annual Report for the Year 1938* (Jerusalem: Government Printing Press, 1938), 89.

[11] Samuel Kurland, *Cooperative Palestine: The Story of Histadrut* (New York: Sharon Books, 1947), 112; Nira Reiss, *The Health Care of the Arabs in Israel* (Boulder, CO: Westview, 1991), 35; *A Survey of Palestine: Prepared in December 1945 and January 1946 for the Information of the Anglo-American Committee of Inquiry* (Jerusalem: Government Press, 1946), 614.

[12] Niederland, "Hashpa'at ha-rof'im"; "Hoda'ot rishmiyot 'al 'edut ha-'Aravim," *Davar*, January 17, 1937, 4.

agricultural settlements, and its annual expenditure was double that of the government's health services.[13]

Jewish Doctors – Arab Patients, Arab Doctors – Jewish Patients

There is no need to discuss the value of medical aid to the Arabs by Kupat Holim for our neighbors' wellbeing and for fostering good neighborly relations ... The Yishuv is interested in providing medical assistance to the Arabs not only for humanitarian reasons but also for sanitary ones and out of necessity – the healing of the land would be impossible without treatment by Kupat Holim of all patients, regardless of nationality or creed. This should be done systematically, and where Jews and Arabs come into close contact.[14]

This statement, taken from a Sick Fund internal memorandum, reflects a Zionist view of their interaction with Arab patients. The Zionist nation-building efforts entailed the formation of multiple medical institutions, which compensated for colonial neglect and targeted mainly Jewish patients.[15] The Zionist healthcare approach toward the Arab population was both an endeavor aimed at facilitating a settler-colonial project and an attempt to strengthen ties with their neighbors. These modes of operation varied between the periphery, where the overwhelming majority of the population was Arab while most doctors were Jewish, and the cities, where Arab patients were treated by both Arab and Jewish doctors, while Jewish patients were almost exclusively treated by Jewish doctors.

The first European Jewish doctors settled in Palestine during the second half of the nineteenth century, parallel to the arrival of missionary medicine and the arrival or return of Palestine's first Arab doctors after medical studies in Beirut or Europe. Whether as refugees, as employees of Jewish philanthropic institutions, as idealist volunteers, or as a combination of the three, they settled mostly in the so-called

13 Reiss, *The Health*, 25–27; Kurland, *Cooperative Palestine*, 108–09.

14 "A Review of Medical Assistance to Arabs in Kupat Holim Institutions," October 8, 1930, Central Zionist Archive (hereafter, CZA), J1/4588.

15 See, e.g., Shifra Shvarts, *The Workers' Health Fund in Eretz YiIsra'el: Kupat Holim, 1911–1937* (Rochester, NY: University of Rochester Press, 2002); Zipora Shehory-Rubin, Shira Shvartz and Yoel Dunhin, *Hadassah li-vri'ut ha-'am: Pe'iluta ha-bri'utit-ha-hinukhit shel Hadassah be-Erets Yisra'el bi-tkufat ha-mandat ha-Briti* (Jerusalem: ha-Sifriya ha-Tsionit, 2003).

Four Holy Cities of Jerusalem, Safad, Hebron, and Tiberias. This medical community expanded gradually since the 1880s with subsequent waves of immigration, as well as geographically with the establishment of the new colonies outside the Old Yishuv's traditional centers. The growing Jewish communities of Jerusalem, Jaffa, and later Tel Aviv became a medical market for these doctors, as were the more remote rural settlements that required local clinics.

The medical relations between Arabs and Jews in late Ottoman Palestine reflected local intercommunal ties and tensions between the two communities. Arab and Jewish doctors treated Jewish and Arab patients, yet the magnitude of this phenomenon varied according to region and class. Usually, Jewish doctors' memoirs underlined a common trope of poor or nonexistent medical facilities and hygiene and narrated their own popularity among the Arab population, particularly the wealthy elite. Dr. Abraham Ticho's clinic, for example, was frequented by the Jerusalem Arab notability; among others, Faidy al-ʿAlami and Haj Amin al-Husayni were treated by the famous Vienna-trained ophthalmologist.[16] Hillel Yoffe was also well known for his treatment of Arabs, and many of them attended his funeral in Haifa.[17]

As mentioned in Chapter 1, the relatively flexible intercommunal borderlines that characterized the late Ottoman period enabled certain medical mobility across communities. A few Arab doctors treated Jewish patients in the moshavot. There is little evidence of Arab doctors treating Jewish patients in the Mandate years, however. Yaʿakov Yehoshua (1905–82), who grew up in Jerusalem, mentions that Dr. Canaan treated many of the city's Jews.[18] Dr. ʿIzaat Tanous recalls his Jewish patients in his Old City clinic.[19]

Jewish doctors usually lived and worked in Jewish settlements or in mixed cities. Dr. Schalit, who arrived in Nablus at the turn of the twentieth century, was one of several doctors who worked in Arab

[16] Serene Shahid, *Jerusalem Memories* (Beirut: Naufal, 1999), 273.

[17] See *ha-Refua*'s issue dedicated to the memory of Dr. Yoffe: *ha-Refuʾa* 10, no. 56/2 (February 1936).

[18] Yaʿaov Yehoshuʿa, *Yaldut bi-Yerushalayim ha-yeshana: Pirkke hove mi-yamim ʿavaru* (Jerusalem: R. Mas, 1965), 125.

[19] Izzat Tannous, *The Palestinians: A Detailed Documented Eyewitness History of Palestine under British Mandate* (New York: IGT, 1988), 134–36.

towns.[20] According to his memoir, he gained great popularity among the local elite, yet a payment dispute with a wealthy soap producer distanced the locals from Schalit, who started to miss his family in Rishon LeZion. Except for his servant and a Jewish friend, no one came to bid him farewell when he happily left the city.[21]

Late Ottoman Jaffa is a good example of a mixed city. One of its first Jewish doctors, Dr. Menachem (Marc) Stein, arrived in 1883, gaining popularity among local Arabs. Together with fellow devoutly Zionist doctors, Stein established the Shaʿar Zion Hospital in 1891, which was popular among the city's non-Jewish population as well.[22] The employment of two female Jewish doctors, Alexandra Belkind and Bat-Sheva Yunis-Guttman, enabled the expansion of the hospital's maternity department and made it more accessible to local Arab women.[23]

Belkind opened her own private clinic in 1906 and quickly gained a reputation among women of all denominations.[24] According to one source, she became so popular that the Nablus Municipality offered her the position of municipal doctor, an invitation she declined. In an article published in 1913, Belkind reported that 1,000 women visited her clinic from 1906 to 1912, of whom only 229 were Jewish, 137 Christian, and 634 Muslim, mostly from Jaffa but also from other towns countrywide.[25] Belkind's sister, Olga Hankin, was a trained midwife, and the two would drive south on a horse carriage to visit Bedouin tribes around Lydda and Ramleh.[26] This movement across medical borderlines continued until the end of the Mandate, yet those boundaries became clearly demarcated as the years passed.

Professional institutionalization and unionization were principal catalysts in the formation of intercommunal boundaries. The establishment of the Hebrew Medicinal Society for Jaffa and the Jaffa District in

[20] Dr. Arieh Chernof, who operated a clinic in Jenin since 1913, is another example. Arieh Chernof, "Jenin," *ha-Poʿel ha-Tsaʿir*, January 31, 1913, 14.

[21] Moshe Schalit, *bi-Ntivot hayyay* (Tel Aviv: Y. Golan, 2000), 292–93.

[22] "ha-Asefah ha-torit ha-reviʿit," *Zichronot Devarim*, March 1, 1912; Nissim Levi, *Prakim be-toldot ha-refuʾa be-Erets Yisraʾel, 1799–1948* (Tel Aviv: ha-Kibbuts ha-Meuhad, 1998), 433–34; Shifra Shvarts, "Bet ha-holim 'Shaʿar Tsion' be-Yafo: Bet holim kehilati rishon ba-arets 1891–1921," *Korot* 9, no. 9–10 (1990): 295–308.

[23] Zipora Shehory-Rubin and Shifra Shvarts, *Aleksandrah Belkind: Sippura shel rofʾa ʿIvriyya poretset derekh* (Zikhron Yaʿakov: Itai Bachur, 2012), 75.

[24] Levi, *Prakim be-toldot*, 260; Helena Kagan, *Reshit darki bi-Yerushalayim* (Jerusalem: WIZO, 1965), 39–40.

[25] Shehory-Rubin and Shvarts, *Aleksandrah Belkind*, 76–78.

[26] Ibid., 88.

1912 reflected an ideology and practice of segregation. The minutes of its first meeting stated that Dr. Yehuda Leib Puchovsky, director of Sha'ar Zion, who chaired the meeting, "definitively agreed that only Jews should be admitted to the society, with the possibility of inviting non-Jews to scientific meetings."[27] The society's meetings and lectures were held in Russian and German, and its journal, *Zikhron Devarim*, became the first medical journal in Hebrew.[28] Members of the Jaffa society treated Arab patients, and Arabs' medical well-being was discussed in their meetings.[29] However, Palestine's Arab professionals were excluded from the debate. The following year, Jerusalem's Jewish doctors established the Hebrew-Speaking Physicians' Society. Several doctors protested the differentiation and alienation from European and Arab doctors, but it was decided that only Hebrew-speaking doctors could join the society.[30]

The First Trachoma Congress is an example of the conflict of medical interests between inclusive healthcare and national medicine. The three-day event was held in Jerusalem in March 1914 and included twenty-five Jewish doctors and Hebrew teachers from across Palestine. Focusing primarily on the Jewish colonies and Hebrew schools, the conference also discussed the importance of treatment for the Arab population. One speaker stated that the motivation for such treatment was both humanitarian and utilitarian – gaining Arab support. One of the conference's resolutions stated that "treatment for trachoma would be given to the entire population without differentiating on the basis of religion or nationality."[31]

On the eve of WWI, Jewish doctors became a professional community with a clear national agenda, setting them apart from their Arab counterparts. As a community, they were no longer focused on serving a specific locale or individual but saw themselves as Hebrew doctors, serving primarily the Hebrew or Zionist project.[32] In addition to this

27 Cited in Levi, *Prakim be-toldot*, 151.
28 Shehory-Rubin and Shvarts, *Aleksandrah Belind*, 94–98.
29 "ha-Asifa ha-torit ha-shlishit," February 22, 1912, *Zichronot Devarim* 1, no. 1, September 1912, 18–19.
30 Levi, *Prakim be-toldot*, 152.
31 Orit Navot and Abraham Gross, "ha-Milhama ba-gar'enet: Reshit bri'ut ha-tsibur be-Erets Yisra'el," *Cathedra* 94 (1999), 89–114.
32 About this transition in Arieh Saposnik, *Becoming Hebrew: The Creation of a Jewish National Culture in Ottoman Palestine* (Oxford: Oxford University Press, 2008).

national vision, many of them saw themselves as loyal Ottoman subjects. During the war, many of the Yishuv's doctors either volunteered or were conscripted into the Ottoman army.[33]

The debate over Jewish doctors' responsibility for the Arab population continued after the war. The association "should only consider the Jewish community," noted Dr. Haim Hisin in its 1919 meeting, "and if the Arabs come, we can accept them as well." Although other opinions were voiced, including reference to the members' humanistic calling, Dr. Puchovsky concluded that the association should only treat Jews.[34]

While the bulk of Jewish doctors settled in cities, safeguarding the health and well-being of the Zionist frontier was essential to the Yishuv. In the Zionist vision, it was the frontier that defined and sustained the city. Zionist institutes, the Histadrut's Sick Fund, and the Hadassah Medical Organization invested time, effort, and funding in frontier settlements beyond their share in the Jewish population. In 1926, there were more than 90 Jewish doctors in Jerusalem, 131 in Tel Aviv, 7–8 in Petah Tikvah and Rehovot, and at least 1 doctor in small colonies such as Nahalal, Nesher, and Ein Harod. Surrounded by a rural Arab population, the isolated Jewish settlements used medical treatment to improve their social ties with neighbors and prevent or assuage already apparent national tensions.

The life and work of Professor Gideon Mer (1894–1961) demonstrates this tension. Mer, one of the leading Jewish malariologists of his time, settled in the late 1920s in Rosh Pina, where he operated a laboratory for the study of malaria. The disease had severely affected the region's inhabitants, especially the Hula Valley Bedouins. Mer became famous for his tireless efforts to fight malaria and cure the infected, Jews and Arabs alike.[35] At the same time, he served as chief commander of the Haganah militia in Rosh Pina. The professor was wholeheartedly dedicated to treating the sick, regardless of ethnicity or creed, as well as to the military defense of the Zionist project.

33 Moshe Sherman, "Prakim min he-ʿavar: ha-Rofʾim ha-Yehudiyyim shel ʿAzah," *ha-Refuʾa* 52, no. 4 (1956), 98–100; Shvarts, *The Workers' Health Fund*, 55–57.

34 Protocol of the Society's tenth meeting, March 13, 1919, *ha-Refuʾa, trʿat* (1918–1919), 79–83.

35 Sandra M. Sufian, *Healing the Land and the Nation: Malaria and the Zionist Project in Palestine, 1920–1947* (Chicago: University of Chicago Press, 2007), 204–05; "Rofe, hoker, haluts," *ʿAl ha-Mishmar*, February 7, 1958, 3, 8.

Usually located in remote rural areas and surrounded by an Arab population, kibbutzim often operated clinics in tents, wooden shacks, or concrete buildings, with a medic, nurse, or doctor. The clinics were regulated by the DoH, Hadassah, and Sick Fund and funded by the latter two. In various cases, the clinics offered medical treatment to Arab patients from neighboring villages.[36] Some kibbutzim established separate clinics for Arab patients. The clinic in Ein Harod, for example, treated Arabs from Qumya and other neighboring villages since the 1920s.[37] Located several miles northeast of Gaza, the members of Kibbutz Gvarʿam (est. 1942) established a clinic for neighboring Arab villages, which was active until the 1948 war. The local doctor reported that patients would stop arriving after "political disturbances," only to return a short while afterward. During the 1948 war, Gvarʿam's physician, Dr. Gideon Greenberger, would ride a donkey to neighboring villages and, while treating patients, collect intelligence about the approaching Egyptian army.[38]

At the institutional level, Jewish health organizations reached out to the Arab population in several locales. Hadassah operated clinics in Samakh, Gaza, Hebron, Beersheba, Bisan, Jerusalem, and Haifa.[39] In Gaza, the organization operated a doctor's clinic from 1924 to 1929. During the 1920s, several Jewish doctors worked there along side a pharmacy operated by the small Jewish community.[40]

36 Michal Man, "Statoskop u-mahresha: bi-Ntiv ha-mirpaʾa ba-kibbutsim, hitpathut sherute ha-beriʾut ba-kibbutsim ba-shanim 1910–1948" (PhD dissertation, Ben-Gurion University of the Negev, 2016), 49–54, 149–52.

37 Ibid., 42–43.

38 Ibid., 43; See *Gvarʿam's Journal*, November 29, 1946 (no. 151), January 4, 1947 (no. 153), and April 11, 1947 (no. 159). We thank Roni Garcia from the Gvarʿam archive for sharing these documents.

39 Once a week, a Jewish doctor operated a clinic and would also go to Tiberias. Sanusi Yakhluf (b. 1924), interviewed by Abdel Majeed Dandeis, June 1, 2004, Jordan, www.palestineremembered.com/Tiberias/Samakh/Story1267.html, accessed October 3, 2021; Reuven Gafni, "'Shlihuta shel ha-ahot ha-ʿIvriyya, ha-yodaʿat lehitmasser gam le-ʿezrat ha-shakhen ha-koshel: Sippura shel tahanat tippat halav be-Samakh, 1942–1947," *Erets ha-Kineret* 29 (2020): 43–47; Nissim Levi, *ha-Refuʾa*117 (August 1989): 92; on Hadassah in Hebron, see Yoram Elmakias, "Peʿilut tsioyonit be-Hevron me-reshit ha-meʾa ha-20 ve-ʿad meʾoraʿot tarpa"t" (MA thesis, University of Haifa, 2011), 52–60.

40 Sherman, "Prakim min he-ʿavar," 98–100. About the Hadassah clinic, see CZA, S22/171; about the dentists and pharmacy, see CZA, AK/7661. See also Ibrahim Sukayk, *Sharit al-dhikrayat: ʿAn Ghazza qabla nisf qarn* (Gaza: Dar al-Katib, 1985), 39.

Discussions of a joint Jewish-Arab health station started in Hadassah in late 1940. Its chairman in Palestine, Haim Yaski, envisioned a joint medical staff – preferably an Arab doctor and a Jewish nurse or a Jewish doctor and an Arab nurse. Such ideas were quickly abandoned in favor of what was seen as a more realistic vision – an Infant Welfare Station (IWC) in a kibbutz that would serve both Jewish and Arab families. In early 1941, leading malariologist Israel Kligler (1888–1944) proposed operating three such clinics to serve both Jewish and Arab populations. By November, the discussion's focus had moved to the Hula Valley as having the greatest potential for positive impact.[41] Several settlements were considered for this purpose. Hadassah's delegates visited them and found that most of their representatives wanted a clinic at the settlement's outskirts. Arab peasants, they argued, frequented the settlement's doctor and interfered with his work. Hadassah refused, as such a segregated clinic "would not be in the spirit" of the organization, since it would do nothing to improve the relationship with the Arabs.[42]

In 1945, the Kligler Health Center for Jews and Arabs, established by Hadassah and Sick Fund, was inaugurated in Kibbutz ʿAmir in the Hula Valley. Both Jews and Arabs attended the ceremony, and the speeches underlined the cooperation between the two peoples.[43] To Hadassah's dismay, the clinic was never really a joint one – it served mothers of the neighboring Arab village of Duara, but Jewish mothers kept away from it. It continued operating nevertheless until the outbreak of the war in December 1947.[44]

[41] CZA, J113/1661, Hadassah Emergency Committee. On Kligler's central role in fighting malaria, see Sufian, *Healing*.

[42] CZA, J113/8088, "Shared health centers – Jews and Arabs." For Hadassah's response, see "Excerpts from the Minutes of the 36th Stated Meeting of the HEC, January 20, 1942," CZA J113/2477, Preventive medicine – Samakh; Man, "Hitpathut sherute," 43–44.

[43] "Merkaz briʾut le-Yehudim ve-ʿAravim nehnakh be-Kibbuts ʿAmir," *ʿAl ha-Mishmar*, November 9, 1945, 8; "Merkaz briʾut le-Yehudim ve-ʿAravim ʿal shem profesor Kligler be-ʿEmek ha-Hula," *Haaretz*, November 9, 1945. In 1946, 5,000 Palestinians were listed as Histadrut members, yet only a minority paid membership tax and were thus entitled to Sick Fund's services, Reiss, *The Health*, 28; Yoseph Washitz, *Ha-ʿAravim be-Erets Yisraʾel* (Merhavia: Hakibbutz Haartzi, 1947), 173–75.

[44] CZA, J113/2486, preventive medicine, Kibbutz ʿAmir, J113/2534, Arab-Jewish Health Centers; Man, "Hitpathut sherute," 43–45.

The Hadassah IWC in Samakh was the direct outcome of contacts between a Hadassah nurse in Tiberias, Ahuva Wittenberg-Pazi, and Samakh's women, who frequented the clinic in Tiberias 13 kilometers away from the village. Wittenberg-Pazi visited Samakh in late 1941, talked with the mayor, and presented a proposal to Hadassah's board, which welcomed the initiative. An IWC in Samakh, she maintained, would save young mothers the trouble of walking all the way to Tiberias. The municipality provided the building and cleaning services, and Hadassah paid for the nurse, weekly doctor's visits, and medications. The IWC was inaugurated in January 1942 and shut down in the summer of 1947. Samakh's municipality withdrew its funding, and the mayor apologized, saying that political pressure had left him little choice.[45]

Some doctors operated private clinics in Arab towns, off the institutional grid. Jewish doctors' clinics could be found in towns such as Beit Safafa, Jericho, and Bethlehem. One survey in the town of Beit Jala noted that they were called "shilling doctors" by the locals, as they were not yet formally licensed and charged one shilling per treatment.[46] Jewish treatment of Arab patients continued intermittently until 1948.

Arab Doctors Protest

Since its inception, the Palestinian national movement saw Zionist soft power, mainly manifested in facilitating Zionist economic hegemony over Palestine, as a threat to the vision of self-determination. The Palestinian press was a central platform for these claims, cautioning of the risk and threat of the expansion of Arab workers' employment in Jewish industry or agriculture, as well as Arab consumption of Yishuv products. The threat posed by the Yishuv's medical community was yet another aspect of this struggle. However, it was unique in being tied to the nature of the medical profession, specifically the intimate patient–doctor encounter. This encounter was particularly

[45] CZA, J113/2477 – preventive medicine – Samakh; Reuven Gafni, "Kehila Yehudit ʿal kav gvul: ha-Nokhehut ha-Yehudit ba-ʿayara Tsemah (Samakh) ba-mahatsit ha-rishona shel ha-meʾa ha-ʿesrim," *Mehkarim hadashim shel ha-Galil* 3 (2018): 9–28; Gafni, "Shlihuta," 43–46.

[46] Lajna min abna' Bayt Jala, *Madinat Bayt Jala* (Bethlehem: Madinat Bayt Lahm, 1994), 144.

charged: it introduced the Jewish doctor into Palestinian bodies, homes, and communities, to a degree absent from virtually every other realm of shared living. In addition, the disproportionate number of Jewish doctors and their training in elite European institutions – made competition in this arena particularly fierce.

In 1932, *Filastin* noted the disproportionate figures of immigrant Jewish doctors.[47] In June 1933, *Filastin* warned against the increasing immigration as posing a greater threat to the livelihood of the existing Jewish professional community than to the Arab one. It argued that even Egyptian doctors, who hardly experienced any Jewish immigration, had demanded to block this immigration, and suggested that the Palestinian medical community must follow suit. A complete boycott of Jewish doctors, the author concluded, would make this migration solely a Jewish problem.[48]

The professional threat posed by immigrant doctors to Palestine's medical community, both Arab and Jewish, was a central theme in the Arab doctors in Palestine Congress, held in Haifa in June 1933. Its resolutions included demanding that British authorities stop licensing immigrant doctors, grant licenses only to Palestine-born doctors, and employ only Arab doctors in government service. It also demanded the promotion of Arab doctors to the highest DoH positions.[49] Following the conference, an op-ed in *Filastin* stated that there were so many Jewish doctors that those in Tel Aviv worked as shoeshiners. Jewish doctors themselves, it noted, felt threatened by this immigration but were afraid of protesting because they wished to avoid conflict with the Jewish Agency.[50] *Mir'at al-Sharq* commented sarcastically that the ratio of Jewish doctors in Palestine had reached the point where every Jewish family had its own doctor.[51]

47 "ʿArab al-Hawarith, fawda al-suhuf, tazahum al-atibbaʾ," *Filastin*, February 24, 1932, 1.

48 "Muʾtamar al-atibbaʾ al-ʿArab," *Filastin*, June 21, 1933, 1. On Egyptian doctors' reaction to Jewish doctors' immigration, see Hasan ʿAbd al-Raʾuf, "Hawla hijrat al-Yahud al-Alman ila Misr," *al-Majalla al-Tibbiyya al-Misriyya* 16 (June 1933), 328–30.

49 "Inʿiqad muʾtamar al-atibbaʾ al-ʿArabi fi Hayfa," *Filastin*, June 20, 1933, 7.

50 "Muʾatamar al-atibbaʾ al-ʿArab," *Filastin*, June 21, 1933, 1; "Jamaʿiyyat al-atibbaʾ wa-matalibuha ila al-hukuma," *Flastin*, July 7, 1933, 3; "Muʾtamar al-atibbaʾ yuballigh qararatihi li-l-hukuma," *Filastin*, July 11, 1933, 3.

51 "Hal yusbihu li-kulli ʿaʾila tabib," *Mirʾat al-Sharq*, October 22, 1934, 6.

The Palestinian press urged patients to embrace a boycott. Arab women allegedly started preferring Jewish doctors, partly because they were less embarrassed to expose themselves to foreigners. These were not necessarily better doctors, warned *Mir'at al-Sharq*, and encouraged female readers to trust their Arab doctor and visit a Jewish one only if the former recommended it.[52] The Palestinian peasant was reportedly immune to the threat: according to *al-Difa'*, Shefa-'Amr's residents refused the solicitations of two Jewish physicians and preferred their local Arab doctors.[53] Jewish doctors reportedly charged lower fees, affecting patients' expectations of Arab doctors.[54] In the following months, the Palestinian press published articles on protests by Egyptian, Syrian, and Lebanese doctors against the licensing of Jewish immigrant doctors. While Egypt did witness some Jewish immigration, the petitions of Syrian and Lebanese doctors to their respective high commissioners were largely declarative.[55]

Al-Kifah was more belligerent, accusing Jewish doctors of deceiving Arab peasants. It did, however, also lay part of the responsibility on Arab doctors, who neglected the countryside: "Jewish doctors are now increasingly frequenting Arab villages. They use assumed names; one would pretend to be German, and another – Austrian ... They charge exorbitant fees from the villagers ... our Arab doctors ... need to visit the villages and dedicate several days to their treatment and care."[56]

In March and April 1936, at the very beginning of the Great Arab Revolt, Dr. Anwar al-Shuqayri wrote a series of articles urging fellow doctors to unionize in order to block the Jewish threat to the medical profession. The first assignment of such an association, he argued, would be the establishment of Arab hospitals in the large cities, as well as voluntary dispensaries to be operated in the countryside on a rotational basis. Such an initiative, he argued, would restore the faith of the Palestinian people in its dedicated doctors and contain the damage of

52 "Al-atibba' al-Yahud wa-basatat sayyidatina," *Mir'at al-Sharq*, April 18, 1934, 3.

53 "Al-atibba' al-Yahud fi al-qura al-'Arabiyya," *al-Difa'*, January 24, 1936, 4.

54 "Ila ayna wasalat mihnat al-tibb? Karamat al-atibba' wa-l-mihna, ya hukumat Filastin!" *Filastin*, December 30, 1935, 7.

55 "Hijrat al-atibba' al-Yahud li-Lubnan," *Filastin*, May 27, 1933, 2; "Yu'aqiduhu al-atibba': Qalaq atibba'ina min dukhul al-atibba' al-Alman li-Suriya," *al-Difa'*, August 31, 1934; "Atibba' Yahud yatajawwaluna fi al-shawari' wa-yu'alijuna al-marid bi-khamsat qurush," *Filastin*, November 16, 1934, 3.

56 "al-Atibba' al-Yahud fi-l-qura," *al-Kifah*, February 2, 1936, 3.

the Jewish immigrant doctors. The Jewish doctors, he claimed, were soliciting Arab patients to create a market for their pharmaceutical products. Taxi drivers, he further maintained, were taking patients from the countryside to a Jewish doctor in Tel Aviv or Haifa's Jewish neighborhoods instead of taking them to an Arab doctor, who was more likely to be more familiar with their ailments. He argued that the immigrants' medical knowledge was inadequate: they did not know Palestine's medical conditions, and their research was based only on what they could find in their settlements, with no inkling about the countryside.[57]

The ongoing public debate continued to highlight the absence of Arab doctors and patients' reliance on Jewish ones. In late 1936, *al-Difa'* lamented that there was not a single Arab doctor in the Bisan district and that patients in the town and surroundings frequented Jewish doctors. The newspaper urged Arab doctors to embrace their national and humanitarian duty, give up the comfort and material advantages of city life, and move to Palestine's towns and villages. By abandoning Bisan, *al-Difa'* concluded, Arab doctors had left its residents in the hands of the Jewish doctor – Dr. Joseph Lehrs (unnamed in the article), who was driven by greed rather than a humanitarian mission.[58] Eleven years later, *Filastin* lamented the appointment of his nephew, Dr. Hugo Lehrs, to Beit Safafa's hospital. The doctor, *Filastin* argued, did not speak Arabic and could not communicate with Arab patients, urging the DoH to reconsider the appointment.[59]

Becoming Political

In November 1934, Dr. Rushdi al-Tamimi sent a letter to the Mandate administration on behalf of the Haifa Doctors' Association, protesting the licensing of immigrant doctors and demanding that it be stopped.[60]

[57] Anwar al-Shuqayri, "al-Da'wa ila mu'tamar al-atibba' al-'Arab al-awwal," *al-Difa'*, March 17, 1936, 2; Anwar al-Shuqayri, "Mu'tamar al-atibba' al-'Arab al-awwal," *al-Difa'*, March 22, 1936, 2; Anwar al-Shuqayri, "Awda ila muzahamat al-atibba' al-Yahud," *al-Difa'*, April 5, 1936, 2.

[58] "Tabib Bisan al-'Arabi," *al-Difa'*, November 11, 1936, 6; "Tabib Bisan al-'Arabi," *al-Difa'*, December 27, 1936, 2.

[59] "Ta'yin tabib Yahudi fi mustashfa Bayt Safafa!" *Filastin*, August 6, 1946, 2.

[60] "Hijrat al-atibba' al-Yahud ila Filastin," *Filastin*, November 9, 1934, 5.

In April 1935, he petitioned the League of Nations' Permanent Mandates Commission (PMC) in similar vein. The British authorities replied to the League that a new ordinance issued that year had remedied the situation, aiming to restrict the licensing of Jewish doctors.[61] When discussing the petition at the Commission, the Portuguese member, Count de Penha Garcia, suggested that the influx of immigrant doctors was responsible for reducing the incidence of infectious disease and, therefore, was not an "entirely unmitigated ill." Palestine's attorney general, Harry Trusted, replied that further Jewish immigration would lead to an undesirable saturation of the profession and force doctors "to engage in some other activities to earn a living."[62]

The outbreak of the Arab Revolt in April 1936 further politicized the professional competition. In the testimony of Arab Higher Committee representative, Jamal al-Husayni, before the 1937 Peel Royal Commission of Enquiry, he argued that Jewish doctors did not improve health conditions in Palestine but lowered salaries and threatened the livelihood of their Arab counterparts.[63]

As Sufian showed, Zionist political leadership used anti-malaria research and drainage works to make claims about the vital contribution of the Jewish settlement project to the development of Palestine and the well-being of its entire population. To this Zionist claim, Dr. Tawfiq Canaan responded that Palestinian Arabs – both medical officers and laborers – were instrumental in government anti-malaria work.[64] This debate was not limited to malaria. Whether contributing to or obstructing Arab health in Palestine, for the Arabs, the evident progress of Zionist health services marked another Palestinian realm under threat of takeover.

Palestinian doctors repeatedly rebuffed Zionist claims to their contribution to the country's health.[65] In his *Conflict in the Land of Peace*, a national political manifesto against Zionist claims published during

[61] The League of Nations, Permanent Mandate Commission, *Minutes of the Twenty-Ninth Session, Held at Geneva from May 27th to June 12th, 1936* (Geneva: League of Nations, 1936), 192.

[62] Ibid., 163–64.

[63] Palestine Royal Commission, *Minutes of Evidence Heard at Public Sessions* (London: His Majesty's Stationery Office, 1937), 325–26.

[64] Sufian, "Re-imagining," 378–80.

[65] Frances S. Hasso, *Buried in the Red Dirt: Race, Reproduction, and Death in Modern Palestine* (Cambridge: Cambridge University Press, 2021), 73–77.

the first months of the Arab Revolt, Dr. Canaan stated that "[S]tatistics show clearly that the Jews have received infinitely more medical help from non-Jewish institutions than non-Jews have received from Jewish institutions. Despite these facts, the Jews continue to boast of the great medical help extended to non-Jews," ignoring all the work done by the DoH and forgetting that their wars against malaria, for example, were fought primarily for their own settlement interests.[66] In his testimony before the Anglo-American Committee (1946), representing the Palestinian Medical Association, Canaan similarly argued that improvements in the medical state of Palestine's Arabs should be credited neither to the British Mandate authorities, which neglected their duties, nor to the Jews, who treated exclusively their own.[67]

This debate, which questioned the moral grounds of Zionist colonization, continued until 1948. Itzhak Kanievsky of the Sick Fund responded to criticism of the numerical imbalance of Jewish and Arab doctors by pointing to vital statistics regarding Palestine's Arab population demonstrating a marked increase in life expectancy and a decrease in child mortality, particularly in comparison to neighboring Arab countries. Aside from these statistics, Kanievsky tried to rebut the Arab case by arguing that Arab patients resorted to Jewish doctors. The elite, including Arab doctors themselves, consulted Jewish specialists, while the lower classes used the Yishuv's free clinics: villagers traveled to nearby Jewish settlements for treatment, and hundreds of Arab workers unionized under the Histadrut were also treated in its Sick Fund. Echoing Palestinian claims, he added that the Arab doctor did not concern himself with the countryside and concluded that the Arab attempt to block licenses to immigrant doctors only exacerbated the peasants' predicament.[68]

In May 1947, *The Lancet* published a short piece about medicine in Palestine, based on Hadassah's medical organization report for the years 1942–44. The piece described the report as bringing "a little

[66] Tawfiq Canaan, *Conflict in the Land of Peace* (Jerusalem: Syrian Orphanage Press, 1936), 84–88.

[67] "'Edut mle'at stirot shel rofe 'Aravi," *Ha-Mashkif*, March 22, 1946, 1.

[68] Y. Kanievsky, "Hana'a mi-kan ve-hasata mi-kan," *Davar*, October 5, 1945, 2. See also "Ha-'Aravim ma'adifim lismokh 'al mumkhiyut ha-rof'im ha-Yehudim," *Ha-Boker*, May 7, 1946, for *al-Difa'* editor's choice to take his son to *Hadassah* hospital in Tel Aviv; and another report in the Jewish press that Canaan preferred Jewish doctors: "Dr. Kan'an mitrape etsel rofe Yehudi," *ha-Tzofe*, March 28, 1946, 4.

light into the present darkness of Palestine." It listed Hadassah's preventive work and achievements, described its neurosurgical center as attracting patients from all over the Near East, and then mentioned the Jewish-Arab cooperation around the abovementioned Samakh clinic.[69] Mahmud Tahir al-Dajani was outraged by the British medical journal's disregard for the Arab medical profession and even the DoH. In an article published in the Palestine Arab Medical Association's journal in July 1947, he criticized the article for ascribing medical progress in Palestine solely to Hadassah. "What about our Arab medical community, which has grown from ten doctors in 1918 to about 300-strong today? What about our medical association and its continuous health propaganda efforts? What about Arab initiatives and government investment, and their role in improving health in the country?" The blame, he concluded, lay partly with Arabs themselves, who preferred Jewish doctors without realizing that this preference would later be used for Zionist propaganda. The public should therefore boycott Jewish doctors and prefer their equally competent Arab counterparts.[70]

Growing Arab demand for healthcare and the Yishuv's increasing ability to meet it prevented a simple political measure such as a boycott. Especially in the countryside, the gap in healthcare provision between the Yishuv and Palestinians persisted until the Mandate's end. Perhaps more than his fear of Zionists using healthcare as propaganda, Dajani expressed concerns and frustration of his medical community, outnumbered and less organized than its professional rival.

Arab Doctors through Zionist Eyes

For the Yishuv, the Palestinian educated elite during the Mandate represented the ultimate national Other, and their cultural, physical, and material affinities with Jewish urbanites constituted a threat. The Palestinian *effendiyya* symbolized the country's cultural and social mobility and had a clear voice and a firm claim. They also led the Palestinian national movement and articulated anti-Zionist vocabulary. Representing the best educated and ablest members of their

[69] "Medicine in Palestine," *The Lancet* 249, no. 6453 (1947): 621.

[70] Mahmud Tahir al-Dajani, "Kalimat al-ʿadad," *al-Majalla al-Tibbiyya al-ʿArabiyya al-Filastiniyya* 2, no. 5 (July 1947): 83.

community, Palestinian doctors manifested all of the above. The involvement of many doctors in the national movement helped color the entire Arab medical community as anti-Zionist and anti-Jewish. The Arab doctors' portrayal in various Hebrew texts was a mirror image of the fraudulent and greedy characteristics attributed to Jewish doctors in the Palestinian press, which was sometimes spiced with antisemitic tropes.

The fact that most of Palestine's Jews never met or even heard of Arab doctors helped create this image. They read about a select few, whom the Jewish press usually framed as ardent nationalists whose opposition to the Zionist project clouded their professional judgement. In early 1930, for example, journalist David Tidhar reported that a very senior official at the DoH in Jerusalem was an ardent nationalist and had told him personally that all the Jews should have been murdered in the 1929 riots.[71] Drs. Fu'ad Dajani and Husayn Fakhri al-Khalidi reportedly refused to incorporate Jewish doctors in an autopsy of Jewish corpses.[72] As shown earlier, balancing between professional calling and national loyalty was gradually becoming impossible.

During the Great Arab Revolt, Hebrew readers learned that the Germanophile physician Dr. Canaan had published a fifteen-page anti-Zionist pamphlet and distributed it among British officials. At the time and in the years to come, Canaan's anti-Zionism was increasingly framed as pro-Nazism.[73] Rushdi al-Tamimi was likewise noted for his anti-Zionist testimony to the Peel Commission in 1937.[74] In 1946, the Yishuv also learned about Arab doctors' decision to boycott Jewish pharmaceutical products.[75]

Far from the public sphere of the Hebrew press, the Haganah's Intelligence Service (*Shai*) tried to obtain more intimate knowledge of Palestine's Arab physicians as part of a larger effort to collect data on Palestinians.[76] Often written by volunteer personnel of different

71 David Tidhar, "mi-Sdare ha-administratsia be-Erets Yisra'el," *Do'ar Hayom*, January 5, 1930, 3.

72 "Rofe 'Aravi nokem ve-noter," *Davar*, January 27, 1930, 1; "Halal bi-Yerushalayim," *Davar*, April 3, 1932, 1.

73 "Mekorav el ha-hugim ha-Natsim menahel ta'amula 'Aravit bein ha-Anglim," *Davar*, June 30, 1936, 7.

74 "Rofe 'Aravi ya'id?" *Davar*, January 18, 1937, 1.

75 "Nobody Asked the Patients," *Palestine Post*, July 25, 1946, 3.

76 Asa Lefen, *ha-Shai, sherut ha-yedi'ot: Shorasheha shel kehillat ha-modi'in ha-Yisra'elit* (Tel Aviv: ha-Merkaz le-toldot koah ha-magen - ha-hagana, 1997);

professions and localities or by Arab agents, the *Shai* files offer a snapshot of what the Yishuv's leadership knew or thought it knew about Palestinians. The bulk of this data was collected after the Revolt and was meant to serve the Haganah in future conflicts. The personal *Shai* files, a massive collection of biographical data, contain detailed insights on many hundreds of Palestinians, ranging from peasants who participated in the Revolt, whom the Haganah considered a direct security threat, activists in the national movement who were considered a political threat, and also details on the Palestinian professional and cultural elite.[77]

Around forty personal *Shai* files were devoted to Palestinian doctors. The longest, most detailed reports were dedicated to leaders or activists in the national movement who expressed anti-Zionist views or were suspected of being Nazi sympathizers.[78] The report on Dr. Husam al-Din Abu al-Saud, for example, noted that he distanced himself from political matters and belonged to the political opposition to the Mufti, but also mentioned that he was a member of the National Committee in Jerusalem during the Revolt and that he treated wounded rebels.[79] Dr. Tahir al-Khatib's file contained information on his affiliation with the rebels, donations to the "gangs," and service as militia leader Fawzi al-Qawuqji's advisor. Dr. Nadim Amin, it was reported, treated the rebels free of charge.[80] Dr. Mufid ʿAbd al-Hadi was mentioned as an enemy of Zionism with Nazi contacts. Dr. Ahmad Tahir was also reported to be a Nazi sympathizer, proclaiming that Hitler would win the war and free the East from the British.[81] Other doctors were

Hillel Cohen, *Army of Shadows: Palestinian Collaboration with Zionism, 1917–1948* (Berkeley: University of California Press, 2008).

77 Yoni Furas, *Educating Palestine: Teaching and Learning History under the Mandate* (Oxford: Oxford University Press, 2020), 70–97.

78 In reality, Palestinian contribution to British war effort during WWII was much greater than the limited, often little more than rhetorical support for the Nazis. Thousands volunteered for the British Army, while others continued to serve in government departments. See Mustafa Abbasi, "Falastinim nilhamim ba-Natsim: Sippuram shel ha-mitnadvim ha-Falastinim be-milhemet ha-ʿolam ha-sheniyyah," *Catedra* 128 (2019), 125–47; Joseph Nevo, "ha-Tnuʿa ha-leʾumit haʿArvit ha-Falestinit be-milhemet ha-ʿolam ha-shniya," in *Hatnuʿa ha-ʿAravit ha-Falestinit: Mi-ʿimut le-hashlama?*, eds. Moshe Maʿoz and Binyamin Zeʾev Kedar (Tel Aviv: Misrad ha-bitahon – ha-hotsaʿa la-or, 1996), 93–114.

79 File 5, series B, letters N, H, W, Y, 914, Truman Library Archive (hereafter, TLA).

80 File 3, 241–390, Biari-bashar, 427, TLA.

81 File 3, 241–390, Biari-bashar, 435, TLA.

reported to be spreading Nazi propaganda[82] or helping Gestapo agents infiltrate the country.[83] At the same time, Palestinian doctors continued working for the DoH, and some were recommended by its director for the Defense Medal in honor of their wartime work.[84]

The *Shai* depicted some doctors favorably. Sulayman Katkhuda was reported to have helped a Jewish refugee obtain employment and to support a binational solution. His virtues were also mentioned in the report: "refuses to take a bribe. Ready to help any man, goodhearted and a first-class gentleman."[85] Naif Hamzeh was reported as being interested in his personal career and as distancing himself from politics.[86]

The detailed report on Rushdi al-Tamimi noted that he was "active in Haifa's social and economic life, gives speeches, a writer, friendly, a Freemason, a senior Rotary member, … who likes to brag his nationalism," and stated that he was suspected of contacts with Nazi sympathizers. Although he appeared to be "a loyal and extreme nationalist," "an agitator during the 1929 riots," and had treated wounded rebels during the Revolt, it was also reported that "some say he did that only out of fear" and that he was "not dangerous" because he had no followers. In April 1945, the report stated that Tamimi's nationalism was not genuine and that he was "secretly in contact with the British."[87] A report such as this on such a central figure in the doctors' community must have cast a shadow over all of its institutions and organizations.

Whether involved in the national movement or not, a collaborator with the British or a Mufti sympathizer, doctors were targeted by Yishuv's intelligence. In that sense, they were no different from teachers, lawyers, merchants, or any notable figure in Palestinian society. The *Shai*'s records, which examined them in terms of potential political threats, portrayed them as enemies for the most part, or as people who ought not to be trusted. Presumably, this was a mirror

82 File 1, letters A, B, T, Th, J, H, 17, 119, TLA; File 4/B, 786, TLA.
83 File 4, series B, 603–839, ʿAlayan-Nashashibi, 676, TLA.
84 Director of Medical Services to Chief Secretary, Government Office, Jerusalem, February 6, 1947, "Nominal Roll of Persons Eligible for the Award of the Defense Medal," TNA, CO 733/625.
85 File 4, series B, 603–839, ʿAlayan-Nashashibi, 705, TLA.
86 File 4, series B, 603–839, ʿAlayan-Nashashibi, 625, TLA.
87 File 1, letters A, B, T, Th, J, H, 40, TLA.

image of how they thought of themselves and how their community thought of them.

Facing Intercommunal Violence

As active and notable community members, Palestinian and Jewish doctors were affected by the waves of intercommunal violence during the Mandate. The number of assassinations and assaults on doctors underlines their place and role within their communities. Doctors were intimately engaged in intercommunal and colonial violence as the ones responsible for treating the wounded.

Doctors' national affiliations were amplified during and immediately after waves of violence, forcibly connecting their professional and national commitments. Such was the case during the 1929 riots, the bloodiest events the country had seen in decades. Reports or rumors of Arab DoH doctors who did not fulfill their duties toward Jewish victims and the fact that Fu'ad Hijazi, a DoH employee in Safad, was convicted for his participation in the massacre there deepened the Yishuv's suspicions toward Arab employees.[88] This problem was acknowledged by the DoH: "In no case" during the riots, DoH director Colonel George Heron reported, "were Arabs and Jews admitted to the same hospital, except as a temporary measure to receive first aid."[89]

The exhumation of the Jewish victims of the Hebron massacre in 1929, followed by an autopsy by Jewish doctors, encapsulated the professional complexities at stake in turbulent times. The physicians were to prove or refute accusations of abuse or mutilation. Taking place a few weeks after the riots, this effort involved high-ranking Arab, Jewish, and British doctors. The Arab delegation, sent to inspect the work of the Jewish doctors, included Tawfiq Canaan, Husam al-Din Abu al-Saʿud, and Husayn Fakhri al-Khalidi. The Jewish delegation included a surgeon from Shaʿare Zedek Hospital and the head of Hadassah Hospital's pathology department. Once exhumed, the

[88] Hillel Cohen, *1929: Year Zero of the Arab-Israeli Conflict* (Waltham, MA: Brandeis University Press, 2015), 241.

[89] DoH to Chief Secretary, "Record of Casualties in Recent Disturbances," October 17, 1929, in: Colonial Office, *Palestine Commission on the Disturbances of August 1929, vol. 1, Evidence Heard during the 1st to 29th Sittings* (London: HMSO, 1930), 1031–32.

bodies were examined separately by Jewish doctors, and, if there was evidence of mutilation, they were passed over to Arab doctors for further examination.[90] The gruesome task ended inconclusively. The bodies' decomposition made it impossible to prove or negate abuse.[91] It did result in clear professional division along national lines, however. One could not imagine a more graphic reflection of the conflict's ability to cement the separation and suspicion between Arab and Jewish doctors, unable or refusing to jointly resolve a medical issue. Apparently, Jewish suspicions toward Arab doctors' integrity continued until the end of the Mandate, particularly when it came to autopsies of Jewish corpses when the suspected reason for death had a nationalist connection.[92]

The three years of the Great Arab Revolt once again fleshed out this connection between professional and national. Thousands of wounded rebels and civilians required medical treatment and several doctors gained fame for their clandestine support of the Revolt, at risk to their lives and licenses.[93] Some would travel to the hinterland, secretly guided into the rebels' whereabouts, and in severe cases, they would treat the wounded in their clinics. Fuʾad Daʿdas and Adib Khartabil both worked in Tulkarem and were known for treating wounded rebels. Disguised as a milkmaid, Daʿdas personally treated ʿAbd al-Rahim Hajj Muhammad, the commander of the Revolt's armed forces.[94]

The British did not take kindly to doctors treating rebels. In June 1939, British police raided Dr. Dajani's hospital and shot to death one of its patients. Shaken by the raid, Fuʾad al-Dajani surrendered his honorary medals (both MBE and MC) and requested that his name be erased from the recipients' list. The subsequent British investigation concluded that the patient had been mistakenly identified

90 The Supreme Muslim Council, *Report of Arab Doctors on Examination of the Bodies of the Jewish Corpses Exhumed at Hebron, on September 11th, 1929* (Jerusalem: Bayt al-makdis Press, 1929).

91 DoH to Chief Secretary, "Record of Casualties in Recent Disturbances."

92 "Rofeʾ ʿAravi nokem ve-noter," *Davar*, January 27, 1930, 1.

93 A few notable figures include Nadim Amin, File 3, 241–390, Biari-bashar, 427, TLA; Rushdi Tamimi, File 1, letters A, B, T, Th, J, H, 40, TLA; Sabri 'Izz al-Din Qadura, File 4, series B, 603–839, ʿAlayan-Nashashibi, 676, TLA; and Mahdi Tahir al-Husayni, File 1, letters A, B, T, Th, J, H, 119, TLA.

94 ʿIsa al-Sifri, *Filastin al-ʿArabiyya bayna al-intidab wa-l-Sahyuniyya* (Jaffa: Matbaʿat maktabat Filastin al-jadida, 1937), 18, 29; Ahmad Abu Shunnar, *Qabilat al-Tiyaha hadara wa-taʾrikh* (Amman: Dar al-mu'tazz li-l-nashr wa-l-tawzi', 2017), 65.

as a known rebel. Al-Dajani accepted the explanation and retained his medals, and the police compensated the victim's family.[95]

Such compensations were rare, though. The period was characterized by brutal British violence against Palestinians, followed by intra-Palestinian violence. Two physicians fell victim to the fierce rivalry between the Mufti and the opposition. Both were sons of leading opposition figures – Hajj Khalil Taha in Haifa and Sheikh Asʿad al-Shuqayri in Acre. Dr. Taha Khalil Taha was murdered in late January 1937 at around the same spot where his father had been murdered four months previously.[96] Anwar al-Shuqayri was murdered outside his clinic in Acre in June 1939, and his father passed away a few months later. His story would later reverberate in popular memory, featured in the historical TV series that opened the previous chapter and in Iyad Barghouti's 2014 novel *Burdaqana* (An Orange). The motive for the murder is still not clear, and explanations include the Mufti's men targeting the son of their patron's political rival, or personal revenge by a local police officer, who suspected the doctor's involvement with his wife.[97]

Jewish doctors were similarly entangled in the violent events and mobilized to support the Yishuv's militias. A major step forward in the institutionalization process of military medicine in the Yishuv was the establishment of a medical corps (*Sherut Refuʾi*) during the Revolt. This was a cooperation between the Haganah, Sick Fund, the Red Shield of David (the Yishuv's equivalent of the Red Cross), and Hadassah. In 1937, Dr. Avraham Katzenelson, head of the health department of the Jewish National Council, convened delegates from the Haganah, Sick Fund, the Jewish Agency, and Hadassah for the establishment of a medical service for the *Notrim* (or *ghaffirs*, a Jewish police and paramilitary force funded by the British).[98]

[95] Matthew Hughes, *Britain's Pacification of Palestine* (Cambridge: Cambridge University Press, 2019), 327–28; "Colonial Office: Palestine Original Correspondence. Conduct of British Troops and Police. Shooting of Hospital Patient," TNA, CO 733/413/5.

[96] "Tashyiʿ janazat al-marhum al-duktur Taha," *al-Difaʿ*, January 29, 1937.

[97] For example, Ted Swedenburg, *Memories of Revolt: The 1936–1939 Rebellion and the Palestinian National Past* (Fayetteville: University of Arkansas Press, 2003), 160–62. For details about the murder, see Israel State Archives, P-176/56.

[98] Eran Dolev, "Shorshe ha-refuʾa ha-tsvaʾit be-tsahal ʿuvdot ve-tehiyot," in Nir Mann ed., *Refuʾa tsvaʾit: ʿIyunim be-sugiyot refuʾiyot be-toldot koah ha-magen ha-ʿIvri* (Ben-Shemen: Modan, 2018), 39–50; Shlomo Nissan, "Hitpathut sherute ha-refuʾa bi-Yerushalayim bi-tkufat ha-mandat," in *Yerushalayim bi-*

Jewish doctors' mobilization proceeded in tandem with their distancing from Arab patients. Most Jewish private practitioners residing in Arab neighborhoods, cities, and towns had left during the Revolt. The boycott of Jewish services and goods was detrimental to these doctors' livelihood, and several cases of assault and murder of Jewish medical personnel were sufficient to make all others feel unsafe. Dr. Lehrs, for example, immigrated to Palestine in 1933, learned Arabic, and settled with his wife in Bisan. When the Revolt erupted in April 1936, the couple left town, but Lehrs returned in October. He was murdered shortly afterward.[99] Olga Feinberg, who had operated a private clinic in Jericho since 1929, left in 1938 after her house was torched.[100] Two nurses working at Jaffa's Government Hospital were murdered in August 1936. The director of Safad's Government Hospital survived an assassination attempt in March 1939 while driving an ambulance in town.[101] Another doctor was murdered while driving his car in Ramle in September 1938.[102]

As Reuven Gafni notes, these doctors did not view themselves as spearheads of Jewish settlement, but both Zionist and Arab observers sometimes saw them as such.[103] Medical treatment thus became another manifestation of contested interaction between Jews and Arabs. During the Revolt, a drastic decrease was noted in the number of Arab patients treated in the Yishuv's hospitals. For example, while treating more than 20,000 Jewish patients between 1936 and 1938, the internal ward of Hadassah Hospital in Jerusalem treated a mere 15 Arab patients.[104]

tkufat ha-mandat ha-ʿasiya ve-ha-moreshet, ed. Yehoshuʻa Ben-Arieh (Jerusalem: Yad Ben-Tsvi, 2003), 299–323.

99 Avishai Teicher, "Ahayot ve-rofʾim korbanot teror ishi bi-tkufat ha-mandat," *ha-Refuʾa* 139 (2000): 312–13.

100 Reuven Gafni, "Lone Jewish Medical Personnel in Arab Towns: A Conditional Presence in British Mandate Palestine," *Israel Studies* 26 (2021): 206–11; Reuven Gafni, "Rofʾa Yehudiyya be-ʿir ʿAravit: Peʿiluta shel Dr. Olga Feinberg be-Yeriho bi-tkufat ha-mandat," *Korot* 24 (2017/18): 69–86.

101 "Hitnakshut be-doctor Sternberg bi-Tsfat," *Haaretz*, March 7, 1939, 1.

102 "Dr. Avraham Rosenthal," *Davar*, September 15, 1938, 1.

103 Gafni, "Lone Jewish," 206–11; Gafni, "Rofʾa yehudiyya."

104 Moshe Sherman, "ha-Rofʾim be-Erets Yisraʾel bi-tehilat shnat 1938," *ha-Refuʾa* 15, no. 7–8 (October 1938): 77–79; Matti Golan, *Rofe – Mosheh Rachmilevitsh* (Tel Aviv: Zemora Bitan, 1989), 98–99.

Cooperating in the Margins

In the late Ottoman and early postwar years, there were limited efforts to promote medical cooperation between the Arab, missionary, and Jewish doctors. These were always ad hoc and connected to concrete epidemic challenges that crossed communal boundaries. Ever-growing Arab-Jewish tensions during the Mandate pushed this collaboration to the margins of medical activity, turning government hospitals into the main shared working space.

One early context in which Jews and Arabs (would-be) physicians met was medical education. Historian Caroline Kahlenberg showed how the American University of Beirut (AUB) became, particularly during the interwar period, a site of encounter between Jewish and Arab students and between Zionism and Arab nationalism. For students on campus, the rival national movement was not an abstract ideology, but concrete presence. Jews arrived in Beirut to study medicine, dentistry, pharmacy, and nursing. Jewish women enrolled in many of AUB's nursing cohorts and were among the first female doctors and dentists trained in Beirut.[105]

Many of the Jewish medical students who studied in Beirut before World War II (WWII) were born in Palestine or had immigrated there at an early age. At St. Joseph, we can find, already in the 1900s, brothers Baruch and Moise Mani from Hebron, and Jerusalem-born Abraham Abu Shadid graduated from the AUB in 1899. In the 1910s, Anthony Shhadah and Raphael Oplatka studied together at St. Joseph, and both later joined the DoH. Simon Btesh, a native Jerusalemite who graduated from the AUB in 1932, would become, in the 1950s, one of the first directors of the Israeli Ministry of Health.[106] Dozens of such classmates can be traced throughout the period. Particularly at St. Joseph, several men who had started their studies in Central Europe and were expelled following the Nazi takeover immigrated to Palestine and resumed their studies in Beirut. They graduated in the mid 1940s and then settled in Palestine. Campus encounters and possible friendships, however, were at the margins of a greater story of the Jewish

[105] For Jewish nurses at the AUB see, American University of Beirut, *Directory of Alumni*, 213–14, 222, 229, 237–38.

[106] "Yeshivat ha-memshala," *Davar*, February 23, 1953.

medical profession, which was a predominantly immigrant community, composed of doctors born and trained in Europe.

Despite these apparent differences and institutional divisions, the few attempts at rapprochement between certified doctors are worth mentioning. In March 1929, Hebrew newspaper *Do'ar Hayom* reported that the National Doctors' Association of Haifa contacted their Jewish counterparts and suggested a joint meeting to discuss professional and scientific collaboration.[107] Decades later, Dr. Itzkovitch, who worked in the city, recalled a meeting held in his house with four Arab doctors headed by Dr. Rushdi al-Tamimi. Both groups discussed future collaboration and the foundation of a joint union, including the Arab request to support the demand to curtail licensing of immigrant doctors – which Jewish doctors refused. Details of the meeting leaked to the Palestinian press, which, according to Itzkovitch, condemned the "treacherous Arab doctors, who try to reach an agreement with the Jews."[108]

Beyond such sporadic, individual initiatives, international and regional professional conferences allowed a certain degree of cooperation without concessions on the national level. They participated in the 1928 Tropical Medicine Conference in Cairo. Among more than 2,000 listed guests, there were about 20 Palestinian Arab physicians and 120 Yishuv doctors. The numerical gap was much more striking in the speakers' list: a few Yishuv doctors lectured on such topics as malaria and trachoma, while the only lecture by a Palestinian Arab was Tawfiq Canaan's, on leprosy.[109]

Five years later, the Egyptian Medical Association held its sixth annual meeting in the YMCA building in Jerusalem. Palestinian doctors lectured and served on the Executive and Scientific Committees.[110] In addition, the Tel Aviv Medical Association invited delegates to witness the development of the Jewish health system. En route to Tel Aviv, they stopped at the Jewish Convalescent Home at Motza. After greetings by Tel Aviv's mayor Meir Dizengoff and

107 "Bein ha-rof'im ha-'Aravim ve-ha-'Ivrim," *Do'ar Hayom*, March 6, 1929, 4.

108 "Sipuro shel Dr. Y. Itzkovitch," *ha-Refu'a* 61 (1961): 129.

109 *Congrès international de médicine tropicale et d'hygiène: Comptes rendus* (Cairo: Imprimerie Nationale, 1929), I: 48; Dr. Tawfiq Canaan, "Leprosy in Palestine," *Congrès international de médicine tropicale*, V : 263–71; "ha-Ve'ida ha-refu'it be-Kahir," *Haaretz*, December 23, 1928, 2.

110 "Egyptian Medical Association," *al-Kulliyyah* 19, no. 5 (1933): 145–47.

president of the city's Medical Association, they visited the Tel Aviv IWC and Hadassah Hospital and, later in Jerusalem, the Nathan and Lina Strauss Health Centre. Iraqi physician Fa'iq Shakir described the Hadassah infant care and school health services, noting anti-trachoma and anti-syphilis measures. He concluded grimly that the excellent care for infants and children would eventually lead to Zionist victory. The cordial Zionist welcome was offset by Mufti Hajj Amin al-Husayni, who invited the delegates to witness the annual Nebi Musa festival of mass pilgrimage to the burial ground of Prophet Musa.[111]

The Palestinian Arab press particularly noted Dr. Yehudah Rokach's opening speech. The head of Jerusalem's branch of the Palestine Jewish Medical Association delivered it in Hebrew without providing translation, except in English for the High Commissioner. Most of the audience could not follow the speech, as *Filastin* commented, but did notice the recurring term "Land of Israel" (*Erets Yisra'el*), which they found extremely rude and ruinous to the atmosphere of human solidarity. Interestingly, the impressive number of Jewish doctors among the speakers was not deemed worthy of comment. It was Dr. Rokach's political statement that alienated most of those present and upset *Filastin*'s correspondent, rather than Jewish doctors' presence per se.[112]

The colonial institutes remained the only space of professional interaction. Haifa's Government Hospital, a major employer of doctors, nurses, Arab and Jewish alike, is a good example. In 1938, the British relocated the hospital to a much larger facility for the benefit of Haifa's significant British community and as the region's medical center. In its single decade of operation, its personnel reflected Haifa's mixed population. Like all major colonial institutions in Palestine, it was headed by a British official, Dr. John Thompson, while the rest of the senior staff were Arab or Jewish. Naif Hamzeh was Thompson's deputy, and Shafiq Haddad, a native of Haifa, headed the Department of Tropical Diseases. Simon Btesh was also employed there, alongside Dr. Emil Kleinhaus, who was trained in Munich and headed the Radiology Department. The hospital treated mainly the Arab population, but the Jewish population

111 "Egyptian Medical Congress," *Palestine Post*, April 9, 1933, 5; "Egyptian Medical Congress," *Palestine Post*, April 12, 1933, 3. For the Iraqi doctor's account of his visits in Jewish health facilities, see Fa'iq Shakir, *Kitab tadbir al-amrad al-zuhariyya* (Baghdad: Matba'at al-'ahd, 1934).

112 "Iftitah al-mu'tamar al-tibbi fi al-Quds," *Filastin*, April 5, 1933; "Fi al-mu'tamar al-tibbi: Shu'ur insani 'ala hisab al-ghayr," *Filastin*, April 7, 1933.

benefited from its services as well. Despite Haifa's history of violence and the apparent national tensions between the communities, medical coexistence endured until the end of the Mandate.

Physical segregation did exist at the Haifa hospital – between British nurses on the one hand and Arab and Jewish nurses on the other. The former ate in a separate dining room, were served better food, and treated British patients in wards that were off-limits to the other nurses. It was this separation, firm hierarchy, and rigid discipline in the training of nurses that enhanced Arab-Jewish solidarity. In the summer of 1947, Jewish and Arab nurses at Haifa's Government Hospital jointly went on a hunger strike in demand for better food.[113] The shared working environment also enabled scientific cooperation: Dr. Haddad and Dr. Valero coauthored the hospital's first academic publication, published in the prestigious *British Medical Journal* in May 1948.[114]

Conclusion

This chapter placed the protagonists of this book within a relational framework, whose contours included the British Mandate authorities and Arab and Jewish doctors. Often working in shared or proximate urban spaces, the Palestinian professional community was challenged by its Jewish counterpart, making this encounter crucial for understanding its development. The direct and indirect interactions between Jewish and Arab doctors shaped the professional identity of both groups. The unionization of Jewish doctors and the institutionalization of Jewish health services prior to WWI, built on the exclusion of Arab doctors, were crucial factors in shaping relationships between the communities.

This relationship was characterized by professional competition, suspicion, and several isolated instances of collaboration. Competition became fiercer following the 1933 mass immigration of German-Jewish doctors, which shifted numerical balance dramatically

[113] "Nurses Go on Hunger Strike," *Palestine Post*, August 15, 1947, 3; "al-Taʿam li-muwazifi mustashfa Hayfa," *Filastin*, August 15, 1947, 2; "Idrab mumaridat mustashfa Hayfa," *Filastin*, August 16, 1947, 2; "Shvitat raʿav shel 60 ahayot be-by"h ha-memshalti," *ha-Mashkif*, August 17, 1947, 4; "Nistayma shvitat ha-ahayot," *ha-Tzofeh*, August 17, 1947, 4.

[114] Chafiq Haddad and Ahron Valero, "Streptomycin in Bubonic Plague," *British Medical Journal* (May 29, 1948): 1026.

in favor of Jewish doctors. This wave of immigration changed the medical balance of power much more radically than in most other labor markets and politicized the medical field in unprecedented ways. Arab doctors started demanding that Mandate authorities limit the licensing of Jewish immigrant doctors, and it was against this background that they held their first national congress in 1933. This political concern continued to color the relationship between Arab and Jewish doctors until the end of the Mandate. Their political engagement also affected the way the Yishuv came to see Palestinian doctors. As the next chapter shows, however, doctors' political and public engagement was not limited to their political and professional competition with their Jewish counterparts. Chapter 6 will concentrate on these doctors' public writing and their unionization, their relations with the broader Arab medical community, their patients, the Mandate authorities, and the Palestinian countryside.

6 A Republic of Medical Letters and Professional Unity

"I will just say that the era of the barber and quack had ended or is coming to its end," noted Salim Salama (b. 1895, Jaffa) in 1919. Salama's prophecy jumped the gun, as barbers and traditional healers would continue to dominate the medical sphere of rural Palestine for decades to come. More than prophesying, however, Salama's wishful thinking articulated the clear boundaries between the traditional barber and a professional, rational doctor – between himself, a dentistry student at the Syrian Protestant College (SPC), and local charlatans. In his article series "A Doctor's Letters," he expounded the virtues of the medical calling and criticized patients who dared to confuse the barber with the certified doctor and bargain over the cost of treatment while they would not dare haggle for a haircut. Some dentists, Salama lamented, reduced themselves to the ranks of radish vendors. The dentist was underappreciated and treated by his patients as a "garbage collector," while their mouths smelled worse than sewage.[1]

Three decades later, in September 1947, Dr. Ra'fat Faris published "Two Embarrassing Situations," conceding a concealed truth: doctors were human beings. As such, he confessed, they had their embarrassing moments and share of anxieties, and were far from omniscient. Doctors' scandals were kept under wraps to maintain the profession's reputation. In order to demystify the trade, Faris wrote about his own mishaps. He narrated an incident in which an old sick man came to his clinic and confessed his fears that the patient would die right then and there or shortly after, and that he would be blamed for it, terminating his professional career. The patient survived his treatment, but Faris' fear led him to give the patient free house visits.[2] The short article was

[1] Salim Salama, "Rasa'il tabib," *al-Nafayis al-'Asriyya*, December 15, 1919, 153. See also: Salim Salama, "Rasa'il tabib: al-Fam," *al-Nafayis al-'Asriyya*, February 15, 1920, 203–06; Salim Salama, "Rasa'il tabib: Mu'alajat al-asnan fi al-qarn al-sadis 'ashar," *al-Nafayis al-'Asriyya*, March 15, 1920, 345–46.

[2] Ra'fat Faris, "Ahraj mawqifayn," *al-Qafila*, September 5, 1947, 11.

published in *al-Qafila*, a government-funded weekly, alongside articles such as "Arab Woman Fights Disease," "Preventing Illness Everywhere," a report on the inauguration of a Hebron clinic, and a romantic short story titled "The Unknown Doctor."[3]

Three decades separate the two physicians, a period of development and maturation of both Palestine's print industry and its professional community. As for the former, in 1919, roughly a decade after the appearance of the first Palestinian periodicals, several literary journals, weeklies, and biweeklies were published. It would take another decade for the first newspaper in Arabic, *Filastin* (est. 1911), to be published on a daily basis. Centered mainly in Jaffa and Jerusalem, the gradual ascendance of the print industry culminated in the 1940s with several dailies and a proliferation of literary, professional, and educational journals.

These publications contributed to the professionalization and popularization of medicine and health. As shown subsequently, the printed press created new kinds of doctor–patient interactions. Palestinians were gradually becoming literate and thus could become part of medical encounters outside the clinic, with doctors they had never met face-to-face. Printed medical knowledge depersonalized these interactions and created an imagined medical community that expanded in tandem with the growth of the doctors' community.

Scholars offer a typology of four kinds of professional associations, which can coexist: (a) an association that emphasizes the profession's knowledge and is dedicated to knowledge exchange and mutual learning; (b) a lobby on behalf of the profession, affecting legislation and policies; (c) a trade union for negotiating professional conditions; (d) an association that controls entry to the profession.[4] Types (c) and (d) are irrelevant for our case study: since most doctors worked in private practice, there was no single employer to negotiate with, and the medical profession had no control over entry to the profession. What we do see in this case is a type (a) association, with some type (b) characteristics.

3 "al-Mar'a al-'Arabiyya tuharibu al-marad"; 'Ali Tawfiq Shusha Basha, "Mukafahat al-marad fi kul makan li-tahqiq salam da'im"; "al-Qafila tazuru mustawsif Khalil al-rahman"; Najwa Qa'war, "Qissat al-'adad: al-Tabib al-majhul," *al-Qafila*, September 5, 1947, 2, 3–5, 12–13, 14–17 (respectively).

4 Michael Burrage, Konrad Jarausch, and Hannes Siegrist, "An Actor-Based Framework for the Study of the Professions," in *Professions in Theory and History: Rethinking the Study of the Professions*, eds. Michael Burrage and Rolf Torstendahl (London: Sage, 1990), 208.

The latter, however, should be qualified in the colonial and settler-colonial context, for which the original model does not account. Lobbying to the authorities meant interaction with a colonial power that had no intention of consulting the local medical profession and, more importantly, relegating any decision-making powers thereto. In addition, with very few exceptions, the professional organization was split along national lines, and professional lobbying meant making specific claims on behalf of Palestinian Arab doctors – against their Jewish-Zionist counterparts and the latter's political and professional power. The analysis of Palestinian doctors' unionization lies within this conceptual framework.

The first section of this chapter focuses on the authorship and role of Palestinian doctors in the Palestinian printed press. Doctors' publications sought to exercise professional, social, and moral authority and claimed professional status within the medical community. Their texts demonstrate the gaps between the writers' self-image and on-the-ground realities. We first explore three main genres of doctors' writing: medical advice columns, essays on modern Arab medicine and cultural revival, and articles envisioning a new medical reality. It then focuses on the writings of three young doctors who sought to reform their society and professional community.

The second part reviews Palestinian doctors' motivations and challenges in establishing professional associations. Most worked alone, either in private clinics or as MOs across the country. Their experience, expertise, and expressiveness in the press were products of intimate encounters with patients rather than daily routines alongside fellow doctors in large hospitals. Membership in associations connected to the American University of Beirut (AUB) or to region-wide medical associations satisfied their need for professional belonging and was of political significance for inter-Arab networking and solidarity. They formed knowledge-exchange networks and platforms for professional and political claims. This part of the chapter is dedicated to their initial failures and ultimate successes in establishing local and national associations.

Medical Texting: Doctors' Treatment of Words

Historians of the French medical profession have noted the extent to which French doctors became, in the late nineteenth century, prolific writers in multiple genres, ranging from medical advice and policy-oriented public health suggestions to history, politics, and more. The Pasteurian revolution heightened physicians' sociocultural standing and lent doctors credibility and legitimacy in matters beyond their clinical expertise. In addition, the growing number of physicians and intensified competition led doctors to seek out a general reading public. The development of print capitalism and growing literacy rates created new venues for expression. At the same time, admission to medical school continued to require a classical male middle-class training in literature, philosophy, and Latin, and medical schools nurtured students' writing skills. This convergence of factors created the physician-writer, and doctors used the press to address their readers' everyday concerns – with obesity and weight loss, maintaining youth and beauty, hygiene or street cleaning, and healthy morals in healthy bodies.[5]

Doctors' writings on medicine, public health, and more general topics were integral to the Arabic Nahda, or renaissance, from at least the 1860s.[6] Nahda luminaries Yaʿqub Sarruf and Faris Nimr published medical articles in their *al-Muqtataf*, one of the earliest scientific journals in Arabic. There, letters to the editor included medical queries. From the 1860s to the 1880s, medical journals such as *Yaʿsub al-Tibb*, *al-Akhbar al-Tibbiyya*, and *al-Tabib* were published in Cairo and Beirut for short periods. Similar journals, scientific or popular, were published throughout the late nineteenth and early twentieth centuries. They marked interrelated phenomena, which this chapter also aims to explore: doctors' involvement in broad social and political debates and the presence of health- and medicine-related topics in the general press. Doctors advised mothers on how to raise their children and young men on how to cultivate their bodies and manage their sexual lives, advertised their trade, and warned the public against quacks.[7]

5 Joan Tumblety, "Rhetoric, Enterprise and Professional Authority: Dr James-Edward Ruffier and Physician-Writers in Twentieth-Century France," *History* 104 (2019): 127–31.

6 Nicole Khayat and Liat Kozma, "Medicine and Arabic Literary Production in the Ottoman Empire during the Nineteenth Century," *The British Journal for the History of Science* 55 (2022): 515–24.

7 Hibba Abugideiri, *Gender and the Making of Modern Medicine in Colonial Egypt* (London: Ashgate, 2010), 187–220; Hanan Kholoussy, "Monitoring and Medicalising Male Sexuality in Semi-Colonial Egypt," *Gender & History* 22 (2010): 677–91; Liat Kozma, "'We, the Sexologists . . .': Arabic Medical Writing on Sexuality, 1879–1943," *Journal of the History of Sexuality* 22 (2013): 426–45.

The interwar period witnessed the proliferation of medical associations in neighboring countries, each priding itself on its medical journal, as did some medical schools in the region. The bilingual *al-Majalla al-Tibbiyya al-Misriyya* (Egyptian Medical Journal) saw light since 1917, preceding the establishment of the Egyptian Medical Association (EMA) by three years, and the Lebanese Medical Association published *al-Majalla al-Tibbiyya al-ʿIlmiyya* in 1923. The AUB published the short-lived *Medical Society Gazette of the American University of Beirut* (1929–31), the Medical School in Damascus published *Majallat al-Maʿhad al-Tibbi al-ʿArabi* beginning in 1924, and the Iraqi Royal College of Medicine published *Majallat al-Kulliyya al-Tibbiyya* beginning in 1935. The professional community also read and contributed to foreign journals, but the ones published by and for Arab doctors provided a discursive and scientific platform throughout the region.

Physicians' prolific presence in the Palestinian press accompanied it from its inception, offering their medical expertise on issues of broad public concern. In addition, they positioned themselves as public intellectuals whose professional status and education had given them the authority to speak on public questions. Writing in the press, doctors also aspired to enhance their profession's authority in a pluralist and competitive market, which included lay practitioners and foreign doctors. During the Mandate, doctors were not allowed to advertise their trade, only to announce in the press that they had changed their address or working hours.[8] Instead, advice columns and general medical information they published in the press enabled them to market themselves indirectly.[9]

Medical Advice and Moral Vice

Medical advice columns were the most common conduit doctors employed to make a name for themselves. Such columns usually

8 Muhammad ʿAql, *Muʿjam al-atibbaʾ wa-l-sayadila al-Filastiniyyin (1748–1948)* (ʿArʿara: self-published, 2021), vol. 1, 133–34.

9 Philippe Bourmaud, "Experts at Large: Physicians, Public Debate and the Press in Late Ottoman Palestine," *Archív Orientální* 80 (2012): 295–305; Yoni Furas, "'What did the Ottomans ever do for us?' Modern Medicine and Administration in Late Ottoman Jerusalem," in *From the Household to the Wider World: Local Perspectives on Urban Institutions in Late Ottoman Bilad al-Sham*, eds. Yuval Ben-Bassat and Johann Büssow (Tübingen: University of Tübingen Press, 2022), 243–61.

included an introduction about a disease and its symptoms, followed by its broad social causes, usually a combination of ignorance and immoral or unhealthy conduct. The authors would then move on to practical advice on prevention and conclude with personal and societal repercussions. "What is the value of life itself," asks Dr. Mustafa Bek Fakhri, "if we cannot appreciate it with healthy eyes?" It is "lawlessness and permissiveness" that cause venereal diseases that harm the eyes the most, notes the Jaffa ophthalmologist. "Be careful young man, and protect your body from these maladies," he concludes, "as the nation's future and hopes are in your hand."[10] Articles on ocular diseases emphasized the importance of medical treatment, asserting that a patient should be rushed to the doctor to prevent permanent damage. They also advised readers to use sunglasses and avoid touching their eyes and prolonged exposure to dust.[11]

Another major medical issue in Palestine was tuberculosis (TB), which, as elsewhere at the time, was considered a "social disease" whose eradication required comprehensive social reform. Palestinian doctors considered poverty, poor housing, and poor hygiene to be contributory factors and used the daily press to advise the public about prevention and eradication. As in other realms, doctors decried the lack of government investment and gaps between Jewish and Arab patients. Jewish health institutions established clinics and sanatoriums, while Arab patients had no hospitalization options.[12]

More generally, doctors advised readers on what to do in cases of emergency, and no less importantly – what not to do. Dr. Hasan Hindi from Haifa advised readers on how to treat simple bone fractures and severe bleeding before rushing the patient to a hospital. He also cautioned readers not to heed the advice of local healers, who might recommend pouring coffee on an open wound, or that of a *mujabbir* (traditional bonesetter), who would fix a broken limb without

10 Mustafa Fakhri, "al-ʿAynayin wa-taʾthir al-amrad al-zuhriyya ʿalayhima," *Filastin*, November 4, 1934, 5.

11 Hana Habib Qayala, "Amrad al-ʿuyun," *al-Difaʿ*, June 9, 1941, 4; Hana Habib Qayala, "al-Amrad al-multahama," *al-Difaʿ*, July 15, 1941, 4; Wahbi Jabji, "Intishar amrad al-ʿuyun fi al-sayf: Darurat al-wiqaya wa-irshadat hamma li-l-muhafaza," *al-Difaʿ*, August 5, 1938, 7.

12 For example, ʿIsa al-ʿIsa, "Wasaya ʿashr li-ittiqaʾ al-sill," *Filastin*, May 8, 1932, 3; "Bahth sihhi mufid: Maʿlumat ʿan marad al-sill," *al-Difaʿ*, January 26, 1936, 6; Niʿma Nakhu, "Marad al-sill: Bahth tibbi mushab tajibu mutalaʿtuhu," *al-Sirat al-Mustaqim*, September 2, 1941, 2.

knowledge of anatomy.[13] Dentists published columns about dental hygiene, explained how cavities were formed, and instructed patients on what to do about toothaches while waiting for their dental appointment.[14]

From its onset in 1936, the Palestine Broadcasting Service (PBS) initiated a weekly health-related broadcast. Doctors' voices could now be publicly heard, not just read. In 1946, the Palestine Arab Medical Association (PAMA) sponsored a similar initiative.[15] Some of these broadcasts were later published in the press. In Tawfiq Canaan's radio broadcast on child nutrition and hygiene, he advised avoiding sweets and excessive eating, keeping the kitchen clean, and washing fruits and vegetables with clean water.[16] These articles and lectures often included popularized medical knowledge and consistent advice to consult a doctor in case of need.

Regarding child development, Dr. Habib Qattan cautioned his readers that mothers' neglect and ignorance about disease prevention and treatment jeopardized children's health and, hence, the national future. In one of his pieces, he told the story of an infant with severe diarrhea, whose older siblings had died in infancy. Following her neighbors' advice, the mother insisted on feeding the child unadulterated cow's milk instead of breastfeeding. It was her ignorance that led to her baby's death, he concluded. Dr. Qattan recommended breastfeeding children and insisted on fresh milk and sterilized bottles if cow's milk was used.[17]

To ensure the normal development of the fetus and infant, advice to expecting and young mothers included regular visits to the physician. Pregnant women were to wear loose clothes and care for bodily hygiene. Doctors advised mothers to breastfeed their babies at regular intervals and avoid animal milk for as long as possible.[18] Others

13 Hasan Hindi, "Isʿafat awwaliyya fi al-tawariʾ," *al-Muntada*, March 1, 1946, 7.

14 Sami Zuʿrub, "Tasawwus al-asnan," *al-Zahra*, August 1, 1924, 233–38; Kamil Itayim, "Sihhat al-insan fi salamat al-asnan," *al-Muntada*, November 1, 1943, 14 and January 1, 1944, 20; Kamil Itayim, "Alam al-asnan ʿadhab li-l-insan," *al-Muntada*, March 1, 1944, 16.

15 Mahmud Tahir al-Dajani, "al-Tibb fi al-ʿashr sanawat al-madiya wa-taqaddum al-hala al-sihhiyya fi Filastin," *al-Muntada*, April 19, 1946, 10–11.

16 Tawfiq Canaan, "al-Taʿam fi al-sihha," *al-Muntada*, December 6, 1946.

17 Habib Qattan, "al-Wafayat bayna al-atfal," *al-Muntada*, November 1, 1945, 16, 22.

18 Mahmuad Tahir al-Dajani, "al-ʿInaya bi-l-tifl," *Huna al-Quds*, October 21, 1941, 15–16; "Irshadat li-l-sayyidat athna al-haml," *al-Muntada*, March 15,

suggested that childcare, health, and hygiene would be incorporated into the girls' school curriculum. They also entrusted nurses with the responsibility of educating mothers on how to nourish children and care for their hygiene.[19] Others advised mothers about balanced nutrition and warned about diseases caused by specific nutritional ingredients.[20]

A Palestinian Medical Nahda

The doctor's self-perceived role was not restricted to the ability to treat diseases or infections. Doctors often discussed their profession's social position – past, present, and future. "There are two main reasons I chose to study dentistry," wrote Salim Salama in 1919. The first was the country's "dire need" for trained specialists in the field, since "rotten teeth are amongst the widespread diseases of the civilized world." The second reason was "that this profession merges science, one of the most important and broadest sciences, and art, amongst the beautiful and lofty arts."[21] Curing mouth's illnesses, we are told, is not only a scientific endeavor but involves the patient's facial aesthetics and therefore requires the craft of an artist.

Dr. Qaysar Khuri (b. 1893) from Bkassine, in southern Lebanon, settled in Haifa after World War I (WWI) and opened a private clinic. Like Salama, he considered himself a Nahda man, referring to himself as a poet-doctor or doctor-poet.[22] Khuri read and published his own poetry and even combined medical advice with verse. In *al-Zahra*, a literary journal published in Haifa, he dedicated a poem to the symptoms and cures of the Spanish flu and another to the romantic virtues of cigarette smoking.[23] Known for his poetic skills, he even improvised

1946, 15; Hasan Far'un, "Al-'Inaya bi-sihhat al-atfal fi al-qarya," *al-Majalla al-Zira'iyya al-'Arabiyya*, July 1, 1947.

19 Hasan Far'un, "al-Tarbiyya al-sihhiyya fi al-bayt wa-l-madrasa," *al-Muntada*, October 1, 1945, 16.

20 Muhammad 'Izzat Adham, "Amrad al-atfal al-nashi'a 'an su' al-taghdiya," *al-Muntada*, February 15, 1946.

21 Salim Salama, "Rasa'il tabib," *al-Nafayis al-'Asriyya*, December 15, 1919, 153.

22 Qaysar Khuri, *al-Dhikrayat* (Jerusalem: al-Matba'a al-tijariya, 1945), 5.

23 See, for example, Qaysar Khuri, "al-Wafida aw al-huma' al-isba'nyuliyya," *al-Zahra* 2, May 2, 1922, no. 1–2, 65–66; Qaysar Khuri, "Sikarati," *al-Zahra* 2, May 2, 1922, no. 23–24, 493–94.

a *qasida* for fellow doctors at the 1933 Haifa conference, celebrating the historical event.[24]

This Nahda spirit echoed strongly in articles about the Arab and Islamic golden ages, especially in medicine. The doctors imagined a Nahda in which they had a significant role.[25] They celebrated the golden age of Arab sciences and described a subsequent state of decline, followed by modern science as the remedy for social ills. Like other Nahda men, they positioned themselves as harbingers of modernity and sought to enlighten the public. The press served as a major venue for saving the public from the mortal dangers of ignorance, superstition, and neglect and for educating the public about health and hygiene. University of Hamburg graduate Husam Wafa Dajani (b. 1909) contributed several articles to *al-Difa'* on historical Arab scientific innovations and superiority over Western medicine.[26] Another doctor wrote in 1946: "We are entitled to be proud and have the right to bring to life that which was lost."[27]

A correspondence on the pages of the *British Medical Journal* in late 1946 and early 1947 exemplified the importance of Palestinian pride in the past. A paragraph-long review letter published by a British physician argued that "'Arabian' medicine was largely the work of Persians, Jews, and Syrians."[28] In one of the journal's following issues, Jerusalemite dentist Dr. Ibrahim George published a longer review letter defending Arab achievements, listing prominent Arab scientists, and explaining that it was the global Arab system that enabled and supported the role of scholars from different cultures.[29] George's reply letter was then translated into Arabic and published in

24 "In'iqad mu'tamar al-atibba' al-'Arabi bi-Hayfa," *Filastin*, June 20, 1933, 7.

25 Compare Sherene Seikaly, *Men of Capital: Scarcity and Economy in Mandate Palestine* (Stanford: Stanford University Press, 2016), 46–47.

26 Husam Wafa al-Dajani, "Ma'thar al-hadara al-Islamiyya: Muhadara fi al-tibb 'inda al-'Arab," *al-Difa'*, June 12–13, 1935, 6; Husam Wafa al-Dajani, "Yawm kana al-mulq lahum: 'Ilm tahdir al-adwiya' wa-l-nabat 'inda al-'Arab," *al-Difa'*, August 19, 1935; Husam Wafa al-Dajani, "Abu al-Qasim al-Zawahiri: Abu al-jaraha fi al-qurun al-wusta," *al-Difa'*, 12 September, 1935, 6.

27 Nabih Faris, "al-'Alam al-'Arabi wa-mustaqbaluhu," *al-Wahda*, April 13, 1946, 5; see also 'Uthman al-Khamra, "al-Tibb 'inda al-'Arab," *al-Karmil*, February 6, 1927, 4.

28 Anthony Neligan, "Rhazes and Avicenna," *British Medical Journal* 2:4484 (December 14, 1946): 919.

29 Ibrahim George, "History of Arab Medicine," *British Medical Journal* 2:4491 (February 1, 1947): 202.

al-Wahda.[30] This debate over civilizational medical virtues on the pages of a British platform showcased the profession's cultural and political attributes. Doctors also claimed a historical role, finding roots that gave them meaning and a sense of belonging.

Talking Policy: Medical Road Maps

The substantial gap between the availability of medical services in the countryside and the city was another recurrent topic in doctors' publications. The Arab physician's absence from the countryside troubled Palestinian physicians, who voiced concerns in the press and urged colleagues to actively change this situation. In a 1947 interview in *al-Qafila*, three leading medical professionals, Tawfiq Canaan, Mahmud Tahir al-Dajani, and Burhan ʿAbd al-Hadi, were asked about their vision for the future development of Palestine's health services and ways to convince Arab doctors to work in the countryside. Dr. Canaan stated that more national hospitals should be opened in which Arab doctors would serve Arab patients – both in cities and the countryside. Like him, Dr. ʿAbd al-Hadi emphasized that Palestinian doctors should be less reliant on foreign health services. To encourage doctors to work in the countryside, he suggested better means of transportation and hygienic clinics supplied with running water and electricity. Dr. Dajani argued that medical services in the countryside were, first and foremost, the responsibility of the Mandate authorities. The government should pave roads to villages, provide peasants with healthy living conditions, and only after those steps had been taken could it make young doctors' urban practice conditional upon two years of service in the countryside.[31] This interview encapsulated doctors' public advocacy during the Mandate: the need for health propaganda, national hospitals, and medical service in the countryside. It also revealed the professional community's limited ability to solve problems of which they were acutely aware.

Calls for Arab doctors and the Arab community more broadly to take matters into their hands were voiced earlier. In May 1932,

[30] Ibrahim Jurj, "al-Tibb ʿinda al-ʿArab," *al-Wahda*, March 8, 1947, 4.

[31] "al-Qafila tastajwibu atibbaʾ thalatha," *al-Qafila*, May 30, 1947, 5–6; see also Dr. ʿAli ʿAqla, "al-Qarya al-ʿArabiyya, daʾuha wa-dawaʾuha," *al-Muntada*, December 1, 1943, 6–7; ʿAli ʿAqla, "Tabib al-nadi al-ʿArabi bi-Yafa," *al-Difaʿ*, November 27, 1945, 3.

Jaffa-based Dr. Emil Abu Khalil, a recent graduate of the University of Rome, lamented the poor state of Arab medicine in Palestine. He stressed the pressing need for a national hospital – like the one Dr. Fu'ad Dajani had just started building. Hospitals in Palestine were not better than "medieval prisons," he proclaimed, and "it is shameful that we do not have a single Arab hospital, a single Arab maternity ward, a single Arab infant care center, and a single Arab dispensary." Consequently, he concluded, "It is high time that Palestinians understand that there is no nation without men, no men without health, and no health without national hospitals and medical institutions. Yes – national, Palestinian, and Arab."[32] Abu Khalil's call reflected growing public interest in and understanding of the personal and collective benefits of medical self-reliance. It also mentioned Dajani's hospital as an exception. Since its construction, it served as a model institution and a source of inspiration that remained unparalleled until the Nakba.

The public was not only aware of healthcare benefits but also had high expectations of doctors as individuals. In an opinion piece from the late 1930s, an anonymous author (*al-dalil*, "The Guide") accused Palestine's Arab doctors of caring for little but profit and fame, neglecting their duties, and pushing the poor into the hands of charlatans and missionaries. The author describes a doctor who refused to treat the poor and showed little concern for their fate, even when no other doctor was available. Private doctors, The Guide lamented, neglected the poor and squeezed the rich, while government doctors enjoyed a comfortable job and failed to use it to address their society's medical needs.[33]

Palestinian individuals and societies made several calls, plans, and attempts to establish an Arab hospital. Most failed. When the Department of Health (DoH) decided in 1934 to establish a TB hospital in Nazareth, the Palestinian press adamantly objected. Citizens wrote petitions and formed a committee to fight the decision.[34]

32 Emil Abu Khalil, "al-Hala al-sihhiyya wa-l-mustashfayat al-wataniyya fi Filastin," *Filastin*, May 14, 1932, 2. Dr. Abu Khalil started working in al-Dajani's hospital in the 1940s; see also, Al-Nadi al-ʿArabi bi-Yafa, "Amrad al-ʿuyun fi al-qura wa-wasaʾil mukafahatiha," *Filastin*, December 22, 1945, 2.

33 "al-Dalil," "al-Maʿrad al-ʿamm: al-Atibbaʾ," *Filastin*, August 20, 1932, 2.

34 "Hawla mustashfa al-sill fi al-Nasira," *Filastin*, April 7, 1934, 2; "Mustashfa al-sill," *al-Difaʿ*, January 17, 1936, 7.

In response to this public outcry, Dr. Niʿma Nakhu, a native of Nazareth and director of Dahr al-Bashiq Sanatorium east of Beirut, invited *Filastin*'s editor to visit two of Lebanon's TB sanatoriums, and explained why Palestine and Nazareth, specifically, would benefit from such a hospital. He noted that the hospital's foreseen isolated location would prevent mass infection in Palestine and separate TB patients from family and friends. Nakhu added that since TB was droplet-borne rather than airborne, sanatorium workers were rarely infected, and patients could learn basic hygiene rules to protect their surroundings. TB carriers and patients were all around, while hospital patients maintained hygiene routines that kept them safe. Furthermore, the very existence of a sanatorium would raise awareness of the disease and could help identify the illness among friends. Economically, Nakhu added, the hospital would yield income to the host city: it would provide its food and services, while patient guests could sleep and dine in the city.[35] Nakhu's call remained unanswered.

After reviewing several initiatives to establish TB hospitals in neighboring countries, *al-Difaʿ* criticized the colonial government for offering no solution.[36] In May 1946, the Palestine Anti-Tuberculosis Society started raising funds to establish a sanatorium that would treat poor patients for free.[37] The plan failed to materialize.

Doctors continued to advocate for more medical institutions. They addressed both the DoH and the Palestinian public, calling on them to participate in establishing an autonomous medical system or at least independent medical institutions. In November 1943, former DoH physician and long-time politician Husayn Fakhri Khalidi listed the medical institutions the DoH should establish, including infectious disease, government, and mental hospitals. In addition, he called on the Supreme Muslim Council to take responsibility for orphanages, hospices, prenatal and infant care centers, and more.[38] With its roots in

35 "Mustashfa al-sill fi al-Nasira wa-l-fawaʾid al-sihhiyya wa-l-iqtisadiyya al-marjjuwa minhu," *Filasitn*, November 4, 1934, 4. For Nakhu's other publications see in "Dr. Nakhu yatakalamu ʿan marad al-sill," *al-Sirat al-Mustaqim*, August 30, 1941, 2, and September 2, 1941, 2 and Niʿma Nakhu, "Asbab al-mawt 1900 wa-1946," *al-Minbar*, March 1, 1947, 112.

36 "Limadha la tabni al-hukuma mustashfa li-l-sill," *al-Difaʿ*, March 27, 1945.

37 Raʾfat Faris, "Kalima bi-niyaba ʿan ittihad al-jamʿiyyat al-ʿArabiyya li-mukafahat al-sill fi Filastin," *al-Muntada*, May 17, 1946, 12.

38 Husayn Fakhri al-Khalidi, "Mashariʿ al-inshaʾ wa-l-tajdid al-sihhiyya fi Filastin baʿd al-harb," *al-Muntada*, November 1, 1943, 45.

the 1930s, this criticism was voiced until the Mandate ended, with different doctors offering different solutions. The following analysis focuses on three doctors who started their careers during that decade.

The Mandate Generation: Budayri, Dajani, and Shuqayri

The 1930s, especially their latter half, marked a new phase in the social history of Palestine's medical community. The "last Ottoman generation" of doctors became a small minority in a growing community, which gradually absorbed dozens of doctors who were children or adolescents when the British occupied Palestine. This generation graduated from medical faculties during the early 1930s and matured professionally during political and military upheavals. Globally, it was a decade of competing ideologies and rhetorical extremes articulated through novel channels such as the radio, cinema, and above all, the printed press. These were also years of expansion of literacy and the establishment of Arabic dailies alongside an expanding market of scientific books and journals from Palestine and beyond.[39] In Palestine, there were more doctors, more conduits to articulate what was on their minds, and, most importantly, more people who could read and respond to their publications.

The Mandate generation did not join the government sector in similar proportions to its predecessor, and its members were not veterans of any war. The discourse of equality and political rights within an empire while seeking to find a position within it was eclipsed by one of political emancipation and self-determination. Above all, with colonialism deepening its roots, the hegemonic vocabulary for the articulation of these concepts was nationalism. Doctors mobilized the medical discourse for the national cause, and personal health was seen through a collectivist prism. The association of individual health with a strong and sound society in the late Ottoman period gave way to an association with a strong nation.

Three representatives of that generation – Mahmud Tahir al-Dajani (b. 1907), Khalil al-Budayri (b. 1909), and Anwar al-Shuqayri (b. 1909) – typified different approaches. While all three conveyed a deep sense of responsibility toward their community, nation, and

[39] Ami Ayalon, *Reading Palestine: Printing and Literacy, 1900–1948* (Austin: University of Texas Press, 2004), 16–41.

profession, each focused on different societal ills and prescribed different remedies. Dajani viewed hygiene and civilization as pillars of national progress; Budayri emphasized the internationalist struggle for political liberation; and Shuqayri shifted focus inward, writing professional critiques and preaching professional reform.

Dajani, Shuqayri, and Budayri were born into Palestinian prominence. Their families owned land and assets, enjoyed senior positions in the Ottoman civil and religious administration, and played central roles within the political leadership. They enjoyed the best private education their families could buy and grew up among public figures, often even related to famous authors, editors, publishers, and leading intellectuals. Expressing well-articulated views was expected, if not required, of them.

While studying at AUB, Mahmud Tahir al-Dajani was president of the Student Union and head of the Palestinian students' club, giving speeches and leading rallies.[40] After graduating in 1932, he opened a private clinic on Mamila Street in Jerusalem, but his public persona was well-known beyond its walls. Already in October that year, he held a talk in the Arab Sports Club in Jerusalem about the peril of venereal diseases. Syphilis and gonorrhea, he explained, were among the ills brought to Palestine by the West. Dajani recommended early marriage, sports, Boy Scout activities, and avoiding "evil girls." Prostitutes were no more than disease vectors and should be avoided, he warned the Jerusalemite youth.[41]

Although not employed by the DoH, Dajani delivered his later lectures and published articles in British-sponsored forums. Even amid the Arab Revolt's violent years, he broadcasted a weekly talk on PBS titled *Talk on Hygiene*, and many of his later publications appeared in the station's journals: *Huna al-Quds*, *al-Muntada*, and *al-Qafila*.[42] Those were more diplomatic less moralistic or admonishing than the lecture mentioned earlier, yet they maintained a similar collectivist

40 "The Students' Union Opening Meeting," *al-Kulliyyah* 15, no. 7, May 1929, 185; "First University Reception," *al-Kulliyyah* 16, no. 1, November 1929, 7.

41 Mahmud Tahir al-Dajani, "al-Amrad al-zuhariyya wa-turuq al-wiqaya minha," *al-Akhlaq*, October 1, 1932, 371–76.

42 "Wireless Programmes," *Palestine Post*, April 8, 1936, 6; May 26, 1936, 4; July 8, 1936, 5; August 5, 1936, 5; September 2, 1936, 4; October 14, 1936, 4; November 11, 1936, 4; December 23, 1936, 4; January 20, 1937, 6; February 17, 1937, 4; April 28, 1937, 7; May 12, 1938, 6; October 4, 1938, 4.

tone. Dajani underlined Arabs' remarkable achievements in the field of health during the Islamic golden ages and made efforts linking his advice to Islamic traditions. In *Medicine and the Holy Hadith*, he declared that the progress of nations was measured by medical conditions and criticized people's reliance on traditional healers rather than doctors. He then discussed the wrongful interpretation of the Hadith: "Healing is in three things: a gulp of honey, cupping, and branding with fire (cauterizing). However, I forbid my followers to use branding with fire." Instead of forthrightly contradicting the Prophet, Dajani offered an apologetic that affirmed the Hadith's compatibility with modern science. At present, he noted, only doctors could fully interpret the Hadith, while local healers were liable to cause more harm than good.[43] In an article about home cleanliness, Dajani attacked those who refused to follow hygienic rules and succumbed to diseases.[44] For him, the doctor was a soldier fighting diseases, but its prevention was every person's responsibility, "and he who ignores it ruins the [nation's] foundation ... while spreading the poison of disease."[45]

Above all, Dajani's articles articulated moral engagement with the medical profession and the community. His public persona projected devotion to his community's well-being and deep conviction in medicine's contribution to humanity. He brought forward his Arab identity and criticized the DoH, albeit mildly.[46] During World War II (WWII), when PBS and its publications were dedicated to pro-British and anti-Axis propaganda, Dajani wrote about the sacred role of British doctors on both the battle and home fronts, and their scientific medical breakthroughs – in contradiction to all the blood and destruction caused by the war.[47]

Dajani's preference for broadcasting and publishing his articles in colonial platforms was primarily instrumental. PBS was the only

43 Mahmud Tahir al-Dajani, "al-Tibb fi al-hadith al-sharif," *Huna al-Quds*, November 16, 1941, 11–12.

44 Mahmud Tahir al-Dajani, "al-Bayt al-sihhi," *al-Muntada*, April 1, 1943, 17.

45 Mahmud Tahir al-Dajani, "al-Amrad wa-l-harb," *al-Muntada*, May 1, 1943, 21.

46 See his enthusiastic report on the 15th Arab Medical Congress in Cairo, Mahmud Tahir al-Dajani, "al-Mu'tamar al-tibbi al-ʿArabi," *al-Muntada*, February 1, 1944, 17.

47 Mahmud Tahir al-Dajani, "Athr al-tibb fi al-harb," *al-Muntada*, January 1, 1944, 3–5.

available radio station, and its journals published articles by Palestine's leading intellectuals. After establishing PAMA in 1944, Dajani no longer expressed personal views or advice but spoke as a spokesperson for PAMA's vision.

A published correspondence in *al-Wahda* between him and a critic of Palestinian doctors reflects this change. In March 1946, George Khuri Samʿan (signed as J.Kh.S) lamented the lack of medical treatment in villages and argued that Arab doctors' primary motivation was profit rather than humanistic ideals. Foreign doctors, he argued, traveled to distant villages to treat patients, while Arab doctors barely left their cities, and one rarely saw them traveling to a distant village at night to treat a patient for a reasonable price.[48]

Dajani replied the following week, advising Samʿan to address his concerns to PAMA, which would quickly investigate the matter. "Don't you know," Dajani asked him, "that the foreign doctors in Palestine do not treat us for our black eyes" but rather for their own political interests? Arab doctors were leading several initiatives to collect donations to build hospitals across Palestine. In them, Dr. Dajani assured the critic, he would be able to find poor patients treated for the sake of God and not for profit.[49] Samʿan was not satisfied. In the following issue, he argued that the initiators of new hospitals were not doctors, and that he had not heard of any association member (or nonmember) who had opened a clinic in a village.[50]

Dajani's response to Samʿan expressed his conviction that PAMA's various projects were bound to materialize and bear long-awaited fruit. In writing, at least, he was already talking in terms of national-professional responsibility and accountability. A month after the correspondence with Samʿan, he returned to *al-Muntada* and published a long review titled "Medicine during the Past Ten Years and Progress in Health Condition in Palestine." In it, he mentioned the creation of health consciousness and the presence of doctors in places never attended before. Dajani admitted that hospitals still had to be

48 J. K. H. S., "Atibba'una wa-l-mada," *al-Wahda*, March 2, 1946; similar criticism in "al-Turuq al-ʿamaliyya li-inhad al-qarya al-ʿArabiyya," *Filastin*, April 27, 1947, 2.

49 Mahmud Tahir al-Dajani, "Radd ʿala kalima," *al-Wahda*, March 9, 1946, 7.

50 Jurj Khuri Samʿan, "Ila' al-duktur Mahmud al-Dajani," *al-Wahda*, March 30, 1946, 7.

constructed and expressed his optimism "that our near future will witness a glorious civilizational movement."[51]

Budayri marked another trajectory, that of socialism and anti-imperialism, more political and less instructive than Dajani. The son of a notable Jerusalemite sheikh, Budayri experienced the thorns of the British occupation at a young age. He grew up hearing of frequent British interrogations of his cousin for his politics and of his father for his teachings and attended national meetings and conferences. At sixteen, Budayri traveled to Germany to complete his secondary education, witnessed the turbulent early 1920s, and was inspired by Schiller's *William Tell* and his "anticolonial" struggle. He attended both fascist and communist demonstrations. The fascist demonstrations against the English and French, enemies of the Arab cause, were to his liking. Budayri was deeply impressed by German culture and politics but also alarmed by their hatred of and ignorance about Islam and Muslims. He later studied at the American University in Cairo, participating in Egypt's heated political debates. Since the early 1920s, Budayri had published articles in the local Palestinian press.[52] In his mind, he was a cosmopolitan leftist intellectual, a Muslim, a Palestinian, and a doctor.

According to his memoir, Budayri chose to study medicine in Geneva because of the city's international importance as headquarters of the League of Nations. He studied with Syrian, Egyptian, and Lebanese students and continued to read local and foreign press. It was there, through the communist *L'Humanité*, that he became acquainted with socialism, devouring communist literature, attending rallies, and publishing articles in the communist press against French colonialism in Syria.[53] He returned to Jerusalem in 1932, volunteered, and then worked at St. John's Ophthalmic Hospital. Budayri writes that he did not get the job because of his professional qualities but because his employment in a British institution enabled the authorities to keep close watch over him. He accepted the offer despite the poor salary and imperial surveillance because it enabled him to treat as

[51] al-Dajani, "al-Tibb fi al-ʿashr sanawat".

[52] Khalil Budayri, *Sitta wa-sittun ʿaman maʿa al-haraka al-wataniyya al-Filastiniya wa-fiha: Tarikh ma aghfalahu al-tarikh* (Jerusalem: Mansharat Salah al-Din, 1982), 11, 13, 28, 31–32, 38–44.

[53] Ibid., 46–48.

many patients as he could for free.[54] He would continue working there for fourteen years.

In Jerusalem, Budayri bonded with a group of Lebanese socialists and contributed articles to the Damascene left-wing *al-Duhur* ("The Ages") and its successor *al-Taliʿa* ("The Vanguard"). In his mid twenties, having lived in Egypt, Germany, and Switzerland, he dedicated himself to socialism, and his essays spoke for enlightenment and liberation of oppressed masses.[55] While witnessing the popularity of fascism among Palestinian youth, he criticized its deceiving ideology, which preached self-sacrifice of the masses and demanded acceptance of their predicament, offering nothing in return. True nationalism, Budayri noted in 1936, aspired for education of all, the personal development of self, and freedom of will and expression. Rather than experimentation and scientific analysis, he prophesied, fascism propagated myths, and its ideology of racial supremacy and ambitions of world domination was bound to lead to war and destruction.[56]

Budayri was also an anti-imperialist and ardent advocate of a unified Arab front against British-American-Zionist colonialism. In "The Road to Liberation," he criticized the Syrian and Egyptian cooperation with their colonizers, which failed to lead them to independence.[57] In 1946, Budayri noted that all negotiations with the British would practically legitimize Britain's role in Palestine and the Jewish "national home" project. Still, his articles stressed the ability of the United Nations (UN) and international community to force the British to change their policy, advocating engaging in this new world order for the sake of the Palestinian cause and peace.[58] In late April 1947, the socialist doctor joined the Palestinian delegation to the UN.[59] The

54 Ibid., 63–64.

55 Ibid., 68–70. See also Khalil Budayri, "Amraduna al-wahmiyya! al-Taraddud wa-l-talakkuʾ wa-l-hayra," *al-Liwaʾ*, February 25 and 27, 1936, 1. The same article was also published in *al-Taliʿa*, March 1, 1936, 87–89.

56 Khalil Budayri, "al-Fashiyya wa-l-wataniyya," *Filastin*, January 5, 1936, 3.

57 Khalil Budayri, "Sabil al-taharrur," *al-Difaʿ*, January 27, 1936, 1.

58 Khalil Budayri, "Kayfa yumkinuna an natanazalu al-istiʿmar," *al-Ghad*, June 7, 1946, 9–10; Khalil Budayri, "Ittaqu Allah fi anfusikim," *al-Ghad*, June 21, 1946, 9–10; Khalil Budayri, "Hulul muʿaqada tatalaʾamu maʿa ahdaf al-istiʿmar al-nukraʾ," *al-Ghad*, August 2, 1946, 5–6; Khalil Budayri, "Man tufawiduna wa-fi ma tufawidun," *al-Ghad*, August 30, 1946, 11; Khalil Budayri, "wa-l-An … madha nahnu faʿilun?," *al-Difaʿ*, February 23, 1947, 1, 4.

59 "Indimam al-duktur Khalil Budayri, li-wafd ʿArab Filastin," *Filastin*, April 27, 1947, 1.

struggle Budayri advocated was not an armed but a diplomatic one, believing that should the Arabs unify and advocate their cause properly in the international arena, they would convince the rest of the world. The 1948 war ended his two years of failed diplomatic efforts. He had resigned from St. John's in 1946 but returned in 1948, working there until retirement in 1970, a nonpartisan socialist in a missionary hospital.

In 1979, four years before his death, the Jerusalem branch of the Doctors' Association held a celebration commemorating fifty years since Budayri's graduation. The seventy-year-old doctor once again conceptualized the medical profession as part of a greater political emancipatory project, tying well-being and liberation of man and society with physical well-being.[60] Budayri worked for an Anglican missionary institution but openly wrote about a postcolonial reality. Dajani was independently employed but found his platform within the colonial framework. Both signed anti-British leaflets during the Revolt, calling to boycott the government and refuse to pay taxes.[61] Both continued their employment under the British in the following years. Dajani focused on the triangle of civilization, medicine, and progress and Budayri on physical, mental, and political liberation.

By contrast, the attention of Shuqayri, the young doctor from Acre, was directed inward, criticizing shortcomings and envisioning prospects of the medical community. Unlike his Jerusalemite counterparts, in Acre he was not surrounded by government, private, and missionary hospitals. His prism is thus unique, for it represented a peripheral angle. His assassination in 1939 ended a short (and promising) career of a doctor and public intellectual.

Shuqayri's criticism of the Palestinian medical community was adamant. In an article about the competition with Jewish doctors, he argued that Arab doctors shared part of the responsibility for the poor population's preference for Jewish doctors. He further noted that Arab doctors "remain selfish" and criticized their avoidance of the national movement. Shuqayri called upon Arab doctors to unionize for scientific research and public health, as well as against Jewish immigrant doctors who would soon put them out of their jobs. While none of the Arab political or civil organizations engaged in health matters, he wrote, Jews were sending doctors to Arab villages.[62]

[60] Budayri, *Sitta wa-sittun 'aman*, 223–24. [61] Ibid., 82, 84–85.

[62] Anwar al-Shuqayri, "al-Munafasa bayna al-atibba' al-'Arab wa-l-yahud," *al-Difa'*, March 15, 1936, 7; Adam 'Anabusi, "Anwar al-Shuqayri, tabib al-thwara wa-'aqluha," Hebrew University, November 2018, unpublished paper.

Shuqayri also criticized British and Jewish doctors' reliance on foreign medical knowledge. In one of his articles, he commented on a survey conducted by the DoH on typhoid in Haifa, arguing that its prevention and sanitary policies were deficient. Terminating the spread of typhoid could only be achieved by examining its local causes and local nutrition habits, and each neighborhood's latrines, sewage, and flies should be examined separately. He then criticized Arab doctors for neglecting this field and for rarely using government laboratories for autopsies. While working at the Haifa Government Hospital, Shuqayri was inspired by the British health regulation of their soldiers and called to implement the army's mandatory vaccine policy.[63]

Shuqayri's vision of a proper national public health system was persistent. In 1938 he attended the Arab Medical Association Congress in Baghdad and published an article series about his experience. He wrote with admiration of the Iraqi medical Nahda, its progress, and the virtues of its army. In the field of public health, he noted that every district had its head doctor, assisted by other doctors, a big hospital, and small ones in every subdistrict, and highlighted the Royal College of Medicine in Baghdad. More than depicting public health in Iraq, the young doctor drew his vision for public health in Palestine.[64] Shuqayri's roadmap included establishing a training facility in Palestine, forming a solid professional union with clear national goals, and, more broadly, emancipation of the medical community from colonial strains to assume full responsibility for the well-being of all Palestinians. He did not survive to witness it, but a significant step in meeting his call would be taken roughly five years after his death.

The Unionization of Palestine's Arab Doctors

Regional networks predated the autonomous urban and national associations and were also maintained by the circulation of medical texts and the annual EMA meetings. These inspired and encouraged local players. This section maps the evolution of professional unionization until it reached fruition in the mid 1940s.

63 Anwar al-Shuqayri, "Bahth tibbi: Intishar humma al-tayfu'id bi-Hayfa," *al-Difa'*, May 20, 1935, 8.
64 Anwar al-Shuqayri, "Ayam Baghdad: al-Jaysh wa-l-tayyaran," *al-Difa'*, March 24, 1938, 2.

Regional Networking

Chapter 2 discussed AUB's fundamental role in creating a regional cultural, professional, and national network. For most Palestinian doctors, it was there that they gained acquaintance with the region. The intense years of training in the institution formed camaraderie and a sense of empowerment. These social, professional, and political ties would become central for unionization processes in the region. The annual EMA meetings expanded these networks and deepened ties. Since 1928, Palestinian doctors were regular participants in these meetings, held first in Egypt and, beginning in 1931, in neighboring countries. Conferences were no longer under the auspices of a foreign university, which enabled the participation of all community members regardless of their alma mater. For Arab doctors across the region, these gatherings articulated national and professional empowerment, underlining shared challenges and possible solutions.

The Sixth Annual Congress was held in April 1933 at the recently inaugurated YMCA building in Jerusalem, attended by 300 doctors, of whom 182 were Egyptian and 96 Palestinians – including 40 Jews. Palestinian doctors gave lectures and served on the executive and scientific committees, as well as officers of the conference's Scientific Sections.[65]

Palestine's Arab doctors continued to participate in EMA meetings, which in February 1938 were rechristened as Arab Medical Association Conferences. Addressing the Arab Medical Association (AMA) that year in Baghdad, Rushdi al-Tamimi, head of Haifa's Medical Association, equated the Arab homeland to a human body, whose right hand lay in Egypt and its left in Syria, while its neck lay in Palestine, presently at peril that threatened the entire national body.[66] The Egyptian Red Crescent Society heeded Tamimi's call. In December, based on reports of civilian casualties during the Revolt, the organization offered to dispatch a medical mission to assist the injured in hostilities. The British Foreign Office refused to give the green light to a possible precedent, opening the door for further regional intervention in Palestine.[67]

[65] "Egyptian Medical Association," *al-Kulliyyah*, 19, no. 5 (May 15, 1933): 145–47; ʿAql, *Muʿjam al-atibbaʾ*, vol. 1, 121.

[66] "Kalimat al-duktur Rushdi al-Tamimi bek," *al-Majalla al-Tibbiyya al-Misriyya* 21 (1938): 257.

[67] "Colonial Office: Palestine Original Correspondence. Situation in Palestine. Medical Personnel from Egypt," CO 733/372/20, TNA.

The Palestinian question and urgency of the struggle came up regularly in regional medical discourse. The 1945 Cairo Conference took a firm stand: one of its resolutions included a boycott of Zionist pharmaceutical companies, and doctors pledged to refrain from prescribing their products. AMA also promised to help Palestinian doctors establish independent Arab hospitals.[68] In the 1946 Aleppo conference, country representatives pledged £50,000 to that end, as far as we know it was never fulfilled.[69]

AMA conferences were crucial for creating a shared professional ethos. They created a pan-Arab medical vocabulary and sense of shared mission. Fulfilling and empowering as they were, Palestine in general and Palestinian doctors in particular faced challenges that differed from those facing their counterparts in the region.

Urban Associations

City-based medical societies organized sporadically in Palestine since the late Ottoman period. Before WWI, collaborations between Arab, missionary, and Jewish doctors failed to materialize into a countrywide or Arab association. However, apparently, there were several attempts in this direction. In 1912 Jaffa, Dr. Iskandar Halabi and pharmacist ʿAtallah Burdqush established a medical association. The objectives included medical research in a laboratory to be established for this end and discussing Jaffa's health issues.[70] Such attempts might have had parallels in Haifa and Jerusalem, but those were short-lived at best. The Ottoman crackdown on Arab civil society and the mobilization of many of Palestine's doctors during WWI prevented the establishment of such associations until the British occupation.

An International Doctors Association, uniting doctors of all denominations, operated in Jerusalem in the early 1920s, but there is little evidence of its activities. Dr. Hugh Orr-Ewing, a British physician from the English Mission Hospital, was its president, ʿIzzat Tannous served as secretary, and its executive committee included Vahan Kalbian. Uniting foreign and local doctors under one roof was an

68 ʿAql, *Muʿjam al-atibbaʾ*, 158.
69 "al-Muʾtamar al-tibbi al-ʿArabi al-sanawi al-thamin ʿashar al-munʿaqad bi-madinat Halab," *al-Majalla al-Tibiyya al-Misriyya* 29 (1946): 150; "Anbaʾ al-jamaʿiyyat al-tibbiyya," *JPAMA* 2, no. 1 (November 1946): 25–26.
70 "Jamaʿiyya tibbiyya," *Filastin*, May 8, 1912, 3.

"international" project, like the International Society of Pharmacists (est. 1918), which operated in Jerusalem during the same period. Anton Halabi was its president, Jacob Michlin, a Jerusalemite Jew and AUB graduate (1920), served as secretary,[71] and Sulayman Tannous, ʿIzzat's brother, was a member of its executive committee.[72] Established in Jerusalem, the association focused on regulating non-licensed pharmacists in Palestine and on the relationship between doctors and pharmacists.[73] Its meeting minutes included a suggestion to publish a shared medical-pharmaceutical journal and reciprocal invitations to lecture before the different associations.[74]

On its anniversary in December 1920, Kalbian gave the International Doctors Association's blessing, and Canaan gave the closing speech, stating the association's importance and adding that the International Doctors Association would follow its lead. He concluded that the country's health situation and scientific knowledge could only be elevated by the joint work of the two associations.[75] It seems that the association continued its activity well into 1923.[76]

During the same period in Jerusalem, the Academy of Medicine held lectures and meetings and published a journal edited by Orr-Ewing. The academy was also a shared endeavor, and in 1928, its committee included Kalbian, Canaan, Futi Freij, and Jewish members such as Helena Kagan. In 1926–27 alone, it held eleven "scientific meetings" and one "business meeting." Reflecting the colonial support for the academy, the High Commissioner served as honorary president.[77]

[71] Amnon Mikhlin, *Maʿase rokeah* (Tel Aviv: Erets ha-zvi, 1992), 47–64.

[72] "News from Jerusalem," *al-Kulliyyah* 7, no. 4 (February 1921): 63. *Doʾar ha-yom* wrongfully referred it as a doctors' association, "Asefa klalit shel ha-rofʾim ha-musmakhim," *Doʾar ha-yom*, January 8, 1922, 3; "Be-Histadrut ha-rok'him ha-musmakhim," *Doʾar ha-yom*, March 26, 1922, 2–3; "Asefa meshutefet shel rofʾim ve-rok'him," December 3, 1922, 3.

[73] "International Society of Certified Pharmacists in Jerusalem," P-15/2847, ISA.

[74] "Asefa shnatit shel histadrut ha-rok'him," *Doʾar ha-yom*, February 9, 1923, 3; "Histadrut ha-rok'him," *Haaretz*, February 15, 1923, 3.

[75] "bi-Yerushalayim," *Haaretz*, November 18, 1920, 3; "bi-Yerushalayim," *Haaretz*, December 1, 1920, 3; "ha-Asefa ha-shnatit shel rok'he Erets Yisraʾel," *Doʾar ha-yom*, December 5, 1920, 3.

[76] "Ha-veʿida ha-klalit shel rok'hei Erets Yisraʾel," *Doʾar ha-yom*, January 6, 1924, 4.

[77] "Miscellaneous," *al-Kulliyyah* 13, no. 4 (February 1927): 116; "Jerusalem Academy of Medicine," *The Palestine Bulletin*, February 6, 1928, 3; "The Academy of Medicine of Jerusalem," *British Medical Journal* 1, no. 3515

In 1928, Canaan, Kalbian, and other doctors attended the Congress of Tropical Medicine and Hygiene in Cairo as academy representatives.[78]

The Arab Jerusalemite societies failed to extend beyond the city's professional community and were overshadowed by the growing activity of the Yishuv's professional associations. The establishment of the Hebrew University in Jerusalem in 1925 and its exclusion of the Arab scientific community made the academy's vision seem redundant. The optimism and universalism that characterized the academy suffered a severe blow in the violent events of the late 1920s, pulling the two medical communities further apart. These factors, along with the expansion of the professional community, gave rise to calls for national union.[79]

These calls could be heeded mainly in the urban centers, where a big enough community resided, one challenged by a significant Jewish medical community and thus in need to organize. Since it operated in a city with an Arab-Jewish administration and an ever-growing Jewish population, Haifa's Arab medical community pioneered this process. In 1928, it established the National Doctors Association, appointing the elderly Dr. Ibrahim Zuʿrub as honorary president, Dr. Jibraʾil Abyad as its acting president, and Dr. Rushdi Tamimi as secretary. The doctors of the city's German, English, and Italian hospitals also joined the association.[80] In December 1930, they dispatched a telegram to the Committee of Enquiry following the 1929 violent events, stating that the reduction in malaria cases resulted from DoH actions and people's awareness and was not attributable to Yishuv's efforts.[81] In late 1932, they convened to discuss the spread of prostitution and venereal diseases in the city.[82] In the following years, the association sent protest letters against licensing Jewish immigrant doctors, the government's poor medical facilities, and the failing hygienic policy

(1928): 865. An earlier source mentions Canaan as secretary and Kalbian as treasurer, "Alumni News," *al-Kulliyyah* 9, no. 9 (July 1923): 167.

78 "Scores of Palestine Physicians Go to Cairo Congress," *The Palestine Bulletin*, December 13, 1928, 3.

79 "Agudat ha-rofʾim ha-ʿAravim," *Haaretz*, March 23, 1927.

80 "Jamaʿiyyat al-atibbaʾ al-wataniyyin," *al-Yarmuk*, May 25, 1928, 3; "Jamaʿiyyat al-atibbaʾ al-wataniyyin," *al-Yarmuk*, July 13, 1928, 3.

81 "Rofʾim ʿAravim le-vaʿadat ha-hakira," *Davar*, January 15, 1930, 2.

82 "Jamʿiyyat atibbaʾ Hayfa wa-intishar al-bighaʾ," *Filastin*, December 4, 1932, 7.

in Haifa.[83] During the 1936 general strike, they also pledged to treat poor villages for free.[84] However, it is doubtful whether the Haifa association went beyond protests and declarations.

Two other local associations were established in Jaffa and Nablus, but there is little evidence of their activities. Jaffa's doctors established their union in February 1934. Eleven doctors were present, and Drs. Nasukh al-Nabulsi and Amin ʿAwda were its elected head and treasurer.[85] Nablus' doctors followed suit only in June 1944, electing Wasif ʿAbd al-Hadi as chair and Taj al-Din ʿArafat as secretary.[86] The local associations addressed some of the professional issues within the local realm. The more significant issues at hand, mainly an ever-growing influx of immigrant Jewish doctors, gave urgency and relevance to establishing a national association that could combine the efforts of the urban professional communities into a unified front.

National Associations

In the summer of 1933, shortly after the EMA meeting in Jerusalem, the first nationwide Congress of Arab Doctors in Palestine was held in Haifa. It was the unprecedented wave of Jewish doctors' immigration during that spring that triggered this collective stand, merging political and professional agendas. Twenty-seven doctors attended, fifteen from Haifa (including two foreign doctors, an Italian and a German), alongside representatives from Jaffa (3), Jerusalem (2), Nablus (2), Nazareth (2), Safed (1), Tulkarem (1), and Shefa-ʿAmr (1). According to *Filastin*, over thirty-five doctors who failed to attend sent letters of support. The elected board reflected Haifa's leading role in the initiative, nominating elderly Dr. Jibraʾil Abyad as president and Tamimi as secretary, while Dr. Sidqi Malhas of Nablus was elected vice president. The executive committee included representatives from Jaffa and Jerusalem.[87] None of the twenty-five Arab delegates was a government employee, for

83 "Ihtijaj jamʿiyyat al-atibbaʾ bi-Hayfa," *Miraʾt al-Sharq*, November 10, 1934, 5; "Asbab intishar al-humma al-tifuʾidiyya," *Filastin*, April 27, 1935.

84 "Jalsat jamʿiyyat al-atibbaʾ al-wataniyya," *al-Difaʿ*, May 24, 1936.

85 "Taʾlif niqabat al-atibbaʾ," *Mirʾat al-Sharq*, February 28, 1934, 3; "al-Atibbaʾ al-ʿArab," *Mirʾat al-Sharq*, June 8, 1935, 3.

86 "al-Jamʿiyya al-ʿArabiyya al-tibbiyya al-Filastiniyya bi-liwaʾ Nablus," *Filastin*, July 6, 1944, 4.

87 "Inʿiqad muʾtamar al-atibbaʾ al-ʿArab bi-Hayfa," *Filastin*, June 20, 1933, 7; "al-Muʾtamar al-tibbi bi-Hayfa," *al-Jamiʿa al-ʿArabiyya*, June 21, 1933, 6;

obvious reasons: on the one hand, attending an anti-British convention could risk their employment, and on the other, the livelihood of DoH employees was less affected by the influx of Jewish doctors than that of private practitioners. Moreover, most attendees represented the veteran generation of doctors who had graduated before or during WWI, well-established doctors who could take the risk.

The congress resolutions focused on the profession's relationship with colonial authorities and the threat posed by the immigration of Jewish doctors. The participants declared their adherence to the resolutions of the Arab Executive against the national home and Jewish immigration. They demanded freezing licenses to Jewish immigrants, employing only Arab doctors in government posts, opening senior ranks at the DoH to Arab doctors, and including Arab doctors in the Mandate's licensing committee. Tamimi sent these demands to the High Commissioner following the congress.[88]

The Palestine Jewish Medical Association published its response to the petition, requesting the government to reject the "inhumane demands of a handful of doctors" and to accept the persecuted immigrant doctors "with open arms."[89] This equation, the catastrophe of European Jewry with Palestine as its haven on the one hand, and the consequent calamity refugees caused to Palestine's native population on the other, was not only a professional issue.

In September, the executive committee convened and decided to send a delegation of doctors to the High Commissioner.[90] After the meeting failed to materialize, *Filastin* stated that the "doctors' conference is in deep slumber," while foreign Jewish doctors kept flooding the country. According to that report, Tamimi had promised two months earlier that if the meeting failed to convene, the association would organize another conference, but that did not happen.[91] In 1934, the association convened several times and continued to dispatch protest letters to the

"me-Hahlatot have'ida ha-refu'it ha-'Aravit be-Hefa," *Do'ar ha-yom*, June 22, 1933, 2.

88 "In'iqad mu'tamar al-atibba'," *Filastin*; 'Aql, *Mu'jam al-atibba'*, 1: 133–34.

89 "Gilui da'at," *Davar*, July 24, 1933, 3.

90 "Ijtima' lajnat al-atibba'," *al-Jami'a al-Islamiyya*, September 26, 1933, 7; "Neged 'aliyat rof'im," *Davar*, September 27, 1933, 2; "Doctors against Doctors: Arab Physicians' Protest," *Palestine Post*, December 19, 1933, 5.

91 "Mu'tamar al-attibba' fi nawm 'amiq," *Filastin*, December 29, 1933, 6.

government.[92] It finally managed to arrange a meeting with the High Commissioner in August that year to discuss the licensing of immigrant doctors, and the British indeed limited the licensing of Jewish doctors the following year.[93]

The Arab Revolt and early WWII years halted unionizing efforts as colonial violence and political turmoil tore the country apart. The British crackdown on Palestinian leadership drove the national movement and its civil branches into exile or underground, and there is no substantial evidence of the association's activity from mid 1930s until 1944.[94]

The visit of penicillin pioneer Professor Howard Florey to Palestine in 1944 was an opportunity to restart the unionizing project. The renowned Oxford scientist lectured doctors and scientists. The Jerusalem Medical Society hosted one of the lectures at the Palestine Museum Hall and invited delegations from the Nablus, Jaffa, and Haifa societies, along with fellow doctors from other localities.[95] Florey's arrival created quite a stir within both medical communities. Since the convening of Jewish and Arab doctors together was out of the question, the Yishuv's medical community worried that Jewish doctors would not get the chance to hear Florey in person. The solution was to hold two separate events in Jerusalem, the second under the auspices of the Palestine Jewish Medical Association at Hadassah hospital.[96]

In August 1944, PAMA was established, uniting the various local unions. A preliminary meeting convened in Jerusalem included seven representatives from Haifa, Nablus, Jaffa, and Jerusalem.[97] In December, the Haifa branch hosted another meeting, which decided

[92] "Rof'im ʿAravim beʿad mas hakhnasa," February 28, 1934, 4; "Rof'im ʿaravim mohim," *Davar*, March 19, 1934, 7; "Mehaʾat ha-rof'im ha-ʿAravim," *Davar*, November 10, 1934, 1; "Tazkir rof'im ʿAravim la-shiltonot," *Haaretz*, November 12, 1934, 5.

[93] "Rof'im ʿAravim dorshim hagbalot la-rof'im ha-hadashim," *Haaretz*, August 10, 1934, 1.

[94] A meeting was convened in March 1942, "Jalsat al-jamʿiyya al-tibbiyya al-ʿArabiyya wa-muqarraratuha," *al-Difaʿ*, March 25, 1942, 3.

[95] "Ehad mi-mamtsiʾei ha-penitsilin yavo le-Erets Yisraʾel ba-shavuʿa haba," *Haaretz*, March 7, 1944, 4; "Muhadarat al-brufisur Fluri ʿan istiʿmal al-binisilin ka-ʿilaj li-l-jurukh," *al-Difaʿ*, March 16, 1944, 2.

[96] Sławomir Łotysz, "Desert Mould: Witold Odrzywolski and His Work on Crude Penicillin in a Military Hospital in the Middle East in 1944," *Kwartalnik Historyczny* 127 (2020): 77–103.

[97] "Taʾlif al-jamʿiyya al-tibbiyya al-ʿArabiyya," *al-Difaʿ*, August 7, 1944, 2.

to convene a conference in Jerusalem the following May, hold formal meetings every three months, and elect an executive.[98] Canaan was elected president, Tamimi his deputy, Mahmud Tahir al-Dajani as secretary and Sa'id 'Abdallah al-Dajani as treasurer, ensuring representation for the medical communities of Jerusalem, Haifa, and Jaffa.[99] In April 1945, PAMA signed an agreement with the PBS and launched ten-minute weekly lectures on health issues.[100]

The inauguration conference was finally held at the YMCA in Jerusalem on July 6–7, 1945. Over 200 doctors, pharmacists, intellectuals, and religious and public figures, including mayors, foreign consuls, and senior British government officials, attended. Dr. John Macqueen, director of medical services, gave his blessing to the conference and urged the young generation of Arab doctors to address the dire shortage of physicians in Arab villages and towns.[101] Macqueen's presence highlighted the organizers' ambivalence toward the government – critical of its limited achievements in addressing the Arab population's needs and of its support of Zionism, on the one hand, but dependent on its funding and administration and still considering it a relevant partner on the other.

The conference directed several demands, first and foremost at the government. These included sending more Arab doctors for specialized training in British universities, increasing government expenditure on health, and establishing new hospitals and clinics, including a sanatorium for TB patients. They also demanded official recognition of PAMA and that it be consulted regarding new restrictions on licensing Jewish doctors, which they maintained constituted unfair competition, as Jewish doctors treated Arab patients while Jews refused to consult Arab doctors.[102]

98 "Mu'tamar tibbi 'Arabi bi-l-Quds," *Filastin*, December 19, 1944, 3; Tawfiq Canaan and Mahmud Tahir al-Dajani, *al-Jam'iyya al-tibbiyya al-'Arabiyya al-Filastiniyya: Taqrir 'amm 'an juhud al-jam'iyya wa-jihadiha, 1947–1950* (Jerusalem: Matba'at dar al-aytam, 1950), 4; 'Aql, *Mu'jam al-atibba'*, vol. 1, 149–50.

99 Khaled Nashef, "Tawfiq Canaan: His Life and Works," *Jerusalem Quarterly*, no. 16 (2002): 12–26.

100 "Ahadith tibbiyya min al-idha'a," *al-Difa'*, April 24, 1945, 2.

101 "Haflat iftitah wa-ijtima'an: al-Mu'tamar al-tibbi al-'Arabi al-awwal fi Filastin," *Filastin*, July 7, 1945, 1; "Atibba' Filastin fi mu'tamarihim: jalsat al-mu'tamar al-tibbi al-'Arabi al-awwal li-yawmay al-jum'a wa-l-sabt," *al-Difa'*, July 8, 1945, 2.

102 "Muqarrarat al-mu'tamar al-tibbi al-'Arabi al-Filastini al-awwal," *Filastin*, July 20, 1945; Canaan and al-Dajani, *al-Jam'iyya al-tibbiyya*, 4–5. Dajani and

Short-lived, PAMA's achievements remained limited. In 1947, it started raising funds for new hospitals, but efforts were interrupted by the war that was to terminate its activities and the Palestinian nation-building effort in general.[103] PAMA also sought inclusion within the developing pan-Arab vision. It offered a £700 donation to aid neighboring Syria after the French bombardment of its parliament in May 1945.[104] In September 1946, PAMA representatives attended the first meeting of the World Medical Association in London. In September the following year, in its first General Assembly, PAMA became one of its founding members, alongside the Palestine Jewish Medical Association.[105] In October 1947, Palestinian doctors traveled to Egypt to help treat cholera victims.[106]

Competition with the Yishuv's medical community was the focus of attention, however. Canaan's testimony before the Anglo-American Committee of Enquiry marked the Yishuv's medical community as a professional Other and questioned its quality and contribution. PAMA's president claimed that only the Yishuv benefited from its public health services and that Arabs who sought its help were overcharged; if anything, immigrants brought diseases with them rather than health services.[107] PAMA called for a boycott of Jewish doctors, pharmacies, and pharmaceutical products.[108]

Construction Attempts

In early 1942, Amina Badr al-Khalidi dedicated her property as waqf for the construction of a hospital and a dispensary in Jerusalem.

Canaan met Macqueen on July 29, 1945, and discussed the detailed list of demands, ISA M 325/19; ʿAql, *Muʿjam al-atibbaʾ*, vol. 1, 151.

103 Canaan and al-Dajani, *al-Jamʿiyya al-tibbiyya*, 6.

104 Nashef, "Tawfiq Canaan."

105 "Anbaʾ al-jamʿiyyat al-tibbiyya," *JPAMA* 1, no. 5 (July 1946): 103; "Anbaʾ al-jamʿiyyat al-tibbiyya," *JPAMA* 2, no. 5 (July 1947): 103.

106 "Filastin tashtariku maʿa Misr fi mukafahat al-kulira : Tatawwuʿ 4 attibaʾ min al-jamʿiyya al-tibbiyya al-ʿArabiyya," *Filastin*, October 8, 1947, 2.

107 Canaan's testimony received critical responses in the Hebrew press: "Tshuva nehretset le-doctor Kanʿan," *Hamashkif*, April 7, 1946, 4; "Hokhaha la-yekholet ha-kalkalit shel ha-arets," *Haaretz*, March 22, 1946, 1; "Teshuva le-divre hasitna shel doctor Kanʿan," *Haaretz*, March 28, 1946, 3.

108 ʿAql, *Muʿjam al-atibbaʾ*, vol. 1, 159–60; "Nobody asks the patients," *Palestine Post*, July 25, 1946; "Lehahrim et ha-rofʾim ha-Yehudim," *Haboker*, January 17, 1946, 4.

A professional committee was appointed, including British and Palestinian doctors, a site was selected in the Sheikh Jarrah neighborhood for a 100-bed hospital, and a British architect was chosen. Telegrams were sent from Gaza, Majdal, and Hebron to the DoH urging it to support the project, and poet Fadwa Tuqan dedicated a poem to the future national hospital. By mid 1943, plans were submitted to the governor, and preparations for construction were underway. By mid 1947, an attempt was made to raise funds and revive the project, which failed.[109] Mustafa al-Khalidi, former judge and mayor of Jerusalem at the time of Amina's death, did everything he could to prevent the project's materialization. The mayor and his brother were Amina's nephews and claimed to be her rightful heirs. They used their connections to prevent the transfer of funds to the waqf's control. A judicial technicality safely placed the assets in the hands of the Khalidi brothers.[110]

Other initiatives that failed to materialize included a hospital or infirmary in Haifa, planned by the Workers' Association on the upper floor of their office building after raising sufficient funds. The Nablus branch envisioned a similar plan.[111] Another collective action initiated in the 1940s was the anti-TB association established in Jaffa in 1943, raising funds for a local TB clinic. The association printed postcards showing the planned clinic, which it sold for 250 piasters. A designated clinic was never built, but the association did manage to operate one in a rented apartment.[112] Three years later, efforts commenced to form a union with similar associations in Nablus, Haifa, and Jerusalem, with the more ambitious goal of establishing a sanatorium like existing Jewish and Lebanese ones. All they managed to accomplish, however, was to fund the hospitalization of twenty patients in Lebanon. In the

109 "Government of Palestine, Department of Health: Sitt Amineh Khalidi Hospital, Jerusalem," M-21/6553, ISA; "li-Insha' mustashfa al-marhuma al-sayyida Amina al-Khalidi," *Filastin*, November 17, 1942, 3; "Mustashfa Amina al-Khalidi: Abyat li-sha'irat Filastin al-mulhima Fadwa Tuqan," *Filastin*, November 28, 1942, 1; "Al-Bad' bi-tanfidh mashru' al-mustashfa al-khayri," *al-Difa'*, July 19, 1943, 3; "Mashru' mustashfa al-muhsina al-Khalidiyya," *Filastin*, May 21, 1947, 4.

110 'Aql, *Mu'jam al-atibba'*, vol. 1, 292–301.

111 *Al-Difa'*, February 16, 1944 and January 1, 1945.

112 "Mustawsif jama'iyyat mukafahat al-sill fi Yafa," *Filastin*, March 12, 1944; "Nishat jam'iyyat mukafahat al-sill al-'Arabiyya fi Yafa," *Filastin*, February 14, 1946, 4.

summer of 1947, union members also traveled to Syria and Lebanon and convinced the political leaderships there to support the sanatorium project.[113] The plans did not reach fruition but nevertheless attest to ambitions, energy, and mobilization of greater magnitude than those seen in earlier years. The Nakba and PAMA's subsequent dissolution leave little chronological space to determine its ability to turn its vision into reality.

The First Palestinian Medical Journal

Very few Palestinian doctors were engaged in active medical research. One of them was Krikor Krikorian, employed at the Central Government Laboratories in Jerusalem, who also published several articles, particularly with G. Stuart, the laboratories' director. One article series was dedicated to rabies and to experimentation with local virus strains on rats and rabbits. Others described typhus cases and rare complications in rabies vaccination. Case studies were based on patients in government hospitals, whose samples were processed in government laboratories.[114] Krikorian and the few others who conducted research and published in academic journals did so sporadically and under foreign auspices. PAMA's journal (*JPAMA*) sought to transform this reality by providing a national scientific platform that would encourage scholarly debate.

JPAMA, published since late 1945, brought together the people and topics mentioned in this chapter. The editors included Mahmud Tahir al-Dajani, Tawfiq Canaan, and Ahmad Sururi. Muhammad Khalil ʿAbd al-Khaliq, Fuʾad Ghusn, and Jamil Basha Fa'iq al-Tutunji, heads of the Egyptian, Lebanese, and Jordanian associations, respectively, later joined the board. This impressive membership, as well as the journal's content, reflected the high academic standards and pan-Arab ethos *JPAMA* sought to embody. Its editorials promoted the

113 "Jamʿiyyat mukafahat al-sill al-ʿArabiyya tuʿaqqidu muʾtamaraha bi-Yafa," *Filastin*, March 12, 1946, 2; "Suriya wa-Lubnan yuʾayyidan mashruʿ jamʿiyyat mukafahat al-sill," *al-Sirat al-Mustaqim*, August 26, 1947, 3.

114 See, for example, G. Stuart and Krikor Krikorian, "Studies in Anti-Rabies Immunisation," *The Journal of Hygiene* 29, no. 1 (1929): 1–34; Arthur Felix, Krikor Krikorian, and Rudolph Reitler, "The Occurrence of Typhoid Bacilli Containing Vi Antigen in Cases of Typhoid Fever and of Vi Antibody in Their Sera," *The Journal of Hygiene* 35, no. 3 (1935): 421–27.

status of the Palestinian medical profession in relation to Arab society in Palestine, British authorities, medical associations in neighboring countries, and the Jewish medical community. It reflected the maturation of processes that had begun a decade or two earlier. The demand for medical services from the colonial government and fear of the overwhelming presence of Jewish doctors were now supplemented by concrete initiatives to raise funds for independent clinics, hospitals, and a sanatorium. *JPAMA*'s main challenges were lack of funds and a small pool of contributors – which did not grow much throughout its existence.

The first issue, charged with a national sense of purpose, included greetings from the presidents of the Iraqi and Jordanian associations.[115] "For Science, Humanism and Arabism," read the title of an article by ʿAli Ibrahim Basha, former Egyptian Minister of Health, EMA president, and rector of King Fuʾad I University.[116] *JPAMA* was published until the spring of 1948, and while short-lived, it provided a professional academic platform for Palestinian doctors.

Between November 1945 and March 1948, the journal published articles on multiple medical conditions, including miscarriage, anemia, and hypertension, and diseases such as typhoid, TB, and measles. *JPAMA*'s readers also learned of new scientific breakthroughs such as DDT, penicillin, and sulfate[117] and that nuclear radiation had enormous potential for medicine despite its monstrous military usage.[118] Canaan published several epidemiological surveys.[119] In one of these, he explained how leishmaniasis migrated from its

[115] Canaan and al-Dajani, *al-Jamʿiyya al-tibbiyya*, 5.

[116] Donald Reid, *Cairo University and the Making of Modern Egypt* (Cambridge: Cambridge University Press, 2002), 136; Ninette S. Fahmy, *The Politics of Egypt: State-Society Relationship* (Abingdon, Oxon and New York: Routledge, 2012), 133–34. *JPAMA* 1, no. 1 (1945): 2–5.

[117] On penicillin: Ahmad Sururi, "Ikhtibarat ukhra ʿan al-ʿilaj bi-binisilin," *JPAMA* 1, no. 3 (March 1946): 57–60; I. B. George, "Evaluation of Penicillin in Oral Therapy," *JPAMA* 2, no. 5 (July 1947): 125–31. On DDT: Ibrahim Itayim, "al-Hama al-rajiʿa wa-mukafahatuha," *JPAMA* 1, no. 5 (July 1946): 86–94; D. A. Berberian, "The Use of DDT Residual Spray in Malaria Control and Its Effect on General Sanitation in Rural Districts," *JPAMA* 3, no. 3 (March 1948): 49–61.

[118] Jamil Pasha Faʾiq al-Tutunji, "al-Taqa al-dhuriyya wa-l-maqsum al-tibbi," *JPAMA* 3, no. 1 (November 1947): 2–8.

[119] Tawfiq Canaan, "al-Tayfuʾid fi Filastin," *JPAMA* 3, no. 2 (January 1948): 21–26.

origin in Jericho to other localities and asked readers to inform him of other localities for future research.[120] The educator Ahmad Samih al-Khalidi contributed articles on the history of Arab medicine.

Futi Freij contributed an article series on Arabic medical terminology. These articles were preceded by an editorial he authored, which advocated for the importance of developing Arabic as a scientific language rather than relying on foreign terminology. He argued that Arabic had been the language of science in the past and could be once again.[121] In the following issues, Freij actively asked for readers' feedback. Doctors sent their suggestions for new terminology, and he incorporated them into his column and discussed their responses.

A column titled "News of the Medical Associations" included short items on steering committees' elections at PAMA's branches and in medical associations in neighboring countries; news of doctors departing to or returning from advanced medical training abroad; lists of newly graduated doctors; news of the associations' professional, public, and broadcasted lectures; and fundraising initiatives for the foundation of clinics and hospitals.[122] The column fostered a sense of community and gave a sense of continuous activity.

In January 1946, Mahmud Tahir al-Dajani urged his colleagues to concentrate their efforts on establishing national medical institutions that would provide affordable care to Palestine's Arabs – both in cities and the countryside. He explained that efforts were underway in several localities but insisted that voluntary spirit was required to turn them into reality.[123] Ra'fat Faris, for his part, championed the goal of sanatoriums to care for TB patients, protect the public from them, and help educate the public about the disease more broadly. His articles also sought to better inform doctors about TB, which tended to be diagnosed too late.[124]

[120] Tawfiq Canaan, "al-Lishmaniyya fi Filastin," *JPAMA* 2, no. 3 (March 1947): 44–51.

[121] Futi Freij, "Kalimat al-ʿadad," *JPAMA* 1, no. 4 (May 1946): 69–71.

[122] See, for example, "Anbaʾ al-jamʿiyyat al-tibbiyya," in *JPAMA* 1, no. 1 (November 1945): 23–25; *JPAMA* 1, no. 2 (January 1946): 50–53; *JPAMA* 2, no. 3 (March 1947): 63–65; *JPAMA* 2, no. 5 (July 1947): 103.

[123] "Muʾassasatuna al-tibbiyya ramz nahadatina," *JPAMA* 1, no. 2 (January 1946): 34–36.

[124] Raʾfat Faris, "Hajat Filastin al-massa ila masahhat li-marad al-sill," *JPAMA* 1, no. 2 (January 1946): 45–47; Raʾfat Faris, "al-Tashkhis al-bakir li-marad al-sill," *JPAMA* 1, no. 4 (May 1946): 76–79.

In July that year, Dr. Ahmad Sururi listed PAMA's main goals: solidifying ties with Arab doctors in neighboring countries, educating the public and advising it on health issues, and establishing much-needed clinics, sanatoriums, hospitals, X-ray and radium institutes, and laboratories. He stated that Nablus' Watani Hospital and the Dajani Hospital in Jaffa, Amina Khalidi's donation in Jerusalem, and the Abu Khadra sisters' donation in Gaza should serve as models for future initiatives. PAMA, he concluded, should demand its inclusion in decision-making at the DoH and in directing government hospitals. Arab doctors should not settle for complaining about government neglect, he insinuated, but should demand involvement in DoH policymaking.[125]

In November 1947, Dajani noted with satisfaction that *JPAMA* had managed to achieve some important goals: serving the nation, maintaining ties between the medical associations in Palestine's cities, strengthening ties with medical associations in neighboring countries, and proving to fellow doctors elsewhere in the world that "the Arab doctor in Palestine is not less capable of organizing, and is endowed with no less skill and creativity than any other."[126] In the same issue, PAMA prided its medical treatment of poor TB patients, radio broadcasts, lectures in schools, and studies on infant mortality, fertility, leishmaniasis, malaria, and eye diseases.[127]

In early 1948, the journal's last two issues grieved Palestine's most difficult time in history but commended the Arab doctor for his tireless work for his country. In January, Futi Freij urged neighboring countries to send medical equipment and medications to their Palestinian brethren, and in March, Dajani thanked neighboring Arab associations for their help.[128] However, as shown in Chapter 7, and as both doctors knew, Arab medical assistance was meager, and the Palestinian Arab doctor did his best but fought a losing battle.

Conclusion

Considering the similar resolutions, membership, and objectives of the 1933 Haifa association, the decade-long nearly complete freeze of

[125] Ahmad Sururi, "Kalimat al-ʿadad," *JPAMA* 1, no. 5 (July 1946): 85–86.
[126] Mahmud Tahir al-Dajani, "Kalimat al-ʿadad," *JPAMA* 3, no. 1 (November 1947): 1–2.
[127] "Anbaʾ al-jamʿiyyat al-tibbiyya," *JPAMA* 3, no. 1 (November 1947): 18.
[128] Futi Freij, "Kalimat al-ʿadad," *JPAMA* 3, no. 2 (January 1948): 20; Mahmud Tahir al-Dajani, "Kalimat al-ʿadad," *JPAMA* 3, no. 3 (March 1948): 30–31.

activity and subsequent establishment of another national association requires an explanation. The division of labor between the government, different missions, and private clinics made unionizing a challenging endeavor. In 1933, the community was already big enough, and many Palestinian doctors were able and willing to unite behind a national cause. However, the lion's share of this group operated private, primarily small clinics, and professional cooperation was rare. The large body of government employees who did possess more significant structural potential for joint action was out of the equation: the colonial government actively prevented its employees from unionizing.[129] The British policy of excluding Palestinian doctors from leading positions in the state's health administration further compromised national unionization efforts, limiting doctors' empowerment to the local and temporary at best.

Intra-Palestinian politics were yet another explanatory factor. National leadership, primarily the Arab Higher Committee headed by the Mufti, never took real interest in providing medical services. The wealthiest institution, the Supreme Muslim Council, took limited action regarding health services and relied on local charity-based *waqf* and *zakat* revenues. First-aid initiatives in times of violent clashes never went beyond local voluntary enterprise. Only in the 1940s did a few municipalities, mainly Jaffa and Ramallah, start collecting health and welfare taxes.[130]

Once the association was established, lack of funding and the absence of a nationwide collective action prevented it from achieving its goals, mainly to provide health services to all Palestinians. In addition, political factionalism, which tore the national movement apart since the 1930s, also prevented the establishment of a national front. The Arab Revolt not only left the national movement devastated but brought this factionalism to the extreme, turning its latter period into a Palestinian civil war. The violent British counterinsurgency and the exile of Palestinian leadership were only a prelude to the long years of WWII, in which the national impetus and state-building initiatives were put on hold under the shadow of the British war effort. After the

[129] Qaraqra, *al-Khidamat*, 160.

[130] Muhammad Qaraqra, "Maʿarekhet ha-bri'ut ha-mandatorit ve-ha-voluntarit ve-ʿArviye Erets Yisra'el, 1918–1948" (MA thesis, Haifa University, 1992), 261–65; Nira Reiss, *Health Services to the Arab Population in Israel* (Tel Aviv: International Center for Peace in the Middle East, 1988), 38.

war, the Palestinian social body could once again raise its head, but political strife remained destructive, and a united leadership or functional and well-funded national institutions were absent.

Despite these factors, PAMA was established and proved capable of overcoming some of these inherent obstacles. A central factor in the rebirth of this vision was the new generation of doctors who graduated during the 1930s, such as Mahmud Tahir al-Dajani, who injected new energy into the community. Perhaps the leadership of Canaan, whose absence from the earlier association was noticeable, also helped vitalize PAMA. Jerusalem was the center of colonial administration, which might explain its relative marginality in the earlier national association. The organization's recentering in Palestine's capital and the election of Jerusalemites to senior positions were more natural. In its reincarnation as PAMA, the national association not only united a larger community of doctors but also openly strove for medical self-sufficiency. In the regional scene, it reclaimed its voice within the other associations. As discussed in the following chapter, PAMA's inclusion in the regional organizational network would prove relevant during the 1948 war.

7 *Nakba: The Displacement of the Medical Community*

"Late one night," David ha-Cohen recalls, "I heard a knock on the door of my house on Mount Carmel." It was 1950, and the former member of Haifa's municipality and senior Haganah official was then a member of the Israeli Parliament (Knesset). Ha-Cohen opened the door to a "thin unshaven figure, dressed in a worn suit and wearing a cap." Upon seeing him, the man burst into tears, embraced him, and fell on his knees. A longtime friend and fellow council member, the visitor begged for ha-Cohen's help in staying in Israel, as he could no longer bear living in a refugee camp, unable to find work in his profession, and treated as an outcast. Ha-Cohen prepared the man a warm bath, a meal, and a bed for the night, and the following morning took him to Sayf al-Din al-Zuʿbi, a Knesset member from Nazareth. The man was Dr. Othman Khamra. He had crossed the border on foot after setting out from Jenin Refugee Camp and then took a bus to Haifa. According to ha-Cohen, Khamra said he would renounce all claims to personal property if he and his family were allowed to return. He was quickly deported by the authorities and never returned, finally settling in Amman, where he died.[1]

So far, we have discussed the expansion and networking of the Palestinian professional medical community. This chapter discusses its dissolution and its members' different trajectories during and after the 1948 war. Their story is part of the Palestinian Nakba, which entailed the displacement of more than half of Palestine's Arab population. Within a few months, hundreds of Palestinian villages, towns, and city neighborhoods were nearly completely depopulated. These were also the deadliest months the country had seen up to that point, in which a mounting number of casualties burdened a rapidly shrinking

[1] David Hacohen, *Time to Tell: An Israeli Life, 1898–1984* (New York: Cornwall Books, 1985), 208; Majid Khamra, *Margharush: Wamadat min Hayfa* (Haifa: al-Wadi li-l-tibaʿa wa-l-nashr: Jamʿiyyat al-tatwir al-ijtimaʿi, 2004). We thank Dr. Majid Khamra for the information about Dr. Khamrah.

medical infrastructure. During those same months, medical services that British authorities had funded and maintained either disappeared or switched ownership to Yishuv's or Arab hands. Meager as they had been, the Department of Health (DoH) was the main provider of services for Palestinian Arabs, employing hundreds of doctors, nurses, midwives, and auxiliary staff countrywide. Some missionary hospitals continued to operate, but many were closed down during the war. Upon British evacuation, DoH offices were closed down permanently. Yishuv militias, and subsequently the Israeli army, took over clinics and hospitals and looted or confiscated equipment and medical supplies.[2] Together with the rest of the Palestinian population, around 70 percent of doctors lost their homes, clinics, and livelihoods. Within Israel's borders, only about ten Palestinian doctors remained.

The events outlined in this chapter unfolded through the course of months, weeks, or even days. Civil society was mobilized, hospitals continued to operate under fire, women's organizations founded makeshift hospitals, and doctors tried to save as many patients as they could. But the pace of events was overwhelming. Hostilities started in December 1947, and by the following spring, Jaffa and Arab Haifa were doomed. Haifa's Palestinian women's organization founded a hospital that operated for two months at the most before the city's occupation by the Haganah in late April, and a Lebanese Red Cross hospital in Acre lasted half that time before its surrender in May.

Observing the medical profession during the war, we find heroic stories of perseverance. Lacking any state structures, however, these efforts were necessarily localized and short-lived, suffering from a severe lack of supplies. Largely dependent on private practice, the Arab medical profession in Palestine began unionizing only three years before the war and had limited resources of its own. This chapter reviews the resources mobilized to deal with these challenges based on Arab Medical Association reports, Supreme Arab Council documents, Palestinian press, and interviews conducted by historians and journalists with Palestinian refugees from the 1960s onward.

Doctors' experience of the Nakba differed from that of most Palestinians in several respects. First, their profession enabled them to

[2] Arnon Degani, "Both Arab and Israeli: The Subordinate Integration of Palestinian Arabs into Israeli Society, 1948–1967" (PhD diss., University of California Los Angeles, 2018), 141; Muhammad Qaraqra, "Sherute ha-briʾut la-ukhlusiya ha-ʿAravit be-Yisraʾel" (PhD diss., Bar-Ilan University, 2013), 53.

help contain the war's human costs, and many found themselves training nurses, working in makeshift hospitals, or treating refugees. Many had little to no experience in community leadership, but events pushed them to assume this role. Overall, few others had such intimate contact with the everyday suffering of others. Second, their profession made them more mobile than others – their expertise was transferable, and they could find employment more easily than those whose livelihood depended on their field or shop. Doctors were of upper-class origins and could rely on their savings for what they initially believed – as many others did – would be a short-term refuge. Already in February 1948, Palestinian and Jordanian newspapers published appeals to Palestinian doctors to return to their homeland, and the Palestine Radio followed suit. Palestinian doctors were reportedly applying for medical licenses in neighboring countries, thus planning for long-term residence.[3] The story of Palestinian doctors is, therefore, also a story of the Palestinian elite in the face of the catastrophe.

The story of those who were displaced and those who remained, those who assisted in war efforts and those who left, is not only a story of class or individual initiatives. The distinctions outlined throughout the book, as well as the Partition Plan's lines and subsequent events of the Nakba, also affected and sometimes determined doctors' fate. Those who had worked in the DoH were left without salaries in hospitals stripped of their budget virtually overnight, with fewer choices than those in private practice. Doctors in Jaffa and Haifa, both occupied in April 1948, were different from those in Nablus or Ramallah, far from the line of fire, or from those in Nazareth, the only Arab town that remained intact in what became the State of Israel. The medical community that was slowly building up was breaking down along existing and new cracks.

This chapter begins with a short outline of the war events and proceeds chronologically, geographically, and thematically. It takes the reader back to Chapter 3 and describes how the British evacuation affected medical services. It proceeds to the Palestinian geography outlined in Chapter 2 and the ways different locales and communities coped with the double challenge of the withdrawal of medical services

[3] "Ila al-atibba' al-haribin: 'Udu ila Filastin wa-kaffiru," *al-Sarih*, February 17, 1948, 4; "Irgun," in "Hit'argenut rof'im, rok'him, 'orkhe din u-mehandesim," file no. 105/166, 52, June 5, 1948, Haganah Archive (hereafter, HA); "Brihat ha-rof'im ha-'Aravim," *'Al ha-Mishmar*, February 20, 1948, 11.

and mounting war casualties during the war's first months. The chapter shows how connections forged during the Mandate, described in Chapter 6, were desperately mobilized. We focus on Jaffa and Haifa's medical mobilization until the spring of 1948 and on Jerusalem following the declaration of the State of Israel in May. This part of the war also brings us to the Galilee and to the doctors who stayed during the war months. The chapter concludes with the war's aftermath and afterlives of the medical community: the few who remained in Israel, those who worked in refugee camps, the medical community others helped build in Jordan, and the formation of the Palestinian medical diaspora.

Outline of the War

Hostilities between the Palestinian Arab and Jewish communities began following the United Nations (UN) resolution approving the Partition Plan on November 29 and the Higher Arab Executive's declaration of a three-day strike.[4] Violent attacks broke out across the country, and the mixed urban centers of Haifa, Jerusalem, and Tel Aviv-Jaffa were divided into belligerent Arab and Jewish neighborhoods. National Palestinian committees were established in each city to secure the well-being and security of the civilian population and organize, train, and fund fighting forces. In Jaffa and Haifa, the balance of power was in the Yishuv's absolute favor. Caught between the Yishuv's attacks, inner Palestinian political factionalism, and a lack of unified strategy, the local leaderships and their ad hoc administration was short-lived, collapsing before the fall of the cities. Most of their political, professional, and financial elite had fled weeks before this collapse.

[4] For further reading see Adel Manna, *Nakba and Survival: The Story of Palestinians Who Remained in Haifa and the Galilee, 1948–1956* (Oakland: University of California Press, 2022); Benny Morris, *The Birth of the Palestinian Refugee Problem Revisited* (Cambridge: Cambridge University Press, 2004); Avi Shlaim and Eugene L. Rogan, eds., *The War for Palestine: Rewriting the History of 1948* (Cambridge: Cambridge University Press, 2007); Qustantin Zuraiq, *Nakbat 1948: Asbabuha wa-subul 'ilajiha*, ed. Walid Khalidi (Beirut: Mu'assasat al-dirasat al-Filastiniyya, 2009); Arif al-Arif, *al-Nakbah: Nakbat Bayt al-Maqdis wa-l-firdaws al-mafquud: 1947–1949* (Beirut: Mu'assasat al-dirasat al-Filastiniya, 2013).

As we have seen in Chapter 5, the Yishuv's medical institutions were almost fully independent of British funding and administration, had decades-long experience, and abundant professional personnel. Government hospitals depended in part on Jewish doctors, but Jewish hospitals did not rely on Arab or British personnel. Yishuv's hospitals were located inside Jewish cities and continued to operate throughout the war, offering treatment to civilians and combatants.

Haifa's surrender on April 22 after a short battle also involved a mass exodus. Battles over the northern port city reached their climax in mid March, and by April, half of its population had already been displaced. Only around 5,000 out of 70,000 Arabs remained in two neighborhoods in Haifa by May 15.[5] Jaffa's neighborhoods bordering Tel Aviv were emptied during the early stages of the war, and mass exodus began in mid March 1948. In late April, the Haganah occupied Jaffa's rural hinterland and isolated Jaffa. Its residents began departing by sea to Lebanon and Egypt, leading to a complete breakdown of local institutions and services. By May 13, the day of Jaffa's surrender, only around 3,000 out of 70,000 Arabs remained.

In Jerusalem, as in Jaffa and Haifa, violent clashes started in early December. Local committees and associations collected donations, established local headquarters, and mobilized guards. Attacks on roads inside and leading to Jerusalem exacerbated the situation. Jews and Arabs residing in mixed neighborhoods or those bordering Jewish neighborhoods began evacuating to safer places, and the British government retreated to heavily guarded security zones. By late March, the Arab neighborhoods outside the Old City – Musrara, Wadi Joz, and Sheikh Jarrah – were emptied almost entirely of their inhabitants.[6] The depopulation of Qatamon, Baqʿa, and Talbiya began in January/February.[7] Qatamon and Talbiya were occupied by the Haganah in late April/early May, Baqʿa in mid May. Many found refuge in the Old City.[8]

[5] Morris, *The Birth*, 115–16, 163–221; Itamar Radai, *Palestinians in Jerusalem and Jaffa, 1948: A Tale of Two Cities* (London: Routledge, 2015), 168–76.

[6] Radai, *Palestinians*, 15–54.

[7] Donn Hutchison, "Occidental Obsessions: Diary of a Country Doctor," *Jerusalem Quarterly* 28 (2006): 45–61.

[8] Nathan Crystal, "The Fall of the New City 1947–1950," in *Jerusalem 1948: The Arab Neighbourhoods and Their Fate in the War*, ed. Salim Tamari (Jerusalem: Institute of Jerusalem Studies & Badil Resource Center, 1999), 92–146; Radai, *Palestinians*, 73–74.

On April 9, Yishuv's forces attacked the village of Deir Yassin on the western outskirts of Jerusalem and conducted a large-scale massacre. Four days later, seventy-eight Jewish doctors, nurses, students, and professors were massacred in a convoy on its way to Mount Scopus in Jerusalem, a Jewish enclave surrounded by Arab neighborhoods and villages. In response, the Arab Higher Committee and Palestinian Arab Medical Association (PAMA) published, not for the first time, an appeal to respect the immunity of medical personnel and refrain from attacking hospitals, ambulances, and medical doctors – Jews and Arabs alike. PAMA stated its commitment to international law and, hence, to the immunity of medical personnel. The loss of medical personnel is a loss to humanity as a whole, it concluded.[9]

In the Galilee, Yishuv's forces succeeded in defeating and displacing some villages from early 1948. Tiberias fell and was later depopulated in late April, Safad in mid May.[10] Acre and Bisan were occupied in mid May as well – around 5,000 Arabs remained in the former while the latter was depopulated. In July, the Israel Defense Forces (IDF) conducted a large-scale operation, occupying Nazareth and the villages around it. The town's symbolic religious importance and its leadership's decision to surrender saved it from the calamity of all the others. It remained.[11]

Farewell to the Department of Health

On July 15, 1947, the DoH held a conference of hospital superintendents. Among other topics, they discussed the training and salary of nurses and the possibility of training male nurses, the quality of hospital nutrition and the feasibility of employing dietitians, and the absence of updated medical literature for hospital staff.[12] Several months later, the war dramatically changed the lives of many of its attendees. R. H. Bland, acting Director of Medical Services, would leave

[9] "Rijal al-isʿaf hum rasl al-insaniyya," *Filastin*, April 16, 1948, 4; Radai, *Palestinians*, 89–90.

[10] Mustafa Abbasi, "Tsfat bi-tkufat ha-mandat, hebetim hevratiyyim ve-politiyyim" (PhD diss., Haifa University, 1999), 323–61.

[11] Mustafa Abbasi, "Kibush Natseret: ha-ʿIr ha-'Arvit she-sarda et ha-milhama," *'Iyyunim* 20 (2010): 101–21; Morris, *The Birth*, 415–23; Manna, *Nakba and Survival*, 60–92.

[12] Government of Palestine, Department of Health, Conference – Medical Supts'. Hospitals, "Superintendents' Conference on 15 July 1947," August 6, 1947, M-6576/28, ISA.

the country. Two other participants, Dr. Lehrs of Beit Safafa and Dr. Maʿluf of Bethlehem, would be murdered a few days apart. Shimon Btesh, superintendent of HaYarkon Hospital in Tel Aviv, would be appointed General Director of the Israeli Ministry of Health (MoH). Dr. Alexander Malhi, Head of the Government Hospital at Bnei Brak, would become Director of Medical Services to Minorities in MoH. Ibrahim Salim Ayyub, then Superintendent of the Government Hospital in Safad, would flee to Lebanon and start working for the Tripoli branch of the Iraqi Petroleum Company. Dr. Naif Hamzeh, then Superintendent of Haifa's Government Hospital, would flee to Jordan and become Director of Nablus Government Hospital.[13]

The British evacuation plan focused on safeguarding their men and equipment, and medical (among other) services were simply left behind. Dr. Sami Khuri, who arrived at Nablus Government Hospital in early April 1948, testified that he "saw the worst conditions ever seen at a hospital. There were no surgical tools or even sewing string for operations. I was amazed at how the British left the hospital in this sad state."[14]

The UN partition vote initiated two simultaneous processes. On the one hand, escalating hostilities overburdened those hospitals available to the Arab population. At the same time, the British authorities started pulling out of Palestine, denying government hospitals much-needed resources. The main blow to health services was DoH's withdrawal of its annual £1.25 million budget. By February, the administration started closing departments whose safety it could no longer guarantee and withdrew, in practice, from most parts of the country. The main benefactor from this process was the Yishuv, which took over much of the resources the British had left behind.[15]

Medical supplies from the DoH storage facilities, medical stores, and equipment were supposed to be handed to various institutions in Palestine, in accordance with their bed strength.[16] When the

13 Ibid.

14 Talaʿat Shinaʿa, *Ayyam zaman: al-Tarikh al-shafawi li-l-Urdun wa-Filastin* (Amman: al-Ahliyya, 1993), 83.

15 Motti Golani, "The 'Haifa Turning Point': The British Administration and the Civil War in Palestine, December 1947 – May 1948," *Middle Eastern Studies* 37 (2001): 94–120.

16 "Bet ha-holim be-Bet Tsafafa," April 11, 1948, 75, and "Homre refuʾa la-ʿAravim me-ha-memshala," April 19, 1948, 78; "Hitʾargenut rofʾim," file no. 105/166, HA.

Palestinian Arab Senior Medical Officer finally took over the distribution, he found that most medical supplies had already been looted.[17] British withdrawal created an administrative and financial vacuum. Responsibility for hospitals was supposed to transfer to the municipalities, and in some places, this transfer indeed took place – in Nablus, Jaffa, and Gaza, as well as the Bethlehem Mental Hospital.[18] In April 1948, Gaza, Beersheba, and Safad hospitals were handed over to the respective municipalities, as well as an epidemic disease clinic in Hebron. In other places, such as Tulkarem, Qalqilya, and Arraba, local communities were unable to assume responsibility for their IWCs, while villages like Masmiya, Faluja, Dir al-Balah, and Rafah accepted responsibility for these centers.

Whereas previously, Jewish and Arab doctors worked together in the larger government hospitals, by January 1948, their smooth operation became impossible. In December, Jewish doctors and nurses in Haifa's Government Hospital began fearing for their safety. According to Jewish sources, Jewish employees were threatened, and armed Palestinian fighters walked around the hospital, some as visitors and some as guards for higher-ranking fighters.[19] Jewish personnel left the hospital, and Jewish patients were taken out. Two-thirds of the hospital's nurses were Jewish, burdening its operation after their departure. Arab nurses from other hospitals and IWCs in the country, as well as volunteers from Haifa's women's organizations, took their place. Arab doctors managed to run the hospital without their Jewish colleagues yet demanded the DoH's intervention to force their return.[20]

[17] "Colonial Office and Commonwealth Office: Defence Department and successors: Original Correspondence. Palestine: report by Dr H M O Lester on the Palestine Department of Health 1946–1948," 12, CO 968/197, NA (henceforth Lester's report).

[18] Palestinian Arab Medical Association (henceforth PAMA), letter from Dr. Mahmud Tahir al-Dajani to Dr. Husayn Fakhri Bek al-Khalidi, January 4, 1948, P-990/19, ISA.

[19] "Ketsad nidheku ha-ʿovdim ha-Yehudim mi-bet ha-holim ha-memshalti be-Hefa," *ha-Tsofe*, January 22, 1948, 4; "Gam bet ha-holim ha-memshalti be-Hefa naki mi-Yehudim," *Haaretz*, January 23, 1948, 7; "Bet ha-holim ha-memshalti be-Hefa hafakh le-mosad ʿAravi tahor," *Ha-Mashkif*, January 26, 1948, 3.

[20] "al-Mujanaddat al-ʻArabiyyat," *al-Difaʿ*, January 2, 1948, 2; "Benisilin li-isʻaf al-juraha fi Hayfa," *Filastin*, January 4, 1948, 2; "al-Atibbaʾ al-Yahud yahdhuna hadhwa al-mumarridat al-mudarrabat," *al-Difaʿ*, January 4, 1948, 2; "Beʿayat ha-ishpuz etsel ha-ʿAravim," *ha-Tsofeh*, January 15, 1948, 2 Lester's report, 11.

Dr. Sami al-Khuri arrived at Haifa's Government Hospital during the hostilities and left in early April. After the declaration of the Partition Plan, Khuri noted, he saw the streets packed with dancing people, while rivers of beer poured into the crowd. The young doctor mentions seeing only Arab employees, testifying that deaths surrounded him "night and day." After one of the hospital's ambulance drivers was killed while attempting to pick up a sick woman near the hospital, Khuri returned to the same place only to be ambushed as well, successfully dodging the bullets.[21] Haifa was irrevocably divided.

Jaffa's experience was similar. Its doctors operated the Government Hospital after the British withdrawal. The Jewish staff had left the hospital at the beginning of hostilities, leaving it understaffed.[22] According to Dr. Hugh Lester, the DoH director, one of the Jewish nurses was shot while returning from work after her afternoon leave. As a result, the medical staff became anxious for the Jewish nurses' safety, and Arab patients refused to be treated by Jewish nurses. The British authorities transferred all Jewish nurses from the General Hospital to Jaffa's Mental Hospital, while the Arab doctors from the Mental Hospital moved to the General Hospital.[23]

As the countdown to full British evacuation advanced, government employees were less and less secure, especially those whose work required movement through what became hostile areas. The most fatal blow to the DoH was the murders of Lehrs and Maʿluf. The Beit Safafa Infectious Disease Hospital had a Jewish medical superintendent, Dr. Lehrs, an Arab physician, mixed nursing staff, and mostly Arab patients. In late December 1947, the Jewish Irgun militia warned British authorities that the Jewish nurses at the hospital were not safe. Dr. Lehrs received intimidation letters but believed that he would not be harmed, and the District Commissioner asked the neighboring military camp to keep an eye on the hospital. Lehrs was ambushed and murdered on hospital grounds.[24]

News of Dr. Lehrs' murder greatly upset his colleague Dr. Mikhaʾil Maʿluf, the Medical Officer of neighboring Bethlehem and Director of its Mental Hospital. He drove a black Dodge, which carried a red cross

[21] Shinaʿa, *Ayyam zaman*, 83.
[22] "Mandub al-shaʿb fi al-mustashfa al-hukumi," *Filastin*, January 17, 1948, 3.
[23] Lester's report, 10.
[24] Reuven Gafni, "Lone Jewish Medical Personnel in Arab Towns: A Conditional Presence in British Mandate Palestine," *Israel Studies* 26 (2021): 203–5.

and a red shield sign. Fearing retaliation over Dr. Lehrs' murder, Bertha, Ma'luf's wife, begged him to remove them, but he saw no reason to worry – retaliation, he believed, would happen in Jerusalem. A few days later, he was murdered. A pick-up truck drove into Bethlehem that morning and caught up with Dr. Ma'luf on his way to the village of Daheisheh.[25] The identity of the murderers remains unknown.

Following these murders, PAMA and its Jewish counterpart published simultaneous statements in several newspapers in English, Arabic, and Hebrew, as well as on the radio, urging fighting parties to refrain from attacking medical personnel and urging doctors and nurses to clearly mark themselves with a Red Cross, Red Crescent, or Star of David, forbidding the use of these symbols for nonmedical purposes.[26]

Local Medical Mobilization

Immediately after the November 29 UN vote, war casualties forced local communities to devise emergency solutions. PAMA began training emergency units and opening emergency centers. In Haifa and Jaffa, British and Arab doctors established and trained first-aid committees made up of local volunteers.[27] In December 1947, women's organizations, doctors, and schools established urgent care centers in neighborhoods, including in Nazareth and Jerusalem.[28]

From December 1947 to May 1948, civil society participated in local initiatives to treat the wounded and refugees. In January, the Higher Arab Relief Organization was founded. As seen in Figure 7.1, its insignia was a combination of the Red Crescent and Red Cross. It was composed of Dr. Husayn Fakhri al-Khalidi, as a representative

[25] GTM.Gamms315, Box 2, Folder 18, Interviews: Numbered Files, 4a, 1–7 Larry Collins Papers, Georgetown University Library.

[26] See, for example, "Medical Staff Immune," *Palestine Post*, January 6, 1948, 3; "Bayan ra'is al-jam'iyya al-tibbiyya al-'Arabiyya li-l-sha'b al-'Arabi," *al-Difa'*, January 6, 1948, 2; "Kroze ha-rof'im ha-'Ivrim ve-ha-'Arvim 'al hasinut kol 'ovde ha-refu'a," *Ha-Boker*, January 7, 1948, 1.

[27] "Juhud al-jam'iyya al-tibbiyya al-'Arabiyya fi Yafa," *al-Difa'*, December 11, 1947, 3; "Juhud al-jam'iyya al-tibbiyya wa-l-Hilal al-Ahmar fi Hayfa," *Filastin*, December 10, 1947, 2.

[28] "Ta'lif 5 wahadat tibbiyya li-l-is'af al-awwali bi-l-Nasira," *al-Difa'*, December 18, 1947, 2; "Insha' 10 marakiz tibbiyya li-l-tawari' fi al-Quds," *al-Difa'*, December 9, 1947, 4.

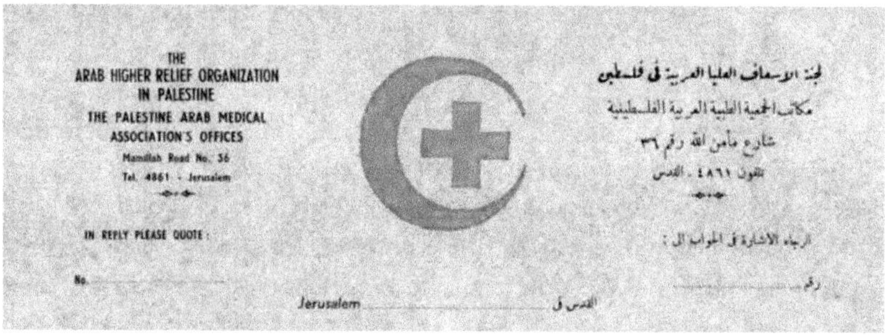

Figure 7.1 Insignia of the Higher Arab Relief Organization.
PAMA, P-990/19, ISA

of the Arab Higher Committee, and Drs. Tawfiq Canaan, Mahmud Tahir al-Dajani, and ʿIzzat Tanus, along with Zulayha Shihabi, Chairwoman of the Palestine Women's Union.[29] Most efforts, however, remained localized.

An emergency committee established in Tiberias in January discussed the possibility of establishing an emergency hospital in the city or its vicinity. Suggestions included converting a hotel into a hospital or using Dr. Rashid al-Tabari's personal home for the purpose and training volunteers from the girls' school.[30] In Safad, the Government Hospital was operated by volunteer nurses.[31] Students of Jenin's secondary school, in league with Dr. Amin Rweiha, decided to establish and equip a twenty-bed hospital in the city and contacted Dr. al-Khalidi for assistance. Jenin's Freemasons' Club served as an emergency clinic.[32] In Jenin and Nablus, women's organizations and students established emergency hospitals.[33] Qalqilya's high-school students turned it into a hospital.[34]

29 "Tashkil al-lajna al-ʿulya li-l-isʿaf wa-tanzim furuʿiha," *al-Difaʿ*, January 28, 1948, 2.
30 "Jalsat lajnat al-isʿaf wa-l-khidamat al-tibbiyya," n.d.; letter from Dr. Rushdi al-Tamimi to the Higher Arab Committee, January 9, 1948, PAMA, P-990/19, ISA.
31 "Bet ha-holim ha-memshalti bi-Tsfat," January 23, 1948, 168, "Hitʾargenut rofʾim," file no. 105/166HA.
32 PAMA, letter from Dr. Mahmud Tahir al-Dajani to Dr. Husayn Fakhri bek al-Khalidi, January 24, 1948, P-990/19, ISA.
33 "Mustashfa al-tulab bi-Nablus li-isʿaf al-munadilin," *al-Difaʿ*, February 29, 1948, 2; "Tajhiz mustashfayayn bi-Jinin," *al-Difaʿ*, March 19, 1948, 2.
34 "Madrasat Qalqilya al-thanawiyya tanshaʾu madrasa li-l-jiraha," *Filastin*, March 12, 1948, 3.

In Lydda, Drs. Mustafa al-Zahlan and Najib Abu Jawdeh provided volunteers with quick training as nurses, and donations were collected for the purchase of medical supplies, equipment, and an ambulance. When casualties kept pouring in, the First Aid Committee managed to turn the CMS boarding school into a sixty-bed hospital, furnishing it to receive patients and conduct minor surgeries.[35]

During these tense months, the Women's Union and its branches took an active part in the furnishing of hospital beds and treating the wounded. A women's union in Tulkarem requested equipment and medications for their hospital and opened a small emergency hospital at Dr. Adib Khartabil's clinic. In Acre, the women's organization opened a hospital in the Ahmedi School.[36] The Palestinian Women's Union branch in Bethlehem, headed by Bertha Ma'luf, along with the local Orthodox Scouts, operated two first-aid centers.[37]

Gaza's PAMA branch met in mid December to divide responsibilities between its members in Gaza, Majdal, Beersheba, Khan Yunis, Rafah, Isdud, and Masmiya – and each doctor was placed in charge of a specific region.[38] Gaza's Orthodox Club turned its building into an emergency hospital, and Dr. Sulayman Qlibu volunteered to offer basic first-aid training, while Dr. Fu'ad Musallam's wife was appointed Head of the Government Hospital.[39] Beit Jala's Everest Café was converted into a hospital as well,[40] and a field hospital was similarly operated in al-Bireh.[41]

Jaffa and Haifa's Fight for Life

Haifa and Jaffa deserve a separate discussion because of their weight in Palestine's medical life. Both cities witnessed the government hospitals'

35 Reja-e Busailah, "The Fall of Lydda, 1948: Impressions and Reminiscences," *Arab Studies Quarterly* 3 (1981): 123–51.
36 "Iftitah mustashfa al-ittihad al-nisa'i fi 'Akka," *al-Difa'*, January 28, 1948, 2.
37 "Lajnat is'af fi Bayt Lahm," *al-Difa'*, March 14, 1948, 3.
38 PAMA, protocol of the Arab Medical Association in Gaza, December 20, 1947, P-990/19, ISA; "Tadabir al-jam'iyya al-tibbiyya bi-Ghazza li-tanzim shu'un al-is'af," *al-Difa'*, December 25, 1947, 3.
39 "Markaz al-is'afat al-awwaliyya bi-Ghazza," *al-Difa'*, January 1, 1948, 3; "Akhbar mukhtalifa," *Filastin*, February 26, 1948, 2.
40 "Bet holim be-Bet Jala," January 5, 1948, p. 60, "Hit'argenut rof'im," 105/166, HA.
41 "Al-Mustashfa li-l-is'af al-awwali bi-l-Birah," *al-Difa'*, February 11, 1948, 3.

inability to survive British defunding and the departure of their Jewish personnel, the collapse of missionary hospitals, and subsequent attempts of civil society mobilization to provide satisfactory medical aid. In both cases, attempts were possible thanks to joint efforts and collaboration between PAMA's representatives and the respective women's association.

In early December 1947, Haifa's National Committee decided to establish a hospital. Twenty beds were purchased and, under the guidance of PAMA and private clinics, were to be converted into first-aid stations. Later that month, PAMA ordered all doctors to provide free treatment to the wounded. In early January, a local medical committee was established to administer medical aid, and the Lebanese government donated 100 beds and surgical equipment.[42] Haifa's Women's Union, led by medical committee member Miryam Khalil ʿAwaida, donated its building and turned it, with the assistance of the Lebanese donation and the local PAMA branch, into an emergency hospital with a surgical unit. They named it Amin Hospital, after national leader Hajj Amin al-Husayni. It was evacuated in late April 1948.[43] Adjacent to it, the women's Red Crescent Society operated the al-Hilal Hospital, led by Dr. Rushdi Tamimi.[44] According to one testimony, Tamimi and his staff continued treating the wounded until the city was occupied.[45] In March, Dr. Michel Jbara converted his three-story house in Wadi Nisnas into a hospital and donated all his

[42] Tamir Goren, *Hefa ha-ʿArvit be-tashah: ʿOtsmat ha-maʾavak u-memade ha-hitmotetut* (Tel Aviv: Ben-Gurion University of the Negev Press, 2006), 179–81, 300–03.

[43] PAMA, letter from Maryam al-Khalil ʿAwaida to the Higher Arab Committee, January 24, 1948, P-990/19, ISA. Dr. Tamimi traveled to Beirut in early January to raise funds for the hospital, "Inshaʾ mustashfa ʿArabi yudahi al-mustashfayat al-ʿaskariyya," *al-Difaʿ*, January 1, 1948, 4; on the Lebanese donation, see "Tabarruʿ Lubnan bi-ghurfat ʿamaliyyat wa-muʿaddat mustashfa kamil," *al-Difaʿ*, January 12, 1948, 1; on its opening, see "Mustashfa 'al-Amin' bi-Hayfa yubashir wajibatahu al-insaniyya," *al-Difaʿ*, February 4, 1948, 2. In mid March it was operative, but lacked supplies, "ʿInayat Mustashfa al-Amin bi-Hayfa bi-jurahaʾ al-nidal," *al-Difaʿ*, March 10, 1948, 2.

[44] This hospital operated at least until early April, "Juhud al-sayyidat al-ʿArabiyyat li-tanshit Mustashfa al-Hillal," *al-Difaʿ*, April 5, 1948, 2.

[45] Rashid al-Haj Ibrahim, *al-Difaʿ ʿan Hayfa wa-qadiyat Filastin: Mudhakkirat Rashid al-Hajj Ibrahim, 1891–1953*, ed. Walid Khalidi (Beirut: Muʾassasat al-dirasat al-Filastiniyya, 2005).

medical equipment. He named it al-Hakim, after the Greek Catholic Bishop, a local patriot.[46]

Jaffa's health services during the war were no better than those of its northern sister.[47] In December 1947, the Jaffa Medical Association sent doctors to the hospitals and helped train women for first-aid assignments.[48] In February 1948, PAMA, the Red Cross and Red Crescent Societies, and women's associations helped turn the CMS hospital, closed in mid 1946, into an emergency hospital and managed to obtain an ambulance.[49] Women's donations enabled the opening of a small Red Cross and Red Crescent hospital.[50]

The Health Committee in Jaffa included Dr. Hasan Far'un, who headed Jaffa's Medical Association. "Life in the city has ceased ..." Far'un recalled. "Only twenty percent of the doctors and hospital employees are still doing their job. The patients' condition is very bleak. We are having problems finding who will bury the dead." The situation in Jaffa, which had become an isolated enclave since early 1948, quickly deteriorated. Far'un reported that during and after the war, hospitals and medical centers were looted.[51] He petitioned Amin al-Husayni, president of the Arab Higher Committee, for medical supplies. We have enough doctors, he emphasized, but lack medical supplies and even food.[52]

Far'un would remain the only Arab doctor in Jaffa's post 1948 Arab enclave, the "Ghetto." As the city was under night curfew, patients who visited him by night sometimes got arrested. Egyptian Dr. Hassan Hathut visited Jaffa in April 1948 and was bewildered by the sight of

46 "Mustashfa 'Arabi jadid fi madinat Hayfa," *al-Difa'*, March 12, 1948, 4; "Mustashfa jadid fi harat wadi al-nisnas bi-Hayfa," *Filastin*, March 12, 1948, 4.
47 Radai, *Palestinians*, 142.
48 "Fi al-zuruf al-khadira: Tadabir tattakhidhuha al-jam'iyya al-tibbiyya al-'Arabiyya bi-Yafa," *Filastin*, December 11, 1947, 2.
49 "Tajhiz al-Mustashfa al-Inglizi," *al-Difa'*, February 29, 1948, 2; "al-Mustashfa al-Inglizi fi Yafa yaftahu abwabahu," *Filastin*, March 9, 1948, 2.
50 "'Ishrun sariran bi-ajhizatiha," *al-Difa'*, March 29, 1948, 2.
51 Imtiyaz Diyyab, *'Atr madinat Yafa* (Beirut: Dar al-fata al-'Arabi, 1991), 67–68.
52 Hasan Far'un to Hajj Amin al-Husayni, January 25, 1948, Muhammad Zuhdi al-Dajani to Husayn Fakhri al-Khalidi, February 1, 1948, and Hasan Far'un to Mahmud Tahir al-Dajani, March 4, 1948, "PAMA," P-990/19, ISA. "Khidmat Mustashfa al-Dajani bi-Yafa wa-a'maluhu," *al-Sha'b*, January 12, 1948, 3; "Ihmal mu'ib natlub min al-hukuma talafihi halan," *al-Sha'b*, January 17, 1948, 3.

the empty city. He visited its hospital and took with him the remaining patients and hospital supplies to the Egyptian hospital in Ramle.[53]

Pleading for Arab Aid

Raising funds for medical care from neighboring countries was a serious challenge. As we have seen in Chapter 6, Palestinian physicians maintained decades-long connections with their peers in Arab countries, and the war proved to be a baptism of fire for Arab medical solidarity. Shortly after the outbreak of hostilities, PAMA sent an urgent appeal to medical associations across the region. In early January 1948, the Egyptian Red Crescent sent first-aid materials that were promptly distributed to emergency care centers in Jerusalem, Jaffa, Haifa, Gaza, and Nablus. Some materials were also dispatched from the Palestine office in Beirut, and two equipped ambulances arrived from the Iraqi Red Crescent Society in Baghdad.[54] The Arab League donated £3,000, which ended up falling into Jewish hands.[55] Other donations reached Palestine from Egypt and Iraq in May 1948, but large sums and medical supplies were confiscated by Jewish forces shortly after the British departure and the Jewish takeover of Jerusalem's Arab neighborhoods.[56] Donations that reached their destination were far too modest to meet wartime medical needs. On January 21, 1948, Dr. Khalidi met government representatives from Lebanon, Jordan, Syria, and Iraq in Amman to discuss Palestine's medical predicament. Arab governments had already pledged the cost of 200 beds – 100 in Amin Hospital in Haifa and 100 in Beit Safafa's hospital. The Amman conference concluded that Palestine needed an additional 375 beds, namely a total of 575, to be equipped by neighboring countries, along with twenty-four equipped

53 Hassan Hathut, *Fi dhikra al-Nakba: Yawmiyyat tabib Misri fi Filastin* (Cairo: Markaz al-iʿlam al-ʿArabi, 2008), 62–72.

54 Tawfiq Canaan and Mahmud Tahir al-Dajani, *al-Jamʿiyya al-tibbiyya al-ʿArabiyya al-Filastiniyya: Taqrir ʿam ʿan juhud al-jamʿiyya wa-jihadiha 1948–1950* (Jerusalem: Matbaʿat dar al-aytam al-Islamiyya al-sinaʿiyya, 1951), 10–11; "Baʿthat tibbiyya ila Filastin," *al-Difaʿ*, January 14, 1948, 2.

55 Letter from Secretary of the Arab Higher Committee to Secretary of the Jordanian Medical Association, January 17, 1948, PAMA, P-990/19, ISA.

56 Canaan and al-Dajani, *al-Jamʿiya*, 11–13.

ambulances and volunteer surgeons and nurses. The Arab Legion also promised to send troops to protect Palestinian hospitals.[57]

Shorter-lived aid arrived from Lebanon: a Red Cross hospital operated by a Lebanese doctor, with nurses and medical equipment, began operating in Acre on April 22, less than four weeks before its surrender. The hospital's personnel found themselves unable to return home and demanded the International Committee of the Red Cross (ICRC) intervention, which managed to secure their safe return in July. Over the next two years, the hospital's equipment was the subject of negotiations between the Lebanese Red Cross, ICRC, and the Israeli government until some compensation and recuperation were secured.[58]

The biggest and longest-standing medical aid arrived from Egypt. In February 1948, a convoy with thirty-one doctors, male nurses, and paramedics, along with several ambulances and twenty-five lorries loaded with medical supplies, reached Palestine from Egypt.[59] The Nile Valley Committee for Palestine Rescue donated the ambulances and supplies.[60] The Egyptian delegation also included high-school girls with first-aid training.[61]

The main beneficiary of Egyptian assistance efforts was the field hospital in Ramle, established in mid February 1948.[62] Ramle-born Dr. Rasim al-Khayri recalled treating three Jewish fighters: one woman who died of hemorrhage and two men whom they managed to save.[63] Dr. Hassan Hathut also mentioned treating both Jewish and Arab combatants, including a young woman, Shoshana Jamil, an Irgun

[57] Ibid.; "al-Qararat allati uttukhidat min qibal mumaththili jama'iyyat al-Hilal wa-l-Salib al-Ahmar al-'Arabiyya bi-jalsatihi 21/1/1948, allati 'uqidat fi 'Amman."

[58] Mission en Palestine, questions spéciales, seizième partie, BG 059/I/GC-114, ICRC archive.

[59] "Istiqbal hafil li-ba'that al-Hilal al-Ahmar al-Misriyya," *al-Difa'*, February 19, 1948, 2.

[60] Canaan and al-Dajani, *al-Jam'iyya*, 11–13; "50 Alf junayh li-shira' adwiya li-'Arab Filastin," *al-Difa'*, February 8, 1948, 2; "al-hay'a al-'Arabiyya wa-imdad Filastin bi-mu'addat al-is'af," *al-Difa'*, February 10, 1948, 4; "Wusul mustashfa al-maydan al-Misri," *Filastin*, February 19, 1948, 2.

[61] "al-Tamrin 'ala al-is'af," *Filastin*, March 17, 1948.

[62] Telegram from 'Adli Basha, Egypt, to the Higher Emergency Council, Jerusalem, February 17, 1948, PAMA, P-990/19, ISA; "Tsror yedi'ot," in "Hit'argenut rof'im," June 1, 1948, 105/166, 83, HA.

[63] Walid al-Khalidi, *al-Ramla tatakallam* (Amman: n.p., 1991), 104–05.

paramedic, who died of severe spinal injuries.[64] In May, the delegation was relocated to Ramallah after having been bombed from the air. Palestinian doctors kept operating the hospital for a few more months.[65]

The Egyptian hospital had a short afterlife in Ramle. In early 1949, Dr. Zahlan still operated its outpatient clinic, as well as two clinics in Lydda, which he frequented once or twice a week. Reports by the Israeli MoH stated that both patients and workers at this hospital verged on starvation, demanding an urgent solution. Dr. Zahlan testified that he was feeding patients with bread and tea, for lack of supplies, and that he was now running out of flour. Although the MoH was able to temporarily grant some aid to Zahlan, working conditions deteriorated in the last months of 1948.[66] The IDF's medical service had already taken over the hospital's equipment, and in early February the Military Governor decided to close it down. Dr. Zahlan, "who had long requested to join his family in Syria," was allowed to do so, and a Jewish doctor replaced him as Ramle's physician.[67]

Jerusalem Burning

Many of Jerusalem's elite, including doctors, lived and worked in its western neighborhoods of Talbiya, Qatamon, and Baqʿa. Villa Kalbian in Talbiya was built for Dr. Vahan Kalbian in the 1920s, and Dr. ʿIzzat Tanous lived on the upper floor of his brother's villa in that neighborhood. Nearby was a hotel owned by Dr. Canaan, alongside the villas

64 He also reported shortage of medication and clean water. Hathut, *Fi dhikra al-Nakba*, 118–24; From the head of the Egyptian medical delegation in Ramle to the Egyptian military headquarters, May 17, 1948, 120, "Hitʾargenut rofʾim," file no. 105/166, HA; *Herut*, October 6, 1946.

65 From the head of the Egyptian medical delegation …, May 17, 1948, 120, "Hitʾargenut rofʾim," file no. 105/166, HA.

66 "Hospitals and Medical Institutions: A Hospital in Ramle (Occupation of Arab Territory)," Dr. K. Lichtig, "The Hospital in Ramle – Protocol," October 6, 1948, ISA; and H. Elishar to Director of the Ministry of Health, "The Hospital in Ramle: Today's Conversation with Dr Lichtig," September 21, 1948; "Hospitals and Medical Institutions: A Hospital in Ramle (Occupation of Arab Territory)," Dr. Emile Moeri, Report no. 24: "Evacuation de l'Hopital de Ramleh," ISA.

67 Dr. Malhi, Director of Services to the Minorities, to Military Governor H. Yavetz, Protocol of Visit to Ramle and Lydda, 15 December 48; minutes of meeting regarding medical services to the minorities, Military Governor Office, Ramle, February 2, 1949.

of Drs. Krikor Krikorian, Ya'qub Nuzha, Tawfiq Baz Haddad, Yousef Hajjar, and Katcher Keshishian. Qatamon was home to Drs. Mahmud Tahir al-Dajani and Futi Freij.[68] The Mamilla area, close to Jaffa Gate, was a commercial and medical hub where Mahmud and Nahil Dajani and Futi Freij's clinics could be found, alongside several Palestinian-owned pharmacies and the dental clinics of 'Isa al-Dajani, Sami Abu Swan, Kamel Itayim, and Burhan Abd al-Hadi.[69] The war made short work of this medical landscape.

The explosion at the Semiramis Hotel in Qatamon on January 5 initiated the population's departure, and the displacement of western neighborhoods was completed in the coming months. The Haganah's bomb killed eighteen people, including dentist Dr. Sami Abu Swan's parents. It awakened Dr. Jirji Mansour's family with terror, shaking the entire house: "We wanted to leave Jerusalem at any cost," he wrote in his diary.[70] On March 10, 1948, Freij's Qatamon house was leveled by a bomb placed by the Stern Gang.[71] George Khuri Farah left his luxurious residence in Upper Baq'a and moved with his four children to the nearby village of Ezariya.[72] Canaan lived in Musrara and was determined to remain there with his sister and wife, despite the bombings. They finally left in early May after a direct hit destroyed their building's third floor. The famous doctor found refuge in one of the Greek Patriarchy's properties in the Old City.[73]

Since early December 1947, youth and women's associations mobilized the community and raised funds. On December 10, posters circulated by PAMA announced the opening of ten emergency clinics around Jerusalem, and four more were added a week later. These were to operate in existing private and public clinics with the help of volunteers who were being trained around the city.[74] With the green

68 Dr. Dajani's house was the subject of Amos Gitai's 1980 documentary film "House"; David Kroyanker, *Shkhunot Yerushalayim: Talbiye, Katamon ve-ha-Moshava ha-Yevanit* (Jerusalem: Mekhon Yerushalayim le-heker Yisra'el: Keter, 2002), 26, 68, 96, 104.

69 Bashir Barakat, *Ta'rikh al-khidamat al-sihhiyya fi Bayt al-Maqdis* (Istanbul: Dar al-nida', 2019), 84–88, 132–33.

70 Hutchison, "Occidental Obsessions."

71 Radai, *Palestinians*, 68.

72 John N. Tleel, *I Am Jerusalem* (Jerusalem: J. N. Tleel, 2007), 98.

73 Laura S. Schor, *Sophie Halaby in Jerusalem: An Artist's Life* (New York: Syracuse University Press, 2019), 105.

74 Radai, *Palestinians*, 23; Letter from Dr. Mahmud Tahir al-Dajani to the Arab Higher Committee, December 8, 1947, PAMA, P-990/19, ISA.

light from the Arab Higher Committee, PAMA, the Women's Association, and the Arab Scouts led the operation. The fourteen centers included, for example, the Arab Women's Union clinic under Dr. Salim Maʿtuq, Dr. Akram Nuri's clinic in Damascus Gate, and the private homes of Drs. Futi Freij and Yaʿqub Nuzha in Qatamon. In Talbiya, a medical center was operated by Drs. Kabian, Tawfiq Haddad, and Emile Khadar. Dr. Mahmud Tahir al-Dajani was in charge of the clinic in PAMA's office in Mamilla, and Dr. Amin Majaj was responsible for the Muslim Brotherhood's center.[75] These initiatives all lacked resources and trained personnel from the outset.[76] More importantly, the doctors and clinics outside the Old City, in the western neighborhoods, probably operated for only a few weeks, challenged by their rapid depopulation and ongoing skirmishes.

Three central medical facilities, the St. John Ophthalmic Hospital, English Mission Hospital, and French Hospital, were located west of the Old City. St. John's was isolated early on, forcing personnel and patients' to evacuate during the first weeks of the war. In January 1948, Vaad Leumi requested Rev. Jones to use the English Mission Hospital as an emergency hospital for Jewish casualties. Their petition stated the hospital was "at present empty, and the staff are standing with nothing to do." In response, the bishop stated it would be wiser to offer the hospital, as well as other mission hospitals, to ICRC.[77] Since early February, Red Shield of David Society operated a first-aid unit in one of the hospital's buildings, later used as a Hadassah clinic.[78] The French Hospital, part of the Notre Dame complex, treated wounded combatants in the early stages of the war. It was occupied by Jewish forces in mid May, while still treating dozens of refugees, patients, and casualties, and employing forty-eight workers.[79]

Following Dr. Lehrs' murder in late December 1947, and as in Haifa and Jaffa's hospitals, the Vaad Leumi ordered all Jewish personnel to leave Jerusalem's Government Hospital, distributing them among

[75] Barakat, *al-Khidamat*, 165. [76] Radai, *Palestinians*, 24.

[77] "English Mission Hospital," M-326/61, ISA.

[78] "Tahanat Hadasha le-ʿezra rishona," *Haaretz*, February 6, 1948, 7.

[79] On French hospitals and treatment of wounded Arabs during the war, "Batei haholim ha-Tsarfatiyyim makom marpe' li-knufiyot," *Ha-Boker*, December 29, 1947; Radai, *Palestinians*, 100.

Jewish hospitals in the city.[80] From early 1948, it was run solely by Palestinian Arab personnel.[81] In late January, the DoH opened a branch at the Government Hospital building in the Russian Compound to enable Arabs to register deaths and births and vaccinate children.[82] The compound was caught in the crossfire of Jewish forces on the neighboring DHO's roof and the Arab Legion soldiers on the Palestine Broadcasting Service's roof.[83] PAMA took over its management, which suffered from a severe lack of medical personnel. When Haganah forces occupied surrounding neighborhoods, an agreement was signed between the DoH, ICRC, and PAMA to maintain the hospital after the British departure. On May 17, it became a Red Cross Hospital, maintained by Arab funds.[84]

Dr. Hasib Bulus worked in the hospital in May 1948, in the early days of the compound's occupation. Fearing Israeli retaliation against wounded Arab soldiers, he took care to evacuate them. He kept telephone contact with Ibrahim Tleel at the Austrian Hospice in the Old City, further discussed later, but was not allowed to rejoin and assist him. On May 23, in one of his attempts to reach the Old City with a nurse and another doctor, he was detained several times by Israeli soldiers. A Jordanian bombardment forced him to return to the compound.[85]

The hospital kept operating for six months under Israeli military control. In July 1948, an Israeli hospital started operating on the building's first floor, using the Government Hospital's facilities and equipment. The former Government Hospital's staff operated a Red Cross Hospital on the second floor. Its patients and staff were not allowed to communicate with anyone outside hospital premises and were prohibited to leave or use its garden, balconies, or roof without the Military Governor's explicit permission. Both the Palestinian and Israeli staff became weary of the deadlock.[86]

80 "Insihab al-atibba᾽ al-Yahud min Mustashfa al-Hukuma," *al-Difa῾*, December 30, 1947, 4.

81 Lester's report, 11–12; "Rofe᾽ Yehudi nirtsah be-vet ha-holim ha-memshalti be-Bet Safafa le-῾ene ῾ozro ha-῾Aravi," *Ha-Boker*, December 29, 1947.

82 "Far῾ jadid li-da᾽irat al-sihha," *al-Sha῾b*, January 28, 1948.

83 Lester's report, 14. 84 Ibid., 12.

85 GTm.Gamms315, Box 4, Doctor Bolous Hassib, 7–11, Georgetown University Library, Larry Collins Papers.

86 "The Red Cross Hospital," G-22/283, ISA, "The Red Cross Hospital in the Russian Compound," 18/7/[1948]; Letter from the military governor to the physician-in-charge, Red Cross Hospital, Russian Compound, August 17, 1948;

In October 1948, Dr. As'ad Bishara, the Palestinian director of Jerusalem's former Government Hospital, negotiated the hospital's surrender to Israeli authorities and the transfer of its staff to the Old City. The Israeli authorities subsequently negotiated the transition of the hospital and former DoH buildings with ICRC representatives. Since most of Hadassah Hospital's equipment remained in the Jewish enclave on Mount Scopus, by then surrounded by Jordanian-controlled territory, the Israelis also requested that they be allowed to use the hospital's equipment.[87] Bishara urged the Red Cross to intervene, but they were preparing to leave Palestine. He was frustrated: "This matter has already dragged beyond anybody's endurance ... This pitiful state of affairs cannot go on forever. We have urgent duties toward ourselves, our families, and our professional consciousness."[88] On November 19, Bishara and his staff left with their equipment in three UN cars and his own private car. The quick departure was enabled by a two-hour truce.[89]

Inside the Old City, the Austrian Hospice was turned into a field hospital.[90] A male nurse working there described the sight of dead and dying combatants as a surreal experience, reminiscent of a *Gone with the Wind* scene he had seen a year before. He circulated a plea for donations, and people indeed brought fuel, items of clothing, food, and bandages. Another nurse, Ra'ifa, described an infernal reality of dead bodies mixed with the severely injured and the dying. She worked closely with Dr. Ibrahim Tleel for six full days, without changing her clothes, hardly eating or sleeping, feeding the doctor with a spoon because he operated twenty hours per day without removing his gloves. Arab Legion soldiers came to the hospital only to be returned to the city walls without being treated. Reinforcement arrived later to help the overworked staff.[91]

Dominique-D Junod, *The Imperiled Red Cross and the Palestine-Eretz-Yisrael Conflict, 1945–1952: The Influence of Institutional Concerns on a Humanitarian Operation* (London: Kegan Paul International, 1996), 152–54.

87 IMA, 1949-959-227.

88 Letter from Dr. Bishara, Medical Superintendent, Government Hospital, Russian Compound, Jerusalem, October 23, 1948, "The Red Cross Hospital," G-22/283, ISA.

89 Barakat, *al-Khidamat*, 188; *Palestine Post*, November 21, 1948, 3.

90 Canaan and al-Dajani, *al-Jam'iyya*, 36–37.

91 Anwar al-Khatib Tamimi, *Ma'a salah al-din fi al-Quds: Ta'ammulat wa-dhikrayat* (Jerusalem: Dar al-tiba'a al-'Arabiyya, 1989), 116–17; Larry Collins Papers, "Aladin et Raifeh Rimawi," 5–8.

Tleel himself was twenty-nine years old in 1948 and operated the emergency hospital at the Austrian Hospice virtually on his own. He had never performed major operations before and was now forced into an around-the-clock operating routine. He telephoned Dr. Hasib Bulus at the Government Hospital, only two years his senior, for advice and consulted his six-volume edition of Love and Bailley's *Emergency Surgery*. He had a room above the operating theater but hardly used it – literally falling asleep on a chair between operations. His operating table used to be a gynecological table, the sterilizer looked like an old washing machine, and the X-ray machine did not work. And yet, he managed to save lives.[92] In April 1949, the Jordanian government signed a contract with the Austrian Church, enabling permanent hospital work at the hospice's compound; its rent was paid until 1967.[93]

Ibrahim's uncle, Nicolas, was a dentist, as were his sons, David and John. While in the Old City, Nicolas asked the Jordanian Military Governor for a permit to cross into the Jewish-controlled zone, reach his clinic, and retrieve some of his medical equipment. He received the permit, crossed the newly created borders, and was escorted by IDF soldiers to his house. With the help of Israeli soldiers, they were able to carry the heavy dental chair to the Old City. It was placed at the St. Nicholas convent, which served the Old City's refugee population.[94]

Another hospital maintained and operated by Palestinian doctors was the former government Infectious Diseases Hospital in Beit Safafa, closed by Mandate authorities in early 1948 following Lehrs' assassination. PAMA assumed responsibility over the hospital under the directorship of Dr. Nahil Habub al-Dajani and a small team of doctors, including her husband, Dr. Mahmud Tahir al-Dajani (see Figure 7.2).[95] Volunteers from the Women's Association cleaned the hospital and prepared it for operation. It was renamed the People's Arab Hospital (*al-mustashfa al-ahli al-ʿArabi*) and opened its doors in

92 "Dr Ibrahim Tlil – Austrian Hospice," 1–5, GTM.Gamms315, Box 4, Larry Collins Papers.

93 Barakat, *al-Khidamat*, 189–90.

94 Tleel, *I Am Jerusalem*, 33–34, 35, 39–40.

95 Lester's report, 11; "al-Jamʿiyya al-tibbiyya al-ʿArabiyya tatawwala mustashfa Bayt Safafa," *al-Difaʿ*, January 14, 1948, 2; "al-Hayʾa al-ʿArabiyya al-ʿUlya tatasalim mustashfa Bayt Safafa," *Filastin*, January 17, 1948, 2; Canaan and al-Dajani, *al-Jamʿiya*, 22–33.

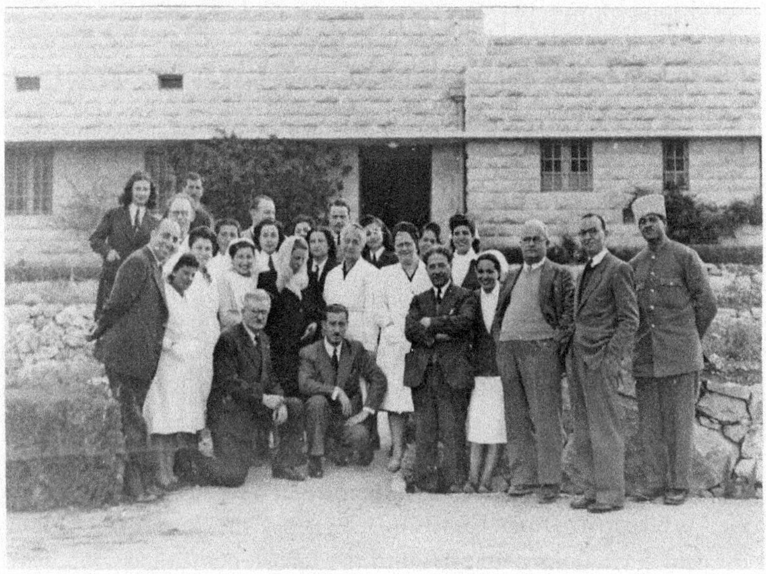

Figure 7.2 Staff of the Beit Safafa Hospital with CICR Doctors, January 30, 1948, Archive CICR, V-P-PS-E-00107.

From left to right: George Atallah, Tawfiq Canaan, and Mahmud Tahir al-Dajani (both kneeling), Nahil al-Dajani (standing wearing glasses), Yousef Hajjar.

mid February. Drs. al-Dajani and Rashid al-Nashashibi moved their practice there. After the British withdrawal, the hospital staff found itself cut off from medical and food supply, but refused to surrender. Protected by Jordanian troops, it kept treating patients. Nurses brought water from a nearby well and food from neighboring Beit Jalla and Bethlehem, carrying Red Cross and Red Crescent flags. During the June ceasefire, some of the wounded were evacuated, and roads were paved to facilitate the provision of food, water, and supplies. A July attack on the hospital wounded some of the nurses and in early August patients and equipment were evacuated to safety in Beit Jalla and Bethlehem. The hospital resumed operation in March 1949.[96]

Jerusalem's medical community had a different fortune than its counterparts in Jaffa and Haifa. After their displacement, the city's geography enabled resettlement and reemployment in the eastern areas

[96] Canaan and al-Dajani, *al-Jamʿiyya*, 31–33.

controlled by Arab forces. PAMA's leadership was centered in Jerusalem and led by Jerusalemite doctors who made great efforts to organize and support the war effort. Old City's churches and convents offered shelter for the wounded and vital spaces for treatment. Many doctors lost their homes and immediate livelihood, but were able to find employment under the Jordanian forces who were quick to take control of what was left of their city.

Northern Exposures: Those Who Remained

Elias Sruji's pediatric career was moving forward satisfactorily. After completing his residency, he opened a private clinic in his native Nazareth. But the young doctor had greater ambitions. He signed a five-year rental lease for a three-story building in Haifa, planning to turn it into a large clinic with two colleagues.[97] But the war moved faster than his plans. Still in Palestinian hands in mid April, he became preoccupied with the refugees and wounded combatants who flooded Nazareth.[98] In June 1948, Sruji left for Beirut to treat his sick father, and returned in late September after learning that the Galilee was in dire need of doctors. He managed to reach Tarshiha and operated a clinic in a former IWC for three weeks, using medical equipment and medications left there, before returning to Beirut for medical supplies.

The journey back to Nazareth began in late October. As it had been occupied since mid July, the plan was to reach Rama, which was still in Arab hands, and cross the no-man's-land at night to his hometown. The plan failed. The route was too mountainous and risky, and the Srujis ended up staying in Rama, which was soon to be occupied as well. After the occupation, the Christians were ordered to pack their possessions and promptly leave the village, but somehow the Srujis were spared. Decades later the doctor found out it was because one of the Israeli officers returned a favor: he was the son of his father's employee, protected by the latter during the 1929 riots.[99] Sruji and

[97] Ilyas Salim Sruji, *Min muruj al-Jalil, mudhakkirat tabib min al-Nasira* (Nazareth: Matbaʿat al-hakim, 2011), 152–53.

[98] Ibid., 158–61.

[99] Elias Srouji, "The Last Days of 'Free Galilee': Memories of 1948," *Journal of Palestine Studies* 33 (2003): 55–67; Elias Srouji, "The Fall of a Galilean Village During the 1948 Palestine War: An Eyewitness Account," *Journal of Palestine Studies* 33 (2004): 71–80; Sruji, *Min muruj*, 182.

his family finally returned to Nazareth under the orders of the famous Colonel-Prof. Gideon Mer, who wanted him to head the anti-smallpox campaign there. IDF cars took the entire family back home.[100] By late 1948, the Galilee came under the jurisdiction of the Israeli MoH and the few remaining Palestinian doctors were hired as its employees. Sruji stayed in his hometown until 1967.

During the last years of the Mandate, thirty doctors are documented as having worked north of Haifa: eight in Nazareth, eight in Acre, seven in Safad, three in Tiberias, and the rest in Bisan, Rama, Kafr Kanna, Tarshiha, and Shefa-ʿAmr. Tiberias, Safad, and Bisan were completely emptied of their Palestinian Arab inhabitants, and only a third of Acre's inhabitants remained. Nazareth remained the only Arab city in the state of Israel, and Tarshiha, Rama, and Kafr Kanna remained populated. The result of this uneven process was that the Galilee boasted the largest number of Palestinian Arab doctors in the young State of Israel – most of them in Nazareth and Acre. Drs. Munir Mishʿalani, Saba Barnick, Mikhaʾil Shammas, Muwaffaq Diab, Yusuf Haddad, Ilyas Dib, and ʻAtallah Shiban remained the main providers of health services to the Galilee's remaining villages. The first three were employed by the MoH, which relied on their DoH experience.[101] Dr. Shammas remained in Nazareth after the war, upon the request of the city's mayor.[102]

The immediate effect of the war for those who remained included both plunder and confiscation of private property – a fate they shared with fellow Palestinians everywhere. The Israeli archives contain several petitions by doctors demanding restitution or compensation.[103] Dr. Saba Barnick tried, through formal and informal channels, to retrieve his confiscated 1946 Hudson car, his entire clinic equipment, and many other personal possessions, missing since the occupation of Acre.[104] MoH Director Dr. Fritz Noak responded that Barnick's car would be taken care of, but as for his losses during and after the war, "he could not express an opinion." "My condition," he wrote, "was

[100] Sruji, *Min muruj*, 188–90.
[101] Tippul refuʾi u-bdikot refuʾiyot, G-155/7, ISA; G154/17, ISA.
[102] 1966-263-1802, IMA; 1952-922-63, IMA; Srouji, *Min muruj*, 192–93.
[103] See, for example, Jaffa-based dentist Gazaros Demirijian, whose clinic has been looted. See 1953-1255-240, IMA.
[104] Typed copy of a letter written by Dr. Barnick, February 15, 1949, "Dr. Barnik," G-298/86, ISA.

much worse than Barnick's" and the damages caused by the enemy in Jerusalem were "much more radical." His own claims, he noted, if that was of any comfort to Barnick, remained unanswered as well. Dr. Barnick, Noak concluded, was appointed "by us" as a government doctor and continued to receive his salary since the war and was thus better off than many Jewish officials. According to available sources, Barnick's Hudson was never returned.[105]

In a similar vein, Dr. Muwaffaq Diab of Shefa-ʿAmr wrote to the Minister of Minorities in August 1948, requesting the return of his car. He was the only Palestinian doctor who stayed in the area between Acre and Nazareth, he explained. About 12,000 people depended on his services, and his ability to reach them depended on this car. We do not know whether the small Chevrolet was returned to its owner, but the Ministry's Director General instructed its district office in Haifa "not to undertake against the Arabs in the country any measures not undertaken against Jews."[106]

Although officially established in October 1948, already in the war months, the Palestinian Arab society that remained in the Galilee was placed under military rule. It was designed to control and monitor the new Arab minority, which the Israeli state saw as a political and security threat, and prevent the return of Palestinian refugees. Depopulated villages were demolished or settled by Jewish immigrants, and villages that remained populated by Palestinians saw most of their lands confiscated, and their inhabitants were subjected to a convoluted system of travel and work permits – that would last until 1966.

The combination of war outcomes, their designation as second-class citizens, and the Military Government led some remaining Palestinian physicians to leave the country. They had found themselves isolated from family and community, with most of their possessions looted or confiscated.[107] One example is Joseph Dawud, the house physician at the French Hospital in Nazareth, who asked permission to leave in 1953 to return to his native Lebanon and reunite with his family. Another is Dr. Naʿim Qutran: his personal possessions were looted during the war, he was denied access to his orchards, and they were

105 Noak to Brin, April 3, 1949, G-3/90, ISA.

106 "Dr M. Diab," G-310/5, Ministry of Minorities, ISA; see also Dr. Sami Abu Swan's claims about his clinic in Mamila, "Dr Sami Abu Swan," G298/7, ISA.

107 Qaraqra, "Sherutei," 128.

ultimately burned down – forcing him to leave the country.[108] Elsewhere, in Lydda, Minister of Minorities Bekhor Shitrit, met Dr. Najib Abu Jawda in July 1949, and recommended granting his request to reunite with his wife and sons, who had already left for Lebanon a few months before.[109]

In spite of the Military Government restrictions and the mortal danger faced by undocumented returnees, thousands of Palestinians managed to return. Several doctors, such as the Sruji brothers and Dr. Manouq Erdekian, managed to return from Lebanon, but these were exceptional cases. Dr. Erdekian was not considered a threat to Israel. According to his grandson, Dr. Leon Erdekian, he spent three years after the Nakba in Lebanon and returned following an authorization from Ben-Gurion himself.[110] On the Day of Independence in 1961, Erdekian was granted an official reward by the Acre Municipality for his devotion and dedication.[111]

In spite of an acute shortage of Arab medical personnel, the Israeli government refused the return of Arab doctors. In March 1951, MoH officials debated the option of granting Israeli medical licenses to "non-Jewish doctors" who had left the country and returned on a tourist visa. According to Dr. Newman from the ministry, mandatory regulations stipulated that the licenses of doctors who did not update their address at the DoH for two years would be revoked, but since no letters had been sent by the MoH to that effect, the policy regarding these doctors should be clarified.[112] About a month later, the Afula District Medical Officer informed the MoH in Jerusalem that the Military Governor had no objection to employing Dr. ʿAziz Sruji in Nazareth. Dr. Sruji, Elias' brother, had just returned from Lebanon, and the MoH decided to allow him to stay and practice.[113]

[108] Sherene Seikaly, "How I Met My Great-Grandfather: Archives and the Writing of History," *Comparative Studies of South Asia, Africa and the Middle East* 38 (2018): 6–20.

[109] 1950-1860-31, IMA.

[110] Telephone interviews with Dr. Leon Erdekian, Yoni Furas, August 8, 2021, 5.

[111] *Maʿariv*, April 24, 1961.

[112] Tippul refuʾi u-bdikot refuʾiyot, Dr. K. Newman to Mr. A. Globus, "Tokef rishyonam shel rofʾim she-ʿazvu et ha-arets," March 7, 1951.

[113] Tippul refuʾi u-bdikot refuʾiyot, Dr. Sever to Dr. Hasis, "Dr. Sruji ʿAziz, Nazareth," April 10, 1951, G155/5, ISA.

The MoH was established in late May 1948.[114] By September, its administration provided services to the Arab population through the mediation of the Ministry of Minorities,[115] with the Histadrut's Sick Fund (HSF) as the main conduit.[116] In December, the Galilee Military Governor reported poor maintenance of health services. Dr. Barnick, he noted, was not given a car, the ambulance was not fixed, cases of malaria and typhus were not treated, and Arab doctors in Acre were not paid.[117] That same month, a special department headed by Dr. Malhi was assigned to provide healthcare for the Arab population. In early January 1949, Malhi reported the establishment of hospitals, permanent and traveling clinics, and IWCs in the Galilee, Haifa, Jaffa, and Ramle.[118] Later that month, the MoH convened a meeting about the state of health services among the "minorities," with delegates from the HSF, Hadassah, and the government. Malhi lamented the challenges in transportation to the villages, the need for the military's approval, and lack of Arabic-speaking personnel.[119] Four Palestinian doctors had already been employed by the MoH, but none attended the meeting.

In the following years, doctors continued to feel the toll of the Military Government, sometimes trying to circumvent its restrictions. Upon Dr. Shammas' request, Dr. Itzkowitz, whom we encountered in Chapter 5 and who was now the Head of the Israeli Medical Association, recognized the Nazareth Medical Association as a branch thereof. Based on this affiliation, both men petitioned the Galilee Military Governor in April 1950 and requested that the handful of doctors remaining in Nazareth be given six-month rather than one-month permits to leave the city and return, so they could attend the

114 Sachlav Stoler-Liss, Shifra Shvarts, and Mordechai Shani, *Liheyot 'am bari be-artsenu: Bri'ut ha-tsibur ba-'aliyya ha-gdolah, 1948–1960* (Beersheba: Ben-Gurion University of the Negev, 2016), 20–21.

115 Avraham Katzenelson to the Ministry of Minorities, September 15, 1948, G-307/55, ISA.

116 Isaac Zusmanovitch to Moshe Aram, September 30, 1948, G-307/55, ISA.

117 Rahav'am Amir to Haifa's Health Department, December 21, 1948, G-307/55, ISA.

118 Malhi to General Director of the Ministry of Health, January 6, 1949, G-307/55, ISA.

119 "Preventive Medicine Amongst the Minorities," meeting minutes, January 18, 1949, G-307/55, ISA.

association meetings, lectures, and library. The governor denied their request.[120]

In April 1949, Dr. Yusuf Haddad asked permission from the Western Galilee Military Governor to return from his temporary residence in Biʿna to Haifa and resume his medical work. His request was granted, as he seemed not to concern himself with "non-medical" issues.[121] In late 1958, the Military Government revoked his medical license due to his membership in the Popular Front and later expelled him from his home in Nazareth.[122] A few months later, during a meeting of the Haifa branch of the Popular Front, Haddad read a *qasida* he had written and later published in *al-Ittihad*. In it, he protested against Israeli tyranny and exalted the Arab awakening in the party branches.[123] "Does a person become a 'security threat' for standing by his people," Haddad lamented in an open letter, "for his wish to live in peace with his Jewish brethren, and his struggle against oppression and discrimination?"[124]

The Refugee Camps

In late June 1948, Elias Sruji traveled to Beirut to treat his father. One day, while driving his car in the city, he was pulled over by a police officer who took his keys, gave him a receipt, and said he could reclaim the car the next day at the central police headquarters. When he arrived there the following day, he found a group of Palestinian doctors who had been rounded up by Dr. Shafiq Haddad. Sruji knew Haddad as a Medical Officer in Nazareth when he himself was still a medical student. Haddad apologized for the unorthodox method of mobilization but explained that doctors had failed to answer calls to volunteer for the refugees. He succeeded in recruiting Sruji and others to work in the newly established camps. When UNRWA took charge of the refugees' healthcare, Haddad became an AUB professor.[125]

[120] 1966-263-1802, IMA; 1952-922-63, IMA.

[121] Ministry of Minorities, "Dr Yusef Haddad," G-1318/35, ISA.

[122] "Raʾiti-shamaʿti," *Haaretz*, November 20, 1958; "Rofe ʿAravi nirdaf al-yede shiltonot ha-mimshal ha-tsvaʾi," *Kol ha-ʿAm*, November 30, 1958, 4.

[123] "Ya jabhat al-shaʿb," *al-Ittihad*, June 30, 1959.

[124] "Mikhtav galui shel rofe ʿAravi ha-toveʿa bitul tsav haglayato," *Kol ha-ʿAm*, July 26, 1959; "al-Duktur Haddad yunashid al-ahrar li-difaʿ ʿan haqqihi fi-l-ʿamal wa-ʿan al-dimuqratiyya al-mahdura," *al-Ittihad*, July 24, 1959.

[125] Sruji, *Min muruj*, 164–65, 168.

Sruji worked for two weeks in Bint Jbeil, next to the border with Israel; he arrived there with dentist Joseph Tamari, who volunteered to assist in general medicine since there was little need for dentists. Tamari and Sruji quickly became close friends. He then worked for two weeks in Baalbek, where he met former patients from the Galilee and was assisted by volunteer nurses, former AUB students. The working conditions were poor and severe cases were sent to Sidon. Sruji was sad and distressed by the refugees' predicament.[126]

Beyond Israel's borders, medical services in Lebanon, Syria, Jordan, and Egypt faced the enormous challenge of hundreds of thousands of refugees – most of them destitute. In the territories of Arab Palestine occupied by Transjordan, for example, the hospital in Hebron and the mental hospital in Bethlehem allocated some beds to refugees. Ramallah transformed a school into an infectious disease hospital. The CMS and the other hospitals also allocated some of their beds to refugees. Across the River Jordan, refugees were treated in a small government hospital in Amman and in a CMS Hospital in al-Salt – at the government's expense. Jordan, Egypt, Lebanon, and Syria inoculated the refugees upon arrival, mainly against typhus. No laboratory services were available for refugees, making epidemic outbreaks difficult to trace.[127]

In Gaza, health services were provided by local doctors serving in the Palestine Public Health Department, who were maintained by the Egyptian Government, with the help of refugee doctors. A completely equipped laboratory was made available through the US Navy. The CMS Hospital and the Government Hospital also made 330 beds available to refugee patients.[128]

As early as mid 1948, several international organizations started providing assistance, including the World Health Organization (WHO), the ICRC, and a UN agency established for this purpose: United Nations Relief for Palestinian Refugees (UNRPR). Palestinian

126 Ibid., 166–69.

127 Anti-Epidemic Action – Assistance to Refugees from Palestine, General Correspondence, H. Mooser, Disaster Relief Project / 1 October 1948, Report on the State of Health and Living Conditions of the Palestinian Refugees, technical questions, 476/1/9, WHO archives, 9.

128 Anti-Epidemic Action – Assistance to Refugees from Palestine, General Correspondence, UNRPR, "Report of the Secretary General on United Nations Relief for Palestinian Refugees," September 30, 1949, technical questions, 476/1/9, WHO archives, 45, 56.

doctors performed much of the work on the ground. In a report to the Director General of WHO on the first six months of UNRPR activities, J. D. Cottrell, WHO Representative and Chief Medical Officer at the UNRPR, stated that there was difficulty recruiting Palestinian doctors as they refused to serve in remote areas and some would not work outside the big cities. Yet, those who were ultimately recruited were dedicated, skilled, and hardworking. Some served for little or no pay when the operation was facing the challenges of scarce medical supplies.[129]

In May 1950, when the United Nations Relief and Works Agency for Palestine Refugees (UNRWA) replaced UNRPR, Palestinian doctors were at its core. Our database lists twenty-eight doctors who worked for UNRWA, including former DoH employees, who were relatively older and had both administrative and medical experience, as well as very young doctors, fresh out of medical school, who appreciated the employment opportunity and the possibility to help their people.

The Palestinian Diaspora

The fate of individual Palestinians who were forced out of Palestine varied by place of origin, country of destination, and class. Those who ended up in Jordan or Syria could be naturalized, while those in Egypt and Lebanon could not even receive a work permit. Palestinian doctors had more opportunities to rebuild their lives and careers than most Palestinian refugees. Jordan and the Gulf States, in particular, were eager for educated bureaucrats and professionals, and some doctors ended up in these countries' public and private sectors. In Jordan, there was much room for integration in state bureaucracy and the economy. Many Palestinian doctors in what became the West Bank of Jordan were not uprooted by the war and remained in their homes in Nablus, Ramallah, and other cities. In Egypt, refugee doctors received Egyptian licenses in 1954, while the vast majority of Palestinian refugees were not allowed to work. Most Palestinian doctors in 1948 were relatively young – educated in the late 1930s and during the 1940s – which

[129] Malaria – assistance to Governments in malaria control – assistance to refugees from Palestine, Technical Question, 453/11/8, WHO archives. "Report to Director General of WHO on the first six months' activities of the United Nations relief for Palestinian Refugees and the operating agencies," J. D. Cottrell, WHO Representative and Chief Medical Officer, U.N.R.P., April 21, 1949, 11.

enabled many to resume practice after their displacement. Older doctors had a much harder time building a new practice and reputation. As many Palestinian doctors hailed from relatively well-to-do families, family fortune and connections enabled some to rebuild their lives.

After annexing the West Bank in 1950, Jordan became the host of the biggest community of Palestinian doctors. Some of them integrated into the Jordanian public health administration. Yaʿqub Abu Ghosh would become a minister in the Jordanian Government, and Mustafa Bushnaq – a member of the Jordanian House of Representatives. Various doctors remained in Jerusalem and many others came to the city after 1948. Mahdi al-Husayni, Muhammad al-Husayni, Vahan Kalbian, Asʿad Bishara, Hasib Bulus, and other Palestinian doctors worked at Augusta Victoria with Raʾfat Amin Faris, who also headed the Tuberculosis Department in Jordan's MoH. Mahmud Tahir al-Dajani served as the ministry's undersecretary while working as head physician at the Spafford Children's Hospital. Dr. Canaan headed Augusta Victoria from 1950 to 1954, and Amin Majaj in the 1980s, after serving as Jordan's Minister of Health.[130]

Yaʿqub Nuzha was employed in Augusta Victoria as well. He lost his house in Qatamon but, like many of his colleagues, remained in Jerusalem, worked at the Austrian Hospice Hospital, and opened a private clinic. At the Hospice, he worked, among others, with Dr. Salim Maʿtuq, a pillar of the Jerusalemite and Palestinian Red Crescent Society until his death in 2007. Maʿtuq was also President of the Red Crescent Hospital (est. 1953).[131] Ophthalmologist Khalil al-Budayri worked in St. John's Hospital until he became a member of the Arab Higher Committee. After the war, the hospital, which was in the Jewish part of the city, reopened in the Old City and Budayri was asked to join its staff. He remained there until his retirement in 1970.[132]

Many doctors joined the national leadership. Futi Freij assumed the role of Minister of Economic Affairs in the short-lived All-Palestine Government formed in exile, and Dr. Husayn Fakhri al-Khalidi was

[130] Julia Shatz, "Governing Jerusalem's Children, Revealing Invisible Inhabitants: The American Colony Aid Association, 1920s–1950s," 423–39; since 1952, Dr. Sami Khouri headed the surgical ward at the hospital after returning from his residency in the United Kingdom, Shinaʿa, *Ayyam Zaman*, 84; Barakat, *al-Khidamat*, 191–93, 236.

[131] Barakat, *al-Khidamat*, 194–95, 228–33, 237.

[132] Ibid., 99, 190–91.

Minister of Health.[133] Khalidi would later become a minister in Jordan. ʿIzzat Tanus and Ahmad Sururi were founding members of the PLO. For the most part, those engaged in national or local politics continued to do so in exile, but the majority either reopened private practices or were absorbed into existing or newly established institutions.

The Next Generation

The classes of 1947 and 1948 at AUB's medical faculty, the last and largest of the Mandate period, exemplified the development of the Palestinian medical community. The diverse origins of over a dozen doctors included Tulkarem, Gaza, Ramle, Kafr Kanna, and Beersheba. Perhaps the most famous of them was George Habash, who would become Secretary General of the Popular Front for the Liberation of Palestine, one of several Palestinian doctors who would assume a leadership role in the post 1948 years. Habash returned to Lydda in July 1948, at the end of his second year of medical studies, and assisted Dr. Zahlan. The sight of the dead and injured, and then the death of his elder sister during the city's occupation shook him deeply and shaped his political worldview. In October, he returned to Beirut to complete his medical studies.[134]

Like Habash, Amin Khatib's political activism started in the Arab Nationalist Movement (*al-Qawmiyun al-Arab*). The war caught him in his third year at AUB. He returned to Jerusalem in June 1948 and joined the Medical Emergency Team of the Army of the Holy War (*al-Jihad al-Muqadas*). Due to his political activism, his return to Lebanon during the second armistice was denied, forcing him to start over at Damascus University.[135] Others graduated and remained in Lebanon,

[133] Muhammad Qaraqra, *al-Khidamat al-sihhiyya al-hukumiyya wa-l-ahliyya li-l-shaʿb al-Filistini aban al-intidab al-Baritani, 1918–1948* (Shefa-ʿAmr: Jamaʿiyyat al-Jalil li-l-buhuth wa-l-khidamat al-sihhiyya, 2017), 331.

[134] Eli Galia, *George Habbash, biographia politit: Ideologia ve-politika ba-maʾavak ʿal Falastin* (Tel Aviv: Resling, 2017), 21–23.

[135] Amin Khatib, "Eyewitness Account: Origins of the Palestinian Health System in the West Bank under Jordanian Rule and the Rise of Non-Governmental Institutions," in *Separate and Cooperate, Cooperate and Separate: The Disengagement of the Palestine Health Care System from Israel and Its Emergence as an Independent System*, eds. Tamara Barnea and Rafiq Husayni (Westport, CT: Praeger, 2002), 31–37.

or immigrated to Jordan, Kuwait, Syria, and the United States – integrating into the large community of Palestinians in exile.

Conclusion

Placing doctors at the center of the 1948 catastrophe and analyzing the war through their eyes and lived experiences adds further layers to our understanding of both the Nakba and the Palestinian community's coping with it. It is, in essence, a bifurcated story of distinctive events, experiences, and fates. Every community was left to fend for itself, and the stories of Haifa, Jaffa, and Jerusalem differed from those of smaller cities and towns. Efforts to continue working were localized, and their success was largely determined by the course of the war, much more than by individual efforts, heroic as they may have been. Those who were left within or outside what became Israel had a different experience from those far from the battleground.

Home to active and organized civil societies and official medical associations, Haifa and Jaffa were relatively quick to mobilize. The doctors who remained played key roles in treating the wounded and administering aid. Nevertheless, the bulk of the two medical communities fled Palestine in the early stages of the war. Literally feeling the pulse of their communities, doctors were far from immune to public anxieties and sought haven as far as possible from war atrocities. Where it was more secure for their families to stay, such as in Jerusalem, doctors were displaced but remained in the Eastern part of the city, dedicating themselves to medical treatment.

The Nakba was also a shared trauma of a professional community that assumed a collective identity and sense of purpose, perceiving itself as a vital organ of its nation. The institutionalization process of the professional community, which culminated on the war's eve, crumbled with the annihilation of urban Palestine. Most doctors, however, were fortunate to continue practicing their professional calling within new traumatic circumstances. This community was relatively young, and since medicine is somewhat of a mobile profession, many of them managed to rebuild a life, becoming members of a professional community in exile. In 1948, Palestine was transformed, and the medical community followed.

Conclusion

The journey toward *Palestinian Doctors* began almost a decade ago, and its intensive writing phase took place during a global pandemic that transformed our generation's engagement with medicine and disease. Palestinian doctors, dispersed regionally and globally, fought the spread of the virus in refugee camps, whether under occupation, under siege in Gaza, or in exile. Many of them, Palestinian citizens of Israel alongside Jewish doctors, were at the forefront of fighting COVID-19 in Israeli hospitals. For many, it was a brief historic moment, a shred of light, an articulation of Jewish-Arab intensive and intimate cooperation.

Since October 2023, this light has turned into petrifying darkness, under which we are still shrouded during the completion of this book. Following Hamas atrocities of October 7, Israel launched an assault on Gaza, resulting in the heaviest death toll and ruination since 1948. Over 53,000 people were killed and many more wounded in a human tragedy that will take years to fully grasp. Pertinent to this book is the targeting of Gaza's starved health system, attacked after a seventeen-year-long siege. All of the Gaza Strip's thirty-six hospitals were attacked, placed under siege, or forced to evacuate at some point during the war. More than 1,400 health workers were killed, and hundreds were arrested. Those who survived are working around the clock, treating tides of trauma patients on the floor, lacking personnel, beds, medications, equipment, or food. Fighting for the worthiest cause, these Palestinian doctors open a new chapter in the annals of this community, which this book attempts to narrate from its inception.

Our point of departure, that of the late 1800s Levant, was a negative image of 2024 Gaza. The entire region was drawn into constantly evolving regional and global routes and networks of commerce, knowledge, and communication, including modern medicine. Picking up on global progress and seeking to counterbalance the growing presence of foreign doctors, local medical schools were established in the region's economic, cultural, and administrative capitals. In parallel, Palestine's urban centers gradually became hubs of modern medicine. Well-connected to these modernization processes and consumers of the evolving medical market, Palestine's urban elite had the means and foresight to demand a leading role. The first generation of Palestinian doctors was far from a monolithic group. They were sons of distinctive families of diverse origins and denominations who chose this professional path. Class played a major role in terms of access to the profession, but the expansion of educated and better-off communities over the decades enabled their entrance into the trade.

In terms of the medical community's expansion and development, British colonial occupation invented no new wheels. Medical training remained, as under the Ottomans, a private familial project conducted outside the country. Public health was on the margins of the Mandate's budgetary interest for most of the period, and its general administration remained in British rather than Palestinian hands. Unlike the loose Ottoman medical control of Palestine, however, the colonial Department of Health (DoH) sought to regulate and at least declaratively improve public health services. Palestinian doctors indirectly benefited from this colonial project, serving as the backbone of the British health system. The British could pay them small salaries, send them wherever they wished, and employ them under Sisyphean working conditions. Palestinian doctors thus constituted mediators between the colonial government and local communities. The greater their exposure to the provision of public health, the greater their demand for its expansion and reach. British inability to provide it led to subsequent disillusionment, frustration, and protest.

The targets of this discontent were twofold: first, the DoH, which failed to meet the population's needs, especially outside the cities; and second, Palestinian doctors themselves, criticized for concentrating almost entirely in the major cities and a few towns. Local medical communities grew and evolved during the Mandate, establishing and enhancing connections between the city and its periphery, a process reaching its apogee toward the Mandate's end.

The community's urban characteristics drew it closer to competition with the Yishuv's medical community. Palestine's largest urban centers were mixed, and the rapid influx of Jewish doctors into the cities, especially since the 1930s, posed a direct threat to Palestinian doctors. The mobilization of the Yishuv's medical community to the national effort made prospects of professional cooperation swing between unlikelihood and impossibility. The occupational threat posed by an organized, larger community and the services it provided to Palestinian patients was a central factor in shaping the Palestinian professional community's unionization and self-image.

This process reached fruition in the mid 1940s, when Palestinian doctors succeeded in unionizing the bulk of the community, articulating its raison d'être and future vision, publishing a journal, and more. PAMA had its roots in local associations and ongoing connections to regional professional networks. Its materialization, however, was made possible by a group of prominent doctors who for more than a decade saw their calling beyond private practice. This group, the founding fathers of the so-called republic of medical letters, constantly accentuated in essays, lectures, meetings, and on the radio the connection between able and strong nations and healthy children, women, and men. The few years separating PAMA's establishment and the 1948 war were years of action and planning, struggling to lay a blueprint for an independent national health system.

Palestinian doctors' experiences during the Nakba did not differ from those of fellow "ordinary" Palestinians. Most of them, living and working in cities and towns displaced by the Yishuv and later Israeli forces, were dispossessed of their homes, land, and social fabric. The book's last chapter tells the story of several doctors who fought heroically to continue saving the lives of war's casualties and thousands of refugees in its immediate aftermath. For a few, PAMA was an organizing principle, but not much more. It had no resources or independent facilities, and it was mainly its idea and vision that mobilized Palestinian doctors to lend their entirety to treatment. Tied with Palestinian tragedy, the catastrophe of the professional community and ensuing demise was also its finest hour, galvanizing a shared sense of meaning, of a present and a future.

At a time of increasing dehumanization, the history of medicine, and the history of Palestinian health and Palestinian medical professionals more specifically, has a humanizing potential. The history of medicine touches the core of our shared humanity, shared vulnerability, and perpetual efforts to find cures and ease suffering. This text was written toward this end.

Bibliography

'Ababinah, Salim. *Ta'rikh al-tibb al-Urduni al-hadith*. Irbid: Dar al-Kitab al-thaqafi, 2019.

Abbasi, Mustafa. "City of Farmers and Merchants: Beisan in the Palestine Mandate Period (1918–1948)." *Journal of Holy Land and Palestine Studies* 14 (2015): 206–09.

"Falastinim nilhamim ba-Natsim: Sippuram shel ha-mitnadvim ha-Falastinim be-milhemet ha-'olam ha-shniyya." *Cathedra* 128 (2019): 125–47.

"Kibbush Natseret: ha-'Ir ha-'Arvit she-sardah et ha-milhamah." *'Iyyunim*, no. 20 (2010): 101–21.

"Mishpahot ha-nikhbadim ha-'Araviyot be-'Ako be-shalhe ha-shilton ha-'Othmani u-bi-tkufat hamandat: Hemshekh o tmura?" *Cathedra* 130 (2008): 51–74.

Tverya ve-toshaveha ha-'Arvim bi-yeme ha-shilton ha Briti, 1918 1948. Jerusalem: Yad Yitshak Ben-Tsvi, 2021.

"The Fall of Acre in the 1948 Palestine War." *Journal of Palestine Studies* 39 (2010): 6–7.

"Tsfat bi-tkufat ha-mandat 1918–1948, hebetim hevratiyyim ve-politiyyim." PhD Dissertation, Haifa University, 1999.

Tsfat bi-Tkufat ha-mandat 1918–1948: 'Arvim vi-Yhudim be-'ir me'or-evet. Jerusalem: Yad Yishak Ben-Tsvi, 2015.

Abou al-Shamat, Hania. "The Religious Educational Divide in Nineteenth Century Lebanon: Institutional Roots of Communal Educational Choices." PhD Dissertation, University of Southern California, 2008.

Abou-Hodeib, Toufoul. *A Taste for Home: The Modern Middle Class in Ottoman Beirut*. Stanford: Stanford University Press, 2017.

Abu Hanna, Hanna. *Dar al-mu'allimin al-Rusiyya fi al-Nasira "al-Siminar" 1886–1914 wa-atharuha 'ala al-nahda al-adabiyya fi Filastin*. Silsilat al-thaqafa. Nazareth: Wizarat al-ma'arif wa-l-thqafa, 1994.

Abu Rabia, Aref. "Bedouin Health Services in Mandate Palestine." *Middle Eastern Studies* 41 (2005): 421–22.

Abu Shunnar, Ahmad. *Qabilat al-Tiyaha hadara wa-ta'rikh*. Amman: Dar al-mu'tazz li-l-nashr wa-l-tawzi', 2017.

Abugideiri, Hibba. *Gender and the Making of Modern Medicine in Colonial Egypt*. London: Ashgate, 2010.

Amir, Gal, and Naama Ben Zeev. "Lawyers in Transition – Palestinian Arab Lawyers in the First Decade of the Jewish State." *Continuity and Change* 35 (2020): 371–92.

Amster, Ellen. "The Many Deaths of Dr. Emile Mauchamp: Medicine, Technology, and Popular Politics in Pre-Protectorate Morocco, 1877–1912." *International Journal of Middle East Studies* 36 (2004): 409–28.

ʿAnabusi, Adam. "Anwar al-Shuqayri, tabib al-thwara wa-ʿaqluha." Hebrew University, November 2018, unpublished paper.

Anderson, Betty. *The American University of Beirut: Arab Nationalism and Liberal Education*. Austin: University of Texas Press, 2011.

ʿAql, Muhammad. *Muʿjam al-atibbaʾ wa-l-sayadilah al-Filastiniyin (1-748-1948)*. Arara: Self-published, 2021.

ʿArif, al-ʿArif. *al-Nakbah: Nakbat Bayt al-Maqdis wa-l-firdaws al-mafquud: 1947–1949*. Beirut: Muʾassasat al-dirasat al-Filastiniyya, 2013.

Arnold, David. *Science, Technology, and Medicine in Colonial India*. Cambridge: Cambridge University Press, 2000.

Arsenian, Hagop, and Arda Arsenian Ekmekji. "Surviving Massacre: Hagop Arsenian's Armenian Journey to Jerusalem." *Jerusalem Quarterly*, no. 49 (2012): 26–42.

ʿAsali, Kamil. *Muqaddima fi taʾrikh al-tibb fi al-Quds mundhu aqdam al-azminah hatta sanat 1918 M*. Amman: al-Jamiʿa al-Urduniyya, ʿImadat al-bahth al-ʿilmi, 1994.

Assaf, Mikhael. *Ha-Yahasim ben Yehudim ve-ʿAravim be-Erets Yisraʾel, 1860–1948*. Tel Aviv: Tarbut ve-hinukh, 1970.

Astafieva, Elena. "La Russie en Terre Sainte: Le cas de la Société Impériale Orthodoxe de Palestine (1882–1917)." *Cristianesimo Nella Storia* 24 (2003): 41–68.

ʿAwda al-Nuʿaimat, Fawwaz. *Nasara al-Quds fi fatrat al-intidab al-Baritani (1917–1948)*. Beirut: Markaz dirasat al-wahda al-ʿArabiyya, 2016.

Ayalon, Ami. *Reading Palestine: Printing and Literacy, 1900–1948*. Austin: University of Texas Press, 2004.

Banko, Lauren. "Migrants, Residents, and the Cost of Illegal Home-Making in Mandate Palestine." *Jerusalem Quarterly* 84 (2020): 47–65.

Bar-El, Yaron and Nissim Levi. "Reshita shel ha-refuʾa ha-modernit be-ʿare ha-Galil, 1860–1900." *Cathedra* 54 (1989): 96–106.

Barakat, Bashir. *Taʾrikh al-khidamat al-sihiyya fi Bayt al-Maqdis*. Istanbul: Dar al-nidaʾ, 2019.

Barel, Dan. *Ruah raʿa: Magefot ha-kolera ve-hitpathut ha-refuʾa be-Erets-Yisraʾel be-shalhe ha-tkufa ha-ʿOthmanit*. Jerusalem: Mosad Byalik, 2010.

Al-Bawwab, ʿAli Hasan. *Mawsuʿat Yafa al-jamila*. Beirut: al-Muʾassasa al-ʿArabiyya li-l-dirasat wa-l-nashr, 2003.

Bayoumi, Soha. "Colonizing and Decolonizing Egyptian Medicine." In *The Oxford Handbook of Modern Egyptian History*, edited by Beth Baron and Jeffrey Culang, 73–88. Oxford: Oxford University Press, 2024.

Bell, Heather. *Frontiers of Medicine in the Anglo-Egyptian Sudan 1899–1940*. Oxford: Clarendon Press, 1999.

Ben Zeev, Naama. "Ben ha-kfar la-ʿir: Hayye mehagrim kafriyyim Falastinim be-Hefa bi-tkufat ha-mandat." PhD Dissertation, Ben Gurion University of the Negev, 2010.

"Civil Associations in Mandatory Haifa: A New Perspective on Palestinian-Arab Political Life." *Middle Eastern Studies* 49 (2013): 958–72.

"'I Came Naïve from the Village': On Palestinian Urbanism and Ruralism in Haifa under the British Mandate." *British Journal of Middle Eastern Studies* 47 (2020): 264–81.

Ben Zeev, Nimrod. "Palestine along the Colour Line: Race, Colonialism, and Construction Labour, 1918–1948." *Ethnic and Racial Studies* 44 (2021): 2190–212.

Ben-Arieh, Yehoshua. *ʿIr bi-reʾi tkufa*. Jerusalem: Yad Ben-Tsvi, 1977.

Ben-Bassat, Yuval and Yossi Ben-Artzi. "Cartographical Evidence of Efforts to Develop Acre during the Last Decades of Ottoman Rule: Did the Ottomans Neglect the City?" *Mediterranean Historical Review* 31 (2016): 65–70.

Bernstein, Deborah. *Constructing Boundaries: Jewish and Arab Workers in Mandatory Palestine*. Albany: SUNY Press, 2000.

Bishara, Nakhle. *Irus Vartani: Sipuro shel bet ha-holim Natseret*. Zikhron Yaʿakov: Itai Bahur, 2011.

Al-Bishawi, Saʿid. *Al-Duktur Ahmad "Mahmud ʿAtalla" al-Sururi: al-Tabib al-insan wa-l-idari al-bariʿ wa-l-siyasi wa-shahadat muʿassirihi, 1336–1408 H / 1908–1988*. Amman: Dar al-ruʿa li-l-dirasat wa-l-nashr, 2021.

Blanchard, Raphael. "La Faculté de Médicine de Beyrouth." *Conférence faite au comité de l'Asie Française, 29.1.1912*. Paris: siège social du Comité de l'Asie Française, 1912.

Blecher, Robert Ian. "Desert Medicine, Ethnography and Colonial Encounter in Mandatory Syria." In *The British and French Mandates in Comparative Perspectives*, edited by Nadine Meouchy and Peter Sluglett, 249–68. Leiden: Brill, 2004.

"The Medicalization of Sovereignty: Medicine, Public Health, and Political Authority in Syria, 1861–1936." PhD Dissertation, Stanford University, 2002.

Bourmaud, Philippe. "'A Son of a Country': Dr. Tawfiq Canaan, Modernist Physician and Palestinian Ethnographer." In *Struggle and Survival in Palestine/Israel*, edited by Mark LeVine and Gershon Shafir. Berkeley: University of California Press, 2012, 104–24.

"Discipline et familiarisation à travers la médecine: Une mission médicale à Gaza (1878–1914)." *Histoire et missions chrétiennes* 21 (2012): 81–102.

"Epidemiology and the City: Communal vs. Intercommunal Health Policy-Making in Jerusalem from the Ottomans to the Mandate, 1908–1925." In *Ordinary Jerusalem, 1840–1940 Opening New Archives, Revisiting a Global City*, edited by Angelos Dalachanes and Vincent Lemire, 440–56. Leiden: Brill, 2018.

"Experts at Large: Physicians, Public Debate and the Press in Late Ottoman Palestine." *Archiv Orientalni* 80 (2012): 295–337.

"Public Space and Private Spheres: The Foundation of St. Luke's Hospital of Nablus by the CMS." In *New Faith in Ancient Lands: Western Missions in the Middle East in the Nineteenth and Early Twentieth Centuries*, edited by Heleen Murre-van den Berg, 133–50. Leiden: Brill, 2006.

"'Ya doktor': Devenir médecin et exercer son art en 'Terre sainte', une expérience du pluralisme médical dans l'Empire ottoman finissant (1871–1918)." PhD Dissertation, Aix-Marseille I, 2007.

Budayri, Khalil. *Sitta wa-sittun ʿaman maʿa al-haraka al-wataniyya al-Filastiniyya wa-fiha: Tarikh ma aghfalahu al-tarikh*. Jerusalem: Manshurat Salah al-Din, 1982.

Bulos, Nassib D. *A Palestinian Landscape*. Beirut: Arab Institute for Research & Publishing, 1998.

Bulus, Rufaʾil. *Kafr Yasif bayna asalat al-madi wa-rawʿat al-hadir*. Kafr Yasif: R.B. Bulus, 2012.

Burrage, Michael, Konrad Jarausch, and Hannes Siegrist, "An Actor-Based Framework for the Study of the Professions." In *Professions in Theory and History: Rethinking the Study of the Professions*, edited by Michael Burrage and Rolf Torstendahl. London: Sage, 1990.

Busailah, Reja-e. "The Fall of Lydda, 1948: Impressions and Reminiscences." *Arab Studies Quarterly* 3 (1981): 123–51.

Büssow, Johann. "Children of the Revolution: Youth in Palestinian Public Life, 1908–14." In *Late Ottoman Palestine: The Period of Young Turk Rule*, edited by Yuval Ben-Bassat and Eyal Ginio, 55–78. London; New York: I. B. Tauris, 2011.

Hamidian Palestine: Politics and Society in the District of Jerusalem 1872–1908. Leiden: Brill, 2011.

"Ottoman Reform and Urban Government in the District of Jerusalem, 1867–1917." In *Urban Governance under the Ottomans: Between*

Cosmopolitanism and Conflict, edited by Ulrike Freitag and Nora Lafi, 97–141. Oxford: Routledge, 2014.

Canaan, Tawfiq. *Conflict in the Land of Peace*. Jerusalem: Syrian Orphanage Press, 1936.

Canaan, Tawfiq and Mahmud Tahir al-Dajani. *Al-Jam'iyya al-tibbiyya al-'Arabiyya al-Filastiniyya: Taqrir 'am 'an juhud al-jam'iyya wa-jihadiha, 1947–1950*. Jerusalem: Matba'at dar al-aytam,1950.

Carmel, Alex. *Ottoman Haifa: A History of Four Centuries under Turkish Rule*. London: I. B. Tauris, 2011.

Charton, Hélène. "L'Homo africanus acadamicus: Les limites de la fabrique d'une élite universitaire africaine en Afrique de l'Est." *Revue Outre-Mer*, no. 394–395 (2017): 15–38.

Chiffoleau, Sylvia. *Médecines et médecins en Egypte: Construction d'une identité professionnelle et projet medical*. Paris: L'Harmattan, 1997.

Cohen, Hillel. *1929: Year Zero of the Arab-Israeli Conflict*. Waltham, MA: Brandeis University Press, 2015.

Army of Shadows: Palestinian Collaboration with Zionism, 1917–1948. Berkeley: University of California Press, 2008.

Collins, Randall. "Market Closure and the Conflict Theory of the Professions." In *Professions in Theory and History: Rethinking the Study of the Professions*, edited by Michael Burrage and Rolf Torstendahl, 24–43. London: Sage, 1990.

Crozier, Anna. *Practicing Colonial Medicine: The Colonial Medical Service in British East Africa*. London: I. B. Tauris, 2007.

Crystal, Nathan. "The Fall of the New City 1947–1950." In *Jerusalem 1948: The Arab Neighbourhoods and Their Fate in the War*, edited by Salim Tamari, 92–146. Jerusalem: Institute of Jerusalem Studies & Badil Resource Center, 1999.

Cuinet, Vital. *Syrie, Liban et Palestine. Géographie administrative, statistique, descriptive et raisonnée*. Paris: Ernest Leroux, 1896.

Da'adli, Tawfiq. "Walking with Ghosts along the Bazaar: Urban Life in Ludd, Palestine, at the Turn of the Twentieth Century." *Palestine/Israel Review* 1(2024), 53–82.

Dajani, Adel. *From Jerusalem to a Kingdom by the Sea*. London: Zuleika, 2021.

Al-Dajani al-Miqdadi, Rabiha. *Ida'at min khibrati wa-turath ummati*. Amman: Dar al-shuruq li-l-nashr wa-l-tawzi', 2010.

Dallasheh, Leena. "Nazarenes in the Turbulent Tide of Citizenships: Nazareth from 1940 to 1966." PhD Dissertation, New York University, 2012.

Davis, Rochelle. *Palestinian Village Histories: Geographies of the Displaced*. Stanford: Stanford University Press, 2011.

"The Growth of the Western Communities, 1917–1948." In *Jerusalem 1948: The Arab Neighbourhoods and Their Fate in the War*, edited by Salim Tamari, 30–66. Jerusalem: Institute of Jerusalem Studies: Center for Jerusalem Studies, 2002.

De Vries, David. *Strike Action and Nation Building: Labor Unrest in Palestine/Israel, 1899–1951*. New York: Berghahn, 2015.

Degani, Arnon. "Both Arab and Israeli: The Subordinate Integration of Palestinian Arabs into Israeli Society, 1948–1967." PhD Dissertation, University of California Los Angeles, 2018.

Deringil, Selim. *The Well-Protected Domains: Ideology and the Legitimation of Power in the Ottoman Empire, 1876–1909*. London; New York: I. B. Tauris, 1999.

Dewachi, Omar. *Ungovernable Life: Mandatory Medicine and Statecraft in Iraq*. Stanford: Stanford University Press, 2017.

Diyyab, Imtiyaz. *ʿAtr madinat Yafa*. Beirut: Dar al-fatah li-l-nashr wa-l-tawziʿ, 1991.

Dodge, Bayard. *The American University of Beirut: A Brief History of the University and the Lands Which It Serves*. Beirut: Khayyat's, 1958.

Dolev, Eran. "Shorshe ha-refuʾa ha-tsvaʾit be-Tsahal ʿuvdot ve-tehiyot." In *Refuʾa tsvaʾit: ʿIyyunim be-sugiyot refuʾiyot be-toldot koah ha-magen ha-ʿIvri*, edited by Nir Mann, 39–50. Ben Shemen: Modan, 2018.

Doumani, Beshara. *Rediscovering Palestine: Merchants and Peasants in Jabal Nablus, 1700–1900*. Berkeley: University of California Press, 1995.

Efron, John. *Medicine and the German Jews: A History*. New Haven, CT: Yale University Press, 2008.

Eizanberg, ʿOvadia. *Mifkad ha-okhlusiya ha-Yehudit be-Hefa – trts"h (5698)*. Haifa: M. Shoham Press, 1940.

El Shakry, Omnia S. *The Great Social Laboratory: Subjects of Knowledge in Colonial and Postcolonial Egypt*. Stanford: Stanford University Press, 2007.

El-Eini, Roza. "Government Fiscal Policy in Mandatory Palestine in the 1930s." *Middle Eastern Studies* 33 (1997): 573–80.

Elmakias, Yoram. "Peʿilut tsioyonit be-Hevron me-reshit ha-meʾa ha-20 ve-ʿad meʾoraʿot tarpa"t." MA Thesis, University of Haifa, 2011.

Fahmy, Khaled. *In Quest of Justice: Islamic Law and Forensic Medicine in Modern Egypt*. Berkeley: University of California Press, 2018.

Fahmy, Ninette S. *The Politics of Egypt: State-Society Relationship*. Abingdon; New York: Routledge, 2012.

Fahoum, Basma. "Tobacco Cultivation and Production in Twentieth-Century Palestine/Israel." PhD Dissertation, Stanford University, 2023.

Fahoum Ghunaym, Siham. *Tahaddiyyat taghayyurat wa-tahawwulat fi ta'rikh al-Nasira*. Nazareth: Matbaʿat al-nahda, 2003.

Falb Kalisman, Hilary. "Schooling the State: Educators in Iraq, Palestine and Transjordan: c. 1890–c. 1960." PhD Dissertation, University of California, Berkeley, 2015.

Teachers as State-Builders. Princeton: Princeton University Press, 2022.

Falk, Edward. "Lyon to Liban: Language, Nation and Faith in the Jesuit Schools of Ottoman Lebanon." In *Entangled Education: Foreign and Local Schools in Ottoman Syria and Mandate Lebanon (19–20th Centuries)*, edited by Julia Hauser, Christine Lindner, and Ester Möller, 163–80. Beirut: Ergon Verlag Würzburg in Kommission, 2016.

Farhan, Sara. *Medical Education and the Making of Iraqi Doctors, 1869–1959*. Edinburgh: Edinburgh University Press, 2025.

Fawaz, Leila. "The Changing Balance of Forces between Beirut and Damascus in the Nineteenth and Twentieth Centuries." *Revue des mondes musulmans et de la Méditerranée* 55–56 (1990): 208–14.

Ferguson, Susanna. "'A Fever for an Education': Pedagogical Thought and Social Transformation in Beirut and Mount Lebanon, 1861–1914." *Arab Studies Journal* 26 (2018): 58–83.

Fleischmann, Ellen. "'Under an American Roof': The Beginnings of the American Junior College for Women in Beirut." *Arab Studies Journal* 17 (2009): 62–84.

The Nation and Its "New" Women: The Palestinian Women's Movement, 1920–1948. Berkeley: University of California Press, 2003.

Fortna, Benjamin C. *Imperial Classroom: Islam, the State and Education in the Late Ottoman Empire*. Oxford: Oxford University Press, 2002.

Furas, Yoni. *Educating Palestine: Teaching and Learning History under the Mandate*. Oxford: Oxford University Press, 2020.

"'What Did the Ottomans Ever Do for Us?' Modern Medicine and Administration in Late Ottoman Jerusalem." In *From the Household to the Wider World: Local Perspectives on Urban Institutions in Late Ottoman Bilad a-Sham*, edited by Yuval Ben-Bassat and Johann Büssow, 247–49. Tubingen: Tubingen University Press, 2022.

Gadelrab, Sherry Sayed. "Medical Healers in Ottoman Egypt, 1517–1805." *Medical History* 54 (2010): 365–86.

Gafni, Reuven. "Kehila Yehudit ʿal kav gvul: ha-Nokhehut ha-Yehudit ba-ʿayara Tsemah (Samakh) ba-mahatsit ha-rishona shel ha-me'a ha-ʿesrim." *Mehkarim hadashim shel ha-Galil* 3 (2018): 9–28.

"Lone Jewish Medical Personnel in Arab Towns: A Conditional Presence in British Mandate Palestine." *Israel Studies* 26 (2021): 206–11.

"Rof'a Yehudiyya be-'ir 'Aravit: Pe'iluta shel Dr. Olga Feinberg be-Yeriho bi-tkufat ha-mandat." *Korot* 24 (2017/18): 69–86.

"'Shlihuta shel ha-ahot ha-'Ivriyya, ha-yoda'at lehitmasser gam le-'ezrat ha-shakhen ha-koshel: Sippura shel tahanat tippat halav be-Samakh, 1942–1947." *Erets ha-Kineret* 29 (2020): 43–47.

Galia, Eli. *George Habbash, biographia politit: Ideologia ve-politika ba-ma'avak 'al Falastin.* Tel Aviv: Resling, 2017.

Gelvin, James L. "The 'Politics of Notables' Forty Years After." *Middle East Studies Association Bulletin* 40 (2006): 19–29.

Ghanayim, Zuhayr. *Liwa 'Akka fi 'ahd al-tanzimat al-'Uthmaniyya, 1281–1337 H / 1864–1918M.* Beirut: Mu'assasat al-dirasat al-Filastiniyya, 1999.

Ghusha, Subhi. *Shamsuna lan taghib.* Jerusalem: al-Matba'a al-'Arabiya al-haditha, 1994.

Giacaman, Rita. *Life and Health in Three Palestinian Villages.* London: Ithaca Press, 1988.

Goebel, Michael. *Anti-Imperial Metropolis: Interwar Paris and the Seeds of Third World Nationalism.* New York: Cambridge University Press, 2015.

Golan, Matti. *Rofe: Moshe Rachmilevitsh.* Tel Aviv: Zemorah, Bitan, 1989.

Golani, Motti. "The 'Haifa Turning Point': The British Administration and the Civil War in Palestine, December 1947–May 1948." *Middle Eastern Studies* 37 (2001): 94–120.

Golz, Avishay. *Refu'at Af-Ozen-Garon be-Erets Yisra'el, 1911–1948.* Zichron Ya'akov: Itai Bahur, 2009.

Goren, Tamir. "Annexation or Separation? The Municipal Status of the Jewish Neighborhoods of Jaffa 1940–1944." *Israel Studies* 21 (2016): 77–101.

Hefa ha-'Arvit be-tashah: 'Otsmat ha-ma'avak u-memade ha-hitmotetut. Tel Aviv: Ben-Gurion University of the Negev Press, 2006.

"Tel Aviv and the Question of Separation from Jaffa 1921–1936." *Middle Eastern Studies* 52 (2016): 473–87.

"The Jewish Neighbourhoods of Jaffa and the Question of Annexation to Tel Aviv at the End of the British Mandate." *Middle Eastern Studies* 52 (2016): 917–37.

"The Jews of Jaffa at the Time of the Arab Revolt: The Emergence of the Demand for Annexation." *Journal of Modern Jewish Studies* 15 (2016): 267–81.

"The Judaization of Haifa at the Time of the Arab Revolt." *Middle East Studies* 40 (2004): 135–52.

"Yihud Hefa bi-tkufat ha-mandat ha-Briti, ha-memad ha-munitsipali." *Ofakim be-geografiya* 73–74 (2009): 77–96.

Greenberg, Zalman. "Bet ha-holim ha-ʿironi ha-Turki bi-Yerushalayim." *Cathedra*, no. 78 (1995): 49–64.

Greenberg, Zalman and Rakefet Zalashik. "Masaʿ mishlahat hever ha-leʾummim le-hakirat ha-malariya be-Erets Yisraʾel bi-shnat 1925." *Cathedra* 134 (2010): 49–64.

Greenwood, Anna and Harshad Topiwala. *Indian Doctors in Kenya 1895–1940, the Forgotten History*. Basingstoke: Palgrave Macmillan, 2015.

Gross, Nachum. *The Economic Policy of the Mandatory Government in Palestine*. Jerusalem: Maurice Falk Institute for Economic Research in Israel, 1982.

Hacohen, David. *Time to Tell: An Israeli Life, 1898–1984*. New York: Cornwall Books, 1985.

Haiduc-Dale, Noah. *Arab Christians in British Mandate Palestine: Communalism and Nationalism, 1917–1948*. Edinburgh: Edinburgh University Press, 2013.

Halevy, Dotan. "The Rear Side of the Front: Gaza and Its People in World War I." *Journal of Levantine Studies* 5 (2015): 44–49.

"Toward a Palestinian History of Ruins: Interwar Gaza." *Journal of Palestine Studies* 189 (2018): 53–72.

Hammuda, Samih. *Sawt min al-Quds: al-Mujahid Dawud Salih al-Husayni min khilal mudhakkiratihi wa-awraqihi*. Ramallah: Manshurat maktabat sar al-fikr, 2015.

Hashash, Yali. "Gender, Religion, and Secularism in the English Mission Hospital of Jerusalem, 1844–1880." *Journal of Levantine Studies* 7 (2017): 9–34.

Hathut, Hassan. *Fi dhikra al-Nakba: Yawmiyat tabib Misri fi Filastin*. Cairo: Markaz al-iʿlam al-ʿArabi, 2008.

Herzstein, Rafaël. "The Foundation of the Saint-Joseph University of Beirut: The Teaching of the Maronites by the Second Jesuit Mission in the Levant." *Middle Eastern Studies* 43 (2007): 749–59.

Hillel, Maayan. "Constructing Modern Identity – New Patterns of Leisure and Recreation in Mandatory Palestine." *Contemporary Levant* 4 (2019): 75–90.

"Cultural Diplomacy in Mandatory Haifa: The Role of Christian Communities in the Cultural Transformation of the City." In *European Cultural Diplomacy and Arab Christians in Palestine, 1918–1948: Between Contention and Connection*, edited by Karène Sanchez Summerer and Sary Zananiri, 127–50. Cham: Palgrave Macmillan, 2021.

Hughes, Matthew. *Britain's Pacification of Palestine*. Cambridge: Cambridge University Press, 2019.

Al-Husayni, Muhammad Yunis. *Al-Tatawwur al-ijtima'i wa-l-iqtisadi fi Filastin al-'Arabiyya*. Jerusalem: Maktabat al-Tahir Ikhwan, 1947.

Al-Hut, Bayan Nuwayhid. *Al-Qiyadat wa-l-mu'assasat as-siyasiyya fi Filastin: 1917–1948*. Beirut: Mu'assasat al-dirasat al-Filastiniyya, 1981.

Hutchison, Donn. "Occidental Obsessions: Diary of a Country Doctor." *Jerusalem Quarterly*, no. 28 (2006): 45–61.

Ibrahim, Rashid al-Haj. *Al-Difa' 'an Hayfa wa-qadiyat Filastin: Mudhakkirat rashid al-hajj Ibrahim, 1891–1953*, edited by Walid Khalidi. Beirut: Mu'assasat al-dirasat al-Filastiniyya, 2005.

İlikan Rasimoğlu, Ceren Gülser. "Boundaries, Education, and License: The Nineteenth Century Ottoman Standardization of Medical Professions." *Trakya Üniversitesi Sosyal Bilimler Dergisi* 19 (2017): 227–46.

"The Foundation of a Professional Group: Physicians in the Nineteenth Century Modernizing Ottoman Empire (1839–1908)." PhD Dissertation, Boğaziçi University, 2012.

Izhaki, Rika. "Hakamato ve-hitpathutu shel bet ha-holim le-mahalot 'enayim St. John." *Cathedra* 67 (1993): 114–35.

Jacobson, Abigail. *From Empire to Empire: Jerusalem between Ottoman and British Rule*. Syracuse: Syracuse University Press, 2011.

Johnson, Ryan. "'An All-White Institution': Defending Private Practice and the Formation of the West African Medical Staff." *Medical History* 54 (2010): 237–54.

Junod, Dominique-D. *The Imperiled Red Cross and the Palestine-Eretz-Yisra'el Conflict, 1945–1952: The Influence of Institutional Concerns on a Humanitarian Operation*. London: Kegan Paul International, 1996.

Kabha, Mustafa. "The Palestinian Exile: Drama Shapes Memory." In *The War of 1948: Representations of Israeli and Palestinian Memories and Narratives*, edited by Avraham Sela and Alon Kadish, 194–202. Bloomington: Indiana University Press, 2016.

Kagan, Helena. *Reshit darki bi-Yerushalayim*. Jerusalem: WIZO, 1965.

Kahlenberg, Caroline. "The Star of David in a Cedar Tree: Jewish Students and Zionism at the American University of Beirut (1908–1948)." *Middle Eastern Studies* 55 (2019): 570–89.

Kalbian, Vicken V. "The Field Hospital of Hafir-El-Auja and US-Ottoman Relations." *Jerusalem Quarterly*, no. 63 (2015): 54–71.

Kana'na, Sharif. *Al-Lajjun*. Bir zayt: Jami'at Bir Zayt, markaz al-watha'iq wa-l-abhath, 1987.

'Ayn Hawd. Bir Zayt: Jami'at Bir Zayt, markaz al-watha'iq wa-l-abhath, 1987.

Kana'na, Sharif and Lubna 'Abd al-Hadi 'Abd al-Hadi. *Lifta*. Bir Zayt: Markaz al-watha'iq wa-l-Abhath, 1991.

Kark, Ruth. *Jerusalem and Its Environs: Quarters, Neighborhoods, Villages, 1800–1948*. Detroit: Wayne State University Press, 2001.

"Pe'ilut 'iriyyat Yerushalayim be-sof ha-tkufa ha-'Othmanit." *Cathedra* 6 (1977): 74–94.

Yafo: Tsmihata shel 'ir, 1799–1917. Jerusalem: Yad Itzhak Ben Tsvi, 1984.

Kass, Amalie M. "Western Medicine in Nineteenth-Century Jerusalem." *Journal of the History of Medicine & Allied Sciences* 44 (1989): 447–61.

Katz, Jonathan G. *Murder in Marrakesh: Émile Mauchamp and the French Colonial Adventure*. Bloomington: Indiana University Press, 2006.

Khater, Insaf As'ad Husayn. "Al-Awda' al-sihhiyya fi Nablus aban al-intidab al-Baritani 1922–1948." MA Thesis, al-Najah University, 2000.

Kelly, Laura. *Irish Medical Education and Student Culture, c. 1850–1950*. Liverpool: Liverpool University Press, 2017.

Kestenian, Hratch Yervant. "A Portrait of Armenian Student Life at the Syrian Protestant College 1885–1920." MA Thesis, the American University of Beirut, 2015.

Khalaf, Issa. *Politics in Palestine: Arab Factionalism and Social Disintegration, 1939–1948*. Albany: State University of New York Press, 1991.

Khalid, Anna and Ryan Johnson. *Public Health in the British Empire Intermediaries, Subordinates, and the Practice of Public Health, 1850–1960*. New York: Routledge, 2012.

Al-Khalidi, Walid. *Al-Ramla tatakallam*. Amman: n.p., 1991.

Khalil, Khalil Ahmad. *Mawsu'at a'lam al-'Arab al-mubd'in fi al-qarn al-'ishrin*, vol. 3. Beirut: al-Mu'assasa al-'Arabiyya li-l-dirasat wa-l-nashr, 2003.

Khamrah, Majid. *Margharush: Wamadat min Hayfa*. Haifa: al-Wadi li-l-tiba'ah wa-l-Nashr : Jam'iyyat al-tatwir al-ijtima'i, 2004.

Khatchadourian, Arpine. *David of Sassoun: An Introduction to the Study of the Armenian Epic*. Eugene: Wipf and Stock Publishers, 2016.

Khatib, Amin. "Eyewitness Account: Origins of the Palestinian Health System in the West Bank under Jordanian Rule and the Rise of Non-Governmental Institutions." In *Separate and Cooperate, Cooperate and Separate: The Disengagement of the Palestine Health Care System from Israel and Its Emergence as an Independent System*, edited by Tamara Barnea and Rafiq Husayni, 31–37. Westport, CT: Praeger, 2002.

Khayat, Nicole and Liat Kozma. "Medicine and Arabic Literary Production in the Ottoman Empire during the Nineteenth Century." *The British Journal for the History of Science* 55 (2022): 515–24.

Kholoussy, Hanan. "Monitoring and Medicalising Male Sexuality in Semi-Colonial Egypt." *Gender & History* 22 (2010): 677–91.

Khoury, Philip S. "The Urban Notables Paradigm Revisited." *Revue des mondes musulmans et de la Méditerranée* 55–56 (1990): 215–30.

Khuri, Qaysar. *Al-Dhikrayat*. Jerusalem: al-Matbaʿa al-tijariyya, 1945.

Kidron, Anat and Shuli Yarkoni. "Hityashvut Yehudim be-ʿarim meʿoravot bi-tkufat ha-mandat: ha-Mikre shel ʿAko." *Israel* 27–28 (2021): 119–22.

Kildani, Hanna. *Modern Christianity in the Holy Land: Development of the Structure of Churches and the Growth of Christian Institutions in Jordan and Palestine*. Bloomington: AuthorHouse, 2010.

Kimmerling, Baruch. "A Model of Analysis of Reciprocal Relations between the Jewish and Arab Communities in Mandatory Palestine." *Plural Societies* 14 (1983): 45–68.

Kimmerling, Baruch and Joel S. Migdal. *The Palestinian People: A History*. Cambridge, MA: Harvard University Press, 2003.

Kobiljski, Aleksandra. "Women Students at the American University of Beirut from the 1920s to the 1940s." In *Gender, Religion and Change in the Middle East: Two Hundred Years of History*, edited by Inger Marie Okkenhaug and Ingvild Flaskerud, 67–84. Oxford: Berg, 2006.

Kozma, Liat. "Health and Nation: The Egyptian Medical Profession under British Rule." In *The Oxford Handbook of Modern Egyptian History*, edited by Beth Baron and Jeffrey Culang, 56–72. Oxford: Oxford University Press, 2024.

"'We, the Sexologists …': Arabic Medical Writing on Sexuality, 1879–1943." *Journal of the History of Sexuality* 22 (2013): 426–45.

Kronfol, Nabil Muhi al-Din. "The Migratory Flow of the Medical Graduates of the American University of Beirut." PhD Dissertation, Harvard University, 1979.

Kroyanker, David. *Rehov ha-neviʾim, shehunat ha-habashim, ve-shehunat Musrara: Sippuro shel makom, dyokana shel ʿir, Yerushalyim, 1850–2000*. Jerusalem: Yad Ben-Tsvi, 2000.

Shekhunot Yerushalayim: Talbiye, Katamon veha-Moshava ha-Yevanit. Jerusalem: Mekhon Yerushalayim le-heker Yisraʾel: Keter, 2002.

Sippur mitham Rotschild: Yerushalayim: Rehov ha-neviʾim, biographiya refuʾit ve-hinnukhit. Jerusalem: Keter, 2001.

Kulick, Amir. "Manhigut ve-hevra be-Hefa: Tsmihata shel elita ʿironit, 1918–1948." PhD Dissertation, Tel Aviv University, 2012.

Kupferschmidt, Uri M. *The Supreme Muslim Council: Islam under the British Mandate for Palestine*. Leiden: Brill, 1987.

Lachenal, Guillaume. *The Lomidine Files: The Untold Story of a Medical Disaster in Colonial Africa*. Baltimore: Johns Hopkins University Press, 2017.

Lajna min abna' Bayt Jala. *Madinat Bayt Jala*. Bethlehem: Madinat Bayt Lahm, 1994.

Lefen, Asa. *Ha-Shai: Sherut ha-yedi'ot: Shorsheha shel kehilat ha-modi'in ha-Yisra'elit*. Tel Aviv: Merkaz le-toldot koah ha-magen ha-"Haganah" : Misrad ha-Bitahon, 1997.

Legrandjacques, Sara. "L'enseignement supérieur en Asie française et britannique. Expériences croisées à l'âge des Empires (années 1850–1930)." *Revue Outre-Mer*, no. 394–395 (2017): 39–59.

Lemire, Vincent. *Jerusalem 1900: The Holy City in the Age of Possibilities*, translated by Catherine Tihanyi and Lys Ann Weiss. Chicago: The University of Chicago Press, 2017.

Ordinary Jerusalem, 1840–1940: Opening New Archives, Revisiting a Global City. Leiden: Brill, 2018.

Levi, Nisim. *Prakim be-toldot ha-refu'a be-Erets Yisra'el*. Haifa: The Technion, 1998.

Likhovski, Assaf. *Law and Identity in Mandate Palestine*. Chapel Hill: University of North Carolina Press, 2006.

Liu, Shiyong. *Prescribing Colonization: The Role of Medical Practices and Policies in Japan-Ruled Taiwan, 1895–1945*. Ann Arbor: Association for Asian Studies, 2009.

Lo, Ming-Cheng M. *Doctors within Borders: Profession, Ethnicity, and Modernity in Colonial Taiwan*. Berkeley: University of California Press, 2002.

Lockman, Zachary. *Comrades and Enemies: Arab and Jewish Workers in Palestine, 1906–1948*. Berkeley: University of California Press, 1996.

"Railway Workers and Relational History: Arabs and Jews in British-Ruled Palestine." *Comparative Studies in Society and History* 35 (1993): 601–27.

Łotysz, Sławomir. "Desert Mould: Witold Odrzywolski and His Work on Crude Penicillin in a Military Hospital in the Middle East in 1944." *Kwartalnik Historyczny* 127 (2020): 77–103.

Mack, Merav. "Orthodox and Communist: A History of a Christian Community in Mandate Palestine and Israel." *British Journal of Middle Eastern Studies* 42 (2015): 384–400.

Mahfuz, Najib. *The History of Medical Education in Egypt*. Cairo: Government Press, 1935.

Mahmoud, Ahmad. "Al-Sihha wa-l-sihha al-'amma fi ta'rikh Hayfa khilal fatrat al-intidab al-Baritani, 1920–1934." MA Thesis, Hebrew University, 2019.

Makdisi, Ussama. *Artillery of Heaven: American Missionaries and the Failed Conversion of the Middle East*. Ithaca, NY: Cornell University Press, 2007.

Malak, Hanna ʿIsa. *Al-Judhur al-Yafiyya*. Jerusalem: Matbaʿat al-sharq al-ʿArabiyya, 1996).

Al-Maliki, Majdi and Salim Tamari, eds. *Al-Madina al-Filastiniyya qadaya fi al-tahawwulat al-hadariyya*. Beirut: Muʾassasat al-dirasat al-Filastiniyya, 2021.

Man, Michal. "ha-Tipul ha-refuʾi ba-kibbutsim ba-shanim 1910–1948." *Alei zait ve-herev* 17 (2018): 95–116.

"Statoskop u-mahresha: bi-Ntiv ha-mirpaʾa ba-kibbutsim, hitpathut sherute ha-briʾut ba-kibbutsim ba-shanim 1910–1948." PhD Dissertation, Ben-Gurion University of the Negev, 2016.

Manna, Adel. *Aʿlam Filastin fi awakhir al-ʿahd al-ʿUthmani (1800–1918)*. Beirut: Muʾassasat al-dirasat al-Filastiniyya, 1995.

Nakba and Survival: The Story of Palestinians Who Remained in Haifa and the Galilee, 1948–1956. Oakland: University of California Press, 2022.

Mansur, Asʿad. *Taʾrikh al-Nasira min aqdam azmaniha ila ayamina al-hadira*. Cairo: Matbaʿat al-Hilal, 1924.

Mansur, Johny. *Al-Madina al-Filastiniyya fi fatrat al-intidab al-Baritani: Tatawwurat wa-tahawwulat ijtimaʿiyya wa-iqtisadiyya wa-thaqafiyya, Hayfa namudhjan*. Ramallah: Al-Ruʿat li-l-dirasat wa-l-nashr, 2009.

Marʿi, Ibrahim Jamil and Salih ʿAbd al-Jawad. *Qaryat Zarʿin*. Bir Zayt: Jamiʿat Bir Zayt, markaz dirasat wa-tawthiq al-mujtamaʿ al-Filastini, 1994.

Marks, Shula. "What Is Colonial about Colonial Medicine? And What Has Happened to Imperialism and Health?" *Social History of Medicine* 10 (1997): 205–19.

Matera, Marc. *Black London: The Imperial Metropolis and Decolonization in the Twentieth Century*. Oakland: California University Press, 2015.

Mikhlin, Amnon. *Maʿase rokeah*. Tel Aviv: Erets ha-zvi, 1992.

Miller, Ylana N. *Government and Society in Rural Palestine, 1920–1948*. Austin: University of Texas Press, 1985.

Al-Minawi, Mahmud. *Hukamaʾ Qasr al-ʿAini*. Cairo: Nahdat Masr, 1999.

Moller, Esther. "'We Do Not Learn for School, But For Life': Alumni Associations at French Schools in Lebanon in the 1930s and 1940s as Privileged Spaces of Sociability." In *Entangled Education: Foreign and Local Schools in Ottoman Syria and Mandate Lebanon (19–20th Centuries)*, edited by Julia Hauser, Christine Lindner and Ester Möller, 265–82. Beirut: Ergon Verlag Würzburg in Kommission, 2016.

Mooreville, Anat. "Oculists in the Orient: A History of Trachoma, Zionism, and Global Health, 1882–1973." PhD Dissertation, UCLA, 2015.

Morgenstern, Abraham. *Tsaraʿat u-metsoraʿim bi-Yerushalayim*. Zikhron Yaʿakov: Itai Bahur, 2019.

Morris, Benny. *The Birth of the Palestinian Refugee Problem Revisited.* Cambridge: Cambridge University Press, 2004.

Mysyrowicz, Ladislas. "Les étudiants 'Orientaux' en médecine à Genève (1876–1914)." *Gesnerus: Swiss Journal of the History of Medicine and Science* 34 (1977): 207–12.

Nadan, Amos. *The Palestinian Peasant Economy under the Mandate: A Story of Colonial Bungling.* Cambridge, MA: Harvard University Press, 2006.

Nashef, Khaled. "Tawfiq Canaan: His Life and Works." *Jerusalem Quarterly*, no. 16 (2002): 12–26.

Navot, Orit and Abraham Gross. "ha-Milhamah ba-gar'enet: Reshit bri'ut ha-tsibur be-Erets Yisra'el." *Cathedra* 94 (1999): 89–114.

Neville Bonner, Thomas. *Becoming a Physician: Medical Education in Britain, France, Germany, and the United States, 1750–1945.* New York: Oxford University Press, 1995.

Nevo, Joseph. "Ha-Tnu'a ha-le'umit ha-'Arvit ha-Falastinit be-milhemet ha-'olam ha-shniya." In *Hatnu'a ha-'Aravit ha-Falastinit: Mi-'imut le-hashlama?* edited by Moshe Ma'oz and Binyamin Ze'ev Kedar, 93–114. Tel Aviv: Misrad ha-bitahon – ha-hotsa'a la-or, 1996.

Niederland, Doron. "Hashpa'at harof'im ha-'olim mi-Germaniya 'al hip-tathut ha-refu'a be-Erets Yisra'el, 1933–1948." *Cathedra* 30 (1984): 111–60.

Nimr, Ihsan. *Ta'rikh jabal Nablus wa-l-Balqa'.* Nablus: Jama'iyyat 'ummal al-matabi' al-ta'awwuniyya, 1975.

Nimr, Sonia. "Sa'id Nimr's Stormy Career from the Dungeons of Istanbul to the Ranks of Faisal's Arab Army." *Jerusalem Quarterly* 30 (2007): 77–87.

Nissan, Shlomo. "Hitpathut sherute ha-refu'a bi-Yerushalayim bi-tkufat ha-mandat." In *Yerushalayim bi-tkufat ha-mandat ha-'asiya ve-ha-more-shet*, edited by Yehoshu'a Ben-Arieh, 299–323. Jerusalem: Yad Ben-Tsvi, 2003.

Nordbruch, Götz. "Arab Students in Weimar Germany – Politics and Thought beyond Borders." *Journal of Contemporary History* 49 (2014): 275–95.

Norris, Jacob. *Land of Progress: Palestine in the Age of Colonial Development, 1905–1948.* Oxford: Oxford University Press, 2013.

The Lives and Deaths of Jubrail Dabdoub: Or, How the Bethlehemites Discovered Amerka. Worlding the Middle East. Stanford: Stanford University Press, 2023.

Ouahes, Idir. *Syria and Lebanon under the French Mandate: Cultural Imperialism and the Workings of Empire.* London: Bloomsbury, 2018.

Panzac, Daniel. "Les docteurs orientaux de la faculté de médecine de Paris au XIXe siècle." *Revue des mondes musulman et de la Méditerranée* 75/76 (1995): 295–303.

Patton, Adell. *Physicians, Colonial Racism, and Diaspora in West Africa*. Gainesville: University Press of Florida, 1996.

Pedersen, Susan. *The Guardians: The League of Nations and the Crisis of Empire*. Oxford: Oxford University Press, 2015.

Penrose, Stephen. *That They May Have Life: The Story of the American University of Beirut 1866–1941*. Beirut: American University of Beirut, 1941.

Perry, Yaron. *British Mission to the Jews in Nineteenth-Century Palestine*. London: Frank Cass, 2003.

"Le-Korot bet ha-holim ha-Briti bi-Tsfat." *Cathedra* 103 (2002): 69–84.

Perry, Yaron and Efraim Lev. *Modern Medicine in the Holy Land: Pioneering British Medical Services in Late Ottoman Palestine*. London: Tauris Academic Studies, 2007.

Political Diaries of the Arab World: Palestine & Jordan. Slough: Archive Editions, 2001.

Provence, Michael. *The Last Ottoman Generation and the Making of the Modern Middle East*. Cambridge: Cambridge University Press, 2017.

Qaʿwar Farah, Najwa. *wa-Kana sabah wa-kana masaʾ: Amali al-dhikrayat*. Amman: Dar al-Bayruni li-l-nashr wa-l-tawziʿ.

Qadura Khartabil, Wadiʿa. *Bahthan ʿan al-amal wa-l-wattan: Sittun ʿaman min kifah imraʾa fi sabil Filastin*. Beirut: Bisan li-l-nashr wa-l-tawziʿ, 1995.

Qalyubi, Tahir Adib. *ʿAʾilat wa-shahsiyyat min Yafa wa-wadaʾiha*. Beirut: al-Muʾassasa al-ʿArabiyya li-l-dirasat wa-l-nashr, 2006.

Qaraqra, Muhammad. *Al-Khidamat al-sihhiyya al-hukumiyya wa-l-ahliyya li-l-shaʿb al-Filastini aban al-intidab, 1918–1948*. Shefa-ʿAmr: Jamaʿiyyat al-Jalil li-l-buhuth wa-l-khidamat al-sihhiyya, 2017.

"Maʿarekhet ha-briʾut ha-mandatorit ve-ha-voluntarit ve-ʿArviye Erets Yisraʾel, 1918–1948." MA thesis, Haifa University, 1992.

"Sherute ha-briʾut la-ukhlusiya ha-ʿAravit be-Yisraʾel." PhD Dissertation, Bar Ilan University, 2013.

Radai, Itamar. *Palestinians in Jerusalem and Jaffa, 1948: A Tale of Two Cities*. London: Routledge, 2015.

Reʾuveni, Yaʿkov. *Mimshal ha-mandat be-Erets Yisraʾel, 1920–1948: Nittuah histori-medini*. Ramat Gan: Bar-Ilan University, 1993.

Reid, Donald. *Cairo University and the Making of Modern Egypt*. Cambridge: Cambridge University Press, 2002.

"Educational and Career Choices of Egyptian Students, 1882–1922." *International Journal of Middle East Studies* 8 (1977): 349–378.

Reiss, Nira. "British Public Health Policy in Palestine, 1918–1947." In *Health and Disease in the Holy Land; Studies in the History and Sociology of Medicine from Ancient Times to the Present*, edited by

Samuel S. Kottek and Manfred Waserman, 301–27. Lewiston, NY: Edwin Mellen Press, 1996.

The Health Care of the Arabs in Israel. Boulder, CO: Westview Press, 1991.

Robson, Laura. *Colonialism and Christianity in Mandate Palestine*. Austin: University of Texas Press, 2011.

Rogel, Nakdimon. " ʿOd ʿal reshit ha-refuʾa ba-Galil" *Cathedra* 63 (1992): 176–83.

Ryzova, Lucie. *The Age of the Efendiyya: Passages to Modernity in National-Colonial Egypt*. Oxford: Oxford University Press, 2014.

Al-Saʿati, Ahmad Muhammad. *Aʿlam min Ghazza, 1876–1967*. Gaza: Matabiʿ markaz Rashad al-Shawwa al-thaqafi, 2005.

Saposnik, Arieh Bruce. *Becoming Hebrew: The Creation of a Jewish National Culture in Ottoman Palestine*. Oxford: Oxford University Press, 2008.

Saruji, Ilyas Salim. *Min muruj al-Jalil, mudhakkirat tabib min al-Nasira*. Nazareth: Matbaʿat al-hakim, 2011.

"The Fall of a Galilean Village during the 1948 Palestine War: An Eyewitness Account." *Journal of Palestine Studies* 33 (2004): 71–80.

"The Last Days of 'Free Galilee': Memories of 1948." *Journal of Palestine Studies* 33 (2003): 55–67.

Savona-Ventura, Charles. "The Hospital of the Order of St. John in Jerusalem." *Historia Hospitalium* 24 (2004): 25–35.

Sayigh, Rosemary. *The Palestinians from Peasants to Revolutionaries*. New York: Zed Books, 2007.

Sayigh, Yusif. *Yusif Sayigh: Arab Economist and Palestinian Patriot: A Fractured Life Story*, edited by Rosemary Sayigh. Cairo: The American University in Cairo Press, 2015.

Schalit, Moshe. *bi-Ntivot hayyay*. Tel Aviv: Y. Golan, 2000.

Schayegh, Cyrus. *The Middle East and the Making of the Modern World*. Cambridge, MA: Harvard University Press, 2017.

Who Is Knowledgeable Is Strong: Science, Class, and the Formation of Modern Iranian Society, 1900–1950. Berkeley: University of California Press, 2009.

Schor, Laura S. *Sophie Halaby in Jerusalem: An Artist's Life*. Syracuse: Syracuse University Press, 2019.

Schumann, Christoph. "The Generation of Broad Expectations: Nationalism, Education, and Autobiography in Syria and Lebanon, 1930–1958." *Die Welt des Islams* 41 (2001): 174–205.

Schwake, Norbert. "Toldot ha-refuʾa bi-Yerushalayim ba-tkufa ha-ʿOthmanit ha-meʾuheret." In *Sefer Yerushalayim be-shilhe ha-tkufa ha-ʿOthmanit (1800–1917)*, edited by Israel Bartal and Haim Goren, 283–300. Jerusalem: Yad Yitzhak Ben-Tsvi, 2010.

Seikaly, May. *Haifa: Transformation of an Arab Society 1918–1939*. London: I. B. Tauris, 2002.

Seikaly, Sherene. "How I Met My Great-Grandfather: Archives and the Writing of History." *Comparative Studies of South Asia, Africa, and the Middle East* 38 (2018): 6–20.

Men of Capital: Scarcity and Economy in Mandate Palestine. Stanford: Stanford University Press, 2015.

"The Matter of Time." *American Historical Review* 124 (2019): 1681–88.

Shahid, Serene. *Jerusalem Memories*. Beirut: Naufal, 1999.

Shahin, Iyad. *Hikayat qarya mudammara, Bashit*. Bir Zayt: Dar ʿAllush li-l-nashr wa-l-tawziʿ, 2002.

Shakir, Faʾiq. *Kitab tadbir al-amrad al-zuhariyya*. Baghdad: Matbaʿat al-ʿahd, 1934.

Shalash, Bilal Muhamad. *Shayʾun ʿaʾbir: Nablus taht al-ihtilal (huzayran/yunyu 1967–adhar/mars 1969)*. Beirut: al-Markaz al-ʿArabi li-l-abhath wa-dirasat al-siyasat, 2023.

Shami, Yehushuʿa. *mi-Zihronot ha-rofe ha-sfaradi ha-Yerushalmi ha-rishon*. Jerusalem: Miryam Kotev, 2015.

Shatz, Julia R. "A Politics of Care: Local Nurses in Mandate Palestine." *International Journal of Middle East Studies* 50 (2018): 676–78.

"Governing Jerusalem's Children, Revealing Invisible Inhabitants: The American Colony Aid Association, 1920s–1950s." In *Ordinary Jerusalem, 1840–1940 Opening New Archives, Revisiting a Global City*, edited by Angelos Dalachanes and Vincent Lemire, 423–39. Brill, 2018.

Shefer-Mossensohn, Miri. *Ottoman Medicine: Healing and Medical Institutions, 1500–1700*. State University of New York Press, 2010.

Shehori-Rubin, Tzipora. *Rofʾot Rishonot be-Erets Israel 1900–1918*. Beersheba: Ben-Gurion University of the Negev Press, 2014.

Shehory-Rubin, Zipora and Shifra Shvarts. *Aleksandrah Belkind: Sippura shel rofʾa ʿIvriyya poretset derekh*. Zikhron Yaʿakov: Itai Bahur, 2012.

Shehory-Rubin, Zipora, Shira Shvartz, and Yoel Dunhin. *Hadassah li-vriʾut ha-ʿam: Peʿiluta ha-briʾutit-ha-hinukhit shel Hadassah be-Erets Yisraʾel bi-tkufat ha-mandat ha-Briti*. Jerusalem: ha-Sifriya ha-Tsionit, 2003.

Shimoni, Yaacov. *ʿArviye Erets ʾYisraʾel*. Tel Aviv: ʿAm ʿoved, 1947.

Shinaʾa, Talaʿat. *Ayyam Zaman: al-Tarikh al-Shafawi lil-Urdun wa-Filastin*. Amman: al-Ahliyya, 1993.

Shlaim, Avi and Eugene L. Rogan, eds. *The War for Palestine: Rewriting the History of 1948*. Cambridge: Cambridge University Press, 2007.

Shtern, Shimon. "Hadar ha-Karmel – merkaz ha-hayim ha-Yehudiyyim be-Hefa." In *Hefa be-Hitpathuta... 1918–1948*, edited by Mordekhai Naor and Yosi Ben Artzi. Jerusalem: Yad Ben Tsvi, 1989, 38–46

"Hitpathut ha-ma'arakh ha-'ironi shel Hefa ba-shanim 1918–1947." PhD Dissertation, the Hebrew University, 1974.
Shvarts, Shifra. "Bet ha-holim sha'ar tsion be-Yafo: Bet holim kehilati rishon ba-arets 1891–1921." *Korot* 9 (1990): 295–308.
"Histadrut nashim le-ma'an imahot be-Erets Yisra'el: Pe'ilutan shel Hadassah, Histadrut Nashim 'Ivriyyot ve-WIZO le-hakamat tahanot em va-yeled be-Erets Yisra'el ba-shanim 1918–1948." *Bitahon Sotsiali* 51 (1998): 57–62.
The Workers' Health Fund in Eretz Israel: Kupat Holim, 1911–1937. Rochester, NY: University of Rochester Press, 2002.
al-Sifri, 'Isa. *Filastin al-'Arabiyya bayna al-intidab wa-l-Sahyuniyya*. Jaffa: Matba'at maktabat Filastin al-jadida, 1937.
Sonbol, Amira. *The Creation of a Medical Profession in Egypt, 1800–1922*. Syracuse: Syracuse University Press, 1991.
Stein, Kenneth W. *The Land Question in Palestine, 1917–1939*. Chapel Hill: University of North Carolina Press, 1985.
Stoler-Liss, Sachlav, Shifra Shvarts, and Mordechai Shani. *Liheyot 'am bari be-artsenu: Bri'ut ha-tsibur ba-'aliyah ha-gdolah, 1948–1960*. Beersheba: Universitat Ben-Guryon ba-Negev, 2016.
Strauss, Johann. *Language and Power in the Late Ottoman Empire*. Abingdon: Routledge, 2016.
Sufian, Sandra. "Arab Health Care during the British Mandate, 1920–1947." In *Separate and Cooperate, Cooperate and Separate: The Disengagement of the Palestine Health Care System from Israel and Its Emergence as an Independent System*, edited by Tamara Barnea and Rafiq Husseini, 9–30. Westport, CT: Praeger, 2002.
Healing the Land and the Nation: Malaria and the Zionist Project in Palestine, 1920–1947. Chicago: University of Chicago Press, 2007.
"Re-imagining Palestine: Scientific Knowledge and Malaria Control in Mandatory Palestine." *Dynamis* 25 (2005): 351–82.
Sukayk, Ibrahim Khalil. *Sharit al-dhikrayat 'an Ghazza qabla nisf qarn*. Gaza: Dar al-Katib, 1985.
Swedenburg, Ted. *Memories of a Revolt: The 1936–1939 Rebellion and the Palestinian National Past*. Minneapolis: University of Minnesota Press, 1995.
Al-Tamam, Bashshar Sa'id. *Baladiyyat Nablus fi al-'ahd al-'Uthmani, 1868–1918*. Nablus: Maktabat baladiyyat Nablus al-'ama, 2012.
Tamari, Salim. *Mountain against the Sea: Essays on Palestinian Society and Culture*. Berkeley: University of California Press, 2008.
The Great War and the Remaking of Palestine. Berkeley: University of California Press, 2017.
Tamimi, Anwar al-Khatib. *Ma' Salah al-Din fi al-Quds: Ta'ammulat wa-dhikrayat*. Jerusalem: Dar al-tiba'a al-'Arabiyya, 1989.

Tamimi, Muhamad and Muhammad Bahjat. *Wilayat Bayrut*, vol. 1. Beirut: Maba'at al-iqbal, 1916.

Tannus, Izzat. *The Palestinians: A Detailed Documented Eyewitness History of Palestine under British Mandate*. New York: I. G. T. Co, 1988.

Taraki, Liza. "Hayat 'adiyya: Usul al-tabaqa al-wusta fi madina saghira fi Filastin fi matl' al-qarn al-'ishrin." In *al-Madina al-Filastiniya qadaya fi al-tahauwulat al-hadariya*, edited by Majdi al-Maliki and Salim Tamari, 147–64. Beirut: Mu'assasat al-dirasat al-Filastiniyya, 2021.

Teicher, Avishai. "Ahayot ve-rof'im korbanot teror ishi bi-tkufat ha-mandat." *ha-Refu'a* 139 (2000): 312–13.

Tibawi, Abdul Latif. *Arab Education in Mandatory Palestine: A Study of Three Decades of British Administration*. London: Luzac, 1956.

Titi, Rihan. *Al-Be'ne 'abr al-ta'rikh*. Be'ne: Majlis al-Be'ne al-mahali, 1997.

Tleel, John N. *I Am Jerusalem*. Jerusalem: J.N. Tleel, 2007.

Tuan Hoang, Van. "L'Université de Hanoi (1906–1945). Un outil de renouvellement des élites et de la culture vietnamiennes?" *Revue Outre-Mer*, no. 394–395 (2017).

Tumblety, Joan. "Rhetoric, Enterprise and Professional Authority: Dr James-Edward Ruffier and Physician-Writers in Twentieth-Century France." *History* 104 (2019): 127–31.

Verdeil, Chantal. "L'empire, les communautés, la France: Les réseaux des médecins ottomans à la fin du xixe siècle." In *Hommes de l'entre-deux: Parcours individuels et portraits de groupes sur la frontière de la méditerranée xvie-xxe siècle*, edited by Bernard Heyberger and Chantal Verdeil, 133–50. Paris: Les Indes savants, 2009.

"Naissance d'une nouvelle élite ottomane. Formation et trajectoires de médecins diplômés de Beyrouth à la fin du XIXe siècle." *Revue des mondes musulmans et de la Méditerranée* 121–122 (2008): 217–37.

Warner, Charles Dudley, ed. *A Library of the World's Best Literature – Ancient and Modern – Vol. II (Forty-Five Volumes); Amiel-Auerbach*. New York: Cosimo, 2008.

Washitz, Yosef. *Ha-'Aravim be-Erets Yisra'el*. Merhavia: al-Kibbuts ha-artsi, 1947.

"Tmurot hevratiyot ba-yishuv ha-'Arvi shel Hefa bi-tkufat ha-mandat ha-Briti: Soharim ve-yazamim aherim." *'Iyyunim* (2003): 393–438.

Watenpaugh, Keith David. *Being Modern in the Middle East: Revolution, Nationalism, Colonialism, and the Arab Middle Class*. Princeton, NJ; Woodstock: Princeton University Press, 2006.

"Middle-Class Modernity and the Persistence of the Politics of Notables in Inter-War Syria." *International Journal of Middle East Studies* 35 (2003): 260–63.

White, Luise. *Speaking with Vampires: Rumor and History in Colonial Africa*. Berkeley: University of California Press, 2000.

Winter, Michael. *Egyptian Society under Ottoman Rule, 1517–1798*. London: Routledge, 1992.

Yazbak, Mahmoud. "Comparing Ottoman Municipalities in Palestine: The Cases of Nablus, Haifa, and Nazareth, 1864–1914." In *Ordinary Jerusalem 1840–1940*, edited by Angelos Dalachanis and Vincent Lemire, 240–61. Leiden: Brill, 2018.

Haifa in the Late Ottoman Period, 1864–1914: A Muslim Town in Transition. Leiden: Brill, 1998.

"Nabulsi Ulama in the Late Ottoman Period, 1864–1914." *International Journal of Middle East Studies* 29 (1997): 71–91.

"The Municipality of a Muslim Town: Nablus 1868–1914." *Archív Orientální* 67 (1999): 339–60.

Yehoshuʿa, Yaʿaov. *Yaldut bi-Yerushalayim ha-yeshana: Pirkke hove mi-yamim ʿavaru*. Jerusalem: R. Mas, 1965.

Young, Elise G. *Gender and Nation Building in the Middle East the Political Economy of Health from Mandate Palestine to Refugee Camps in Jordan*. New York: I. B. Tauris, 2012.

Zaatrai, Ghazi. *Pathology and Laboratory Medicine at the American University of Beirut 1866–2015*. Beirut: American University of Beirut, 2015.

Ziadeh, Nicola A. *Ayyami: Sirah dhatiyya*, vol. 2. London: Hazar, 1992.

Zuʿaytir, Akram. *Yawmiyat Akram Zuʿaytir: Amal al-wahdah wa-alam al-inqisam 1949–1965*. Beirut: al-Markaz al-ʿArabi li-l-abhath wa-dirasat al-siyasat, 2021.

Zuraiq, Qustantin. *Nakbat 1948: Asbabuha wa-subul ʿilajiha*, edited by Walid Khalidi. Beirut: Muʾassasat al-dirasat al-Filastiniyya, 2009.

Index

For EU product safety concerns, contact us at Calle de José Abascal, 56–1°,
28003 Madrid, Spain or eugpsr@cambridge.org.

www.ingramcontent.com/pod-product-compliance
Ingram Content Group UK Ltd.
Pitfield, Milton Keynes, MK11 3LW, UK
UKHW020120250925
463284UK00008B/250